ALLE ZEIT WACH 1842

W. Bleifeld C. W Hamm
E. Braunwald (Eds.)

Unstable Angina

With 75 Figures and 29 Tables

Springer-Verlag
Berlin Heidelberg New York
London Paris Tokyo
Hong Kong Barcelona

WALTER BLEIFELD, Professor Dr.
CHRISTIAN W. HAMM, Privatdozent Dr.
Universitätskrankenhaus Eppendorf
– Kardiologie – Martinistraße 52
2000 Hamburg 20, FRG

EUGENE BRAUNWALD, Professor Dr.
Department of Medicine
Brigham and Women's Hospital
Harvard Medical School
75 Francis Street
Boston, MA 02115, USA

Front cover: Picture of a sun protuberance, taken at the Sacramento Peak Observatory, Sunspot, New Mexico, USA

ISBN-13:978-3-642-64778-9 e-ISBN-13:978-3-642-61288-6
DOI: 10.1007/978-3-642-61288-6

Library of Congress Cataloging-in-Publication Data. Unstable angina / W. Bleifeld, C. W. Hamm, E. Braunwald (eds.), p. cm. Based on a symposium held in Hamburg, June 3–4, 1989. Includes index. ISBN-13:978-3-642-64778-9
1. Angina pectoris–Congresses. I. Bleifeld, W. (Walter) II. Hamm, C. W. (Christian W.) III. Braunwald, Eugene, 1929– [DNLM: 1. Angina Pectoris–diagnosis–congresses. 2. Angina Pectoris–therapy–congresses. 3. Myocardial Infarction–prevention & control–congresses. WG 298 U587 1989] RC685.A6U55 1990
616.1'22–dc20 DNLM/DLC for Library of Congress

Softcover reprint of the hardcover 1st edition 1990

2119/3130-543210 – Printed on acid-free paper

Preface

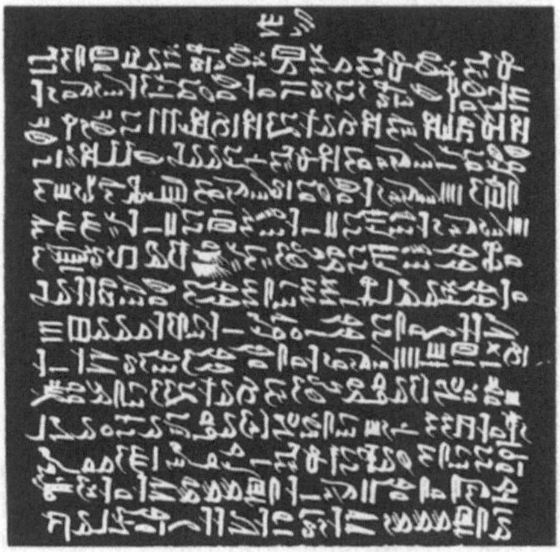

If you find a man
with cardiac discomfort,
with pain in his arms,
at the side of his heart,
death is near.

The Ebers papyrus 2600 B.C.

This is the first document describing what today are termed "acute ischemic syndromes". These syndromes includes acute myocardial infarction, unstable angina, variant angina (Prinzmetal angina), and some forms of sudden death. Modern understanding of the pathophysiology and therapy of the acute ischemic syndromes developed in four stages: Following the initial description of acute myocardial infarction by Herrick in 1912, up to the early 1960s the therapeutic options available were extremely limited and consisted of pain relief, bed rest, and antithrombotic treatment to protect against pulmonary embolism. The second stage was marked by the introduction of coronary care based on external electrical defibrillation and cardiac pacing. Complications resulting from arrhythmias were effectively treated, resulting in a reduction of the in-hospital mortality of acute myocardial infarction from approximately 30% to between 15% and 20%. The third stage began with the initiation of intracoronary thrombolysis during the early 1980s. Early reperfusion of an acutely occluded coronary artery resulted in preservation of left ventricular function and a further reduction of mortality to between 5% and 10%.

The current, fourth phase in the care of patients with acute ischemic syndromes emphasizes the *prevention* of coronary artery occlusion and thereby of acute myocardial infarction, a condition which is often preceded by unstable angina. Although an acute occluding thrombus is present initially in about 90% of acute transmural myocardial infarctions, and although 10% to 15% of patients with unstable angina develop an acute infarction as a result of an occlusive thrombus, the importance of the link between these two conditions has become appreciated only recently. After documentation of the presence of coronary thrombi in many patients succumbing to sudden coronary death, an occluding thrombus complicating plaque rupture was recognized as the principal etiologic mechanism in the majority of patients with acute transmural myocardial infarction. Nonocclusive intracoronary thrombi have been observed at angioscopy and coronary arteriography in patients with unstable angina. Biochemical evidence of coronary thrombosis has been provided by the finding of platelet release products in the blood and urine of patients with acute ischemic syndromes. Finally, aspirin and heparin have been shown to prevent nonfatal myocardial infarction or cardiac death in several randomized, controlled studies of patients with unstable angina.

Thus, substantial evidence is now available to support the position that an alteration of the vessel wall, the complex interaction between the vascular endothelium and the different components of the blood, especially of platelets and fibrinogen, and the reaction of vascular smooth muscle are responsible in various combinations for the development of acute ischemic syndroms including unstable angina.

In a rapidly expanding field in which there is considerable research the scientific issues are often controversial, but such controversy often stimulates important additional investigations. Accordingly, the editors felt that the time was now opportune to bring together current knowledge, both basic and clinical, concerning acute ischemic syndrome. A symposium on "Unstable Angina" was held in Hamburg, June 3–4th, 1989 and the present volume has emerged from that meeting. Our profound thanks go to the participants in the symposium for their lively ideas, their stimulating presentations and discussions, their high level of scholarship, and their cooperation in the production of this monograph. Both conference and publication were made possible by the support given by Pharma Schwarz, ICI Medtronic, and Bayer to the University of Hamburg. Special thanks go to Mrs. Barbara Kratzenberg for her valued assistance in organizing the symposium. Our work as editors was supported enormously by the efforts of Dr. Wolfram Terres and also Dr. Claudia Osthoff from Springer-Verlag

The Editors

Contents

List of Contributors

J. A. Ambrose, M.D., Division of Cardiology, Mount Sinai Hospital, One Gustave L. Levy Place, New York, NY 10029, USA

F. W. Bär, M.D., Cardiologie, Academisch Ziekenhuis Maastricht, Rijksuniversiteit Limburg, Annadal 1, 6201 BX Maastricht, The Netherlands

A. E. Becker, M.D., Vakgroep Pathologie, Academisch Medisch Centrum, Universiteit van Amsterdam, Meibergdreef 9, 1105 AZ Amsterdam Zuidoost, The Netherlands

B. F. Becker, M.D., Physiologisches Institut der Universität, Pettenkoferstraße 12, 8000 München 2, FRG

W. Bleifeld, M.D., Abteilung für Kardiologie, Medizinische Klinik, Universitätskrankenhaus Eppendorf, Martinistraße 52, 2000 Hamburg 20, FRG

E. Braunwald, M.D., Department of Medicine, Brigham and Women's Hospital, Harvard Medical School, 75 Francis Street, Boston, MA 02115, USA

R. Brennecke, M.D., II. Medizinische Klinik und Poliklinik der Universität, Langenbeckstraße 1, 6500 Mainz, FRG

S. Chierchia, M.D., Divisione di Cardiologia, Ospedale San Raffaele, Via Olgettina, 60, 20132 Milano, Italy

P. J. Commerford, M.D., Cardiac Clinic and MRC Liver Research Centre, Department of Medicine, University of Cape Town, Groote Schuur Hospital, Observatory 7925, South Africa

T. Eggeling, M.D., Abteilung Innere Medizin IV, Medizinische Universitätsklinik und Poliklinik, Robert-Koch-Straße 8, 7900 Ulm, FRG

R. Erbel, M.D., II. Medizinische Klinik und Poliklinik der Universität, Langenbeckstraße 1, 6500 Mainz, FRG

E. Gerlach, M.D., Physiologisches Institut der Universität, Pettenkoferstraße 12, 8000 München 2, FRG

G. Gerstenblith, M.D., Division of Cardiology, Johns Hopkins Hospital, 601 N. Wolfe Street, Baltimore, MD 21205, USA

S. O. Gottlieb, M.D., Division of Cardiology, Francis Scott Key Medical Center, 4940 Eastern Avenue, Baltimore, MD 21224, USA

B. K. W. Green, M.D., Cardiac Clinic and MRC Liver Research Centre, Department of Medicine, University of Cape Town, Groote Schuur Hospital, Observatory 7925, South Africa

W. Haerer, M.D., Abteilung Innere Medizin IV, Medizinische Universitätsklinik und Poliklinik, Robert-Koch-Straße 8, 7900 Ulm, FRG

C. W. Hamm, M.D., Abteilung für Kardiologie, Medizinische Klinik, Universitätskrankenhaus Eppendorf, Martinistraße 52, 2000 Hamburg 20, FRG

M. Höher, M.D., Abteilung Innere Medizin IV, Medizinische Universitätsklinik und Poliklinik, Robert-Koch-Straße 8, 7900 Ulm, FRG

V. Hombach, M.D., Abteilung Innere Medizin IV, Medizinische Universitätsklinik und Poliklinik, Robert-Koch-Straße 8, 7900 Ulm, FRG

H. A. Katus, M.D., Abteilung Innere Medizin III, Klinikum der Universität, Bergheimer Straße 58, 6900 Heidelberg 1, FRG

R. E. Kirsch, M.D., Cardiac Clinic and MRC Liver Research Centre, Department of Medicine, University of Cape Town, Groote Schuur Hospital, Observatory 7925, South Africa

M. Kochs, M.D., Abteilung Innere Medizin IV, Medizinische Universitätsklinik und Poliklinik, Robert-Koch-Straße 8, 7900 Ulm, FRG

M. Kottmeyer, M.D., II, Medizinische Klinik und Poliklinik der Universität, Langenbeckstraße 1, 6500 Mainz, FRG

W. Kübler, M.D., Abteilung Innere Medizin III, Klinikum der Universität, Bergheimer Straße 58, 6900 Heidelberg 1, FRG

R. Lorenz, M.D., Medizinische Klinik Innenstadt der Universität, Ziemssenstraße 1, 8000 München 2, FRG

J. Lubsen, M.D., Center for Clinical Decision Analysis, Erasmus Universiteit, P.O. Box 1738, 3000 DR Rotterdam, The Netherlands

J. L. McCans, M.D., Sir Mortimer B. Davis Jewish, General Hospital, 3755 Cote Ste-Catherine Rd., Montreal, Quebec H3T 1E2, Canada

B. J. Messmer, M.D., Abteilung für Thorax-, Herz- und Gefäßchirurgie, Klinikum der RWTH, 5100 Aachen, FRG

J. Meyer, M.D., II. Medizinische Klinik und Poliklinik der Universität, Langenbeckstraße 1, 6500 Mainz, FRG

L. H. Opie, M.D., Heart Research Unit and Hypertension Clinic, University of Cape Town, Observatory 7925, South Africa

P. Ouyang, M.D., Division of Cardiology, Francis Scott Key Medical Center, 4940 Eastern Avenue, Baltimore, MD 21224, USA

T. Pop, M.D., II. Medizinische Klinik und Poliklinik der Universität, Langenbeckstraße 1, 6500 Mainz, FRG

H.-J. Rupprecht, M.D., II. Medizinische Klinik und Poliklinik der Universität, Langenbeckstraße 1, 6500 Mainz, FRG

H. R. Schelbert, M.D., Division of Nuclear Medicine and Biophysics, UCLA School of Medicine, Los Angeles, CA 90024, USA

H. Schmid-Schönbein, M.D., Abteilung Physiologie, Klinikum der RWTH, Pauwelsstraße, 5100 Aachen, FRG

A. Schmidt, M.D., Abteilung Innere Medizin IV, Medizinische Universitätsklinik und Poliklinik, Robert-Koch-Straße 8, 7900 Ulm, FRG

W. Terres, M.D., Abteilung für Kardiologie, Medizinische Klinik, Universitätskrankenhaus Eppendorf, Martinistraße 52, 2000 Hamburg 20, FRG

U. Thadani, M.D., Cardiovascular Section, Department of Medicine, University of Oklahoma, Health Sciences Center, South Pavillion, Room 5SP300, Oklahoma City, OK 73190, USA

S. Wieshammer, M.D., Abteilung Innere Medizin IV, Medizinische Universitätsklinik und Poliklinik, Robert-Koch-Straße 8, 7900 Ulm, FRG

I. Pathophysiology of Unstable Angina

The Vascular Endothelium: Interactions with Hemostatic Mechanisms (Platelets, Coagulation, Fibrinolysis)

E. GERLACH and B. F. BECKER [1]

Introduction

The vascular endothelium, which lines all blood vessels like a continuous sheet, must nowadays be regarded as a rather large tissue compartment of particular functional importance. With respect to its size, one should realize that in a person with 70 kg body weight the endothelial mass amounts to about 1000–1500 g, comparable to the mass of the liver [10]. Even more impressive is the size of the endothelial surface, estimated to be about 800–1000 m^2 [47]. This huge surface is in continuous contact with the 5–6 l of circulating blood, or, in other words, 5–6 ml of blood are on the average exposed to an endothelial area of 0.8–1 m^2. As an interesting consequence, one can calculate that the mean thickness of the blood film covering the endothelial surface amounts to about 5 μm, a value corresponding to the thickness of two red blood cells. These figures are merely intended to illustrate that intimate interactions of the streaming blood and its constituents with the endothelium are readily possible.

Detailed studies on interactions between endothelium and blood have become possible only within the past decade. In this period newly elaborated, sensitive analytical methods, culture techniques as well as suitable in vitro and in vivo vessel preparations have become available. These innovations have enabled an extensive characterization of endothelial cells, particularly with respect to their biochemical, immunological, and physiological properties [13, 18]. The results obtained leave no doubt that the vascular endothelium plays a decisive and active role in the interactions of blood with the vessel wall and the adjacent tissues.

Various Functional Features of the Vascular Endothelium

Some important functional features of the vascular endothelium are summarized in Table 1. First of all, the endothelium controls exchange processes between the intra- and extravascular spaces. The physical barrier function preventing simple passive transfer of blood cells or larger molecules has long

[1] Physiologisches Institut der Universität, Pettenkoferstrasse 12, 8000 München 2, West Germany

W. Bleifeld et al. (Eds.)
Unstable Angina

Table 1. Functional features of the vascular endothelium

Control of exchange processes	
– Physical barrier	
– Metabolic barrier	
Modulation of vascular tone	
– Dilatation:	PGI_2, EDRF (NO), adenosine
– Constriction:	Angiotensin II ↑, bradykinin ↓, endothelin, EDCF
Influence on hemostasis	
– Antithrombogenic surface (physiological state)	
– Thrombogenic surface (perturbed state)	
Participation in inflammatory and immune reactions	
– Leukocyte adhesion, activation, and emigration	
– Antigen presentation, T-lymphocyte activation, binding of complement factors	

been known. The metabolic barrier function, however, was only recently recognized. It applies, for instance, to substances such as ATP and ADP [26, 33] or lipoproteins [12], which become degraded by ectoenzymes at the luminal surface and therefore, as such, cannot cross the endothelial layer. Another example is the nucleoside adenosine. When presented in low but vasoactive concentrations to the luminal surface, for example, of the coronary endothelium, adenosine is rapidly taken up by the endothelial cells, where it becomes fully metabolized [19, 28]. Nevertheless, though it does not reach the smooth muscle cells, adenosine in low concentrations induces coronary dilatation. From these findings it has been concluded that this dilatation must be mediated by the endothelium [27, 29, 30].

A second aspect, receiving widespread attention today, is the role of endothelial cells in modulating vascular tone. Three vasodilating substances are formed and released by the endothelium: prostacyclin (PGI_2), endothelium-derived relaxing factor (EDRF), and adenosine [18]. EDRF has recently been identified as nitric oxide (NO) [31]. Since these substances also affect platelet aggregation, they are discussed in greater detail below. Under certain circumstances endothelial cells can promote vasoconstriction. For instance, angiotensin-converting enzyme, located at the endothelial surface, forms the constrictory angiotensin II; at the same time it degrades dilatory bradykinin to vasoinactive products, thereby potentiating the vasoconstriction (for review, see [18]). Furthermore, endothelial cells are the source of the newly detected polypeptide endothelin, a very potent vasoconstrictor [48]. Finally, endothelial cells of lung and brain vessels appear to be capable of producing another, still unidentified constrictory factor, called EDCF [45]. At present, it is a matter of debate to what extent endothelium-dependent dilatory and constrictory mechanisms contribute to the modulation of general vascular tone, or whether they are only of local importance.

The third functional feature concerns the role of the vascular endothelium in hemostasis. On the one hand, it is well known that under normal physiological conditions the luminal surface of the entire vascular system exhibits antithrombogenic properties [18, 34]. These comprise mechanisms directed against platelet aggregation and blood coagulation as well as mechanisms promoting fibrinolysis. On the other hand, in the past few years evidence has been obtained that the endothelial surface can become thrombogenic. However, this appears to be a phenomenon restricted mainly to areas with a perturbed endothelium, as encountered under various pathological conditions, such as inflammatory and immune reactions as well as during development of arteriosclerotic lesions [9, 11, 35, 41].

Finally, in the course of inflammatory and immune reactions the vascular endothelium may not only develop a thrombogenic surface. As indicated in Table 1, the endothelial cells actively participate in the processes of adhesion, activation, and emigration of leukocytes, in particular of polymorphonuclear neutrophils and monocytes [9, 11]. Under certain conditions the endothelium can take part in antigen presentation and activation of T-lymphocytes [3]. Furthermore, binding sites for factors of the complement system can be expressed [36]. Most of these activities involve an endothelial synthesis of new proteins which subsequently are incorporated into the cell membranes. It should be emphasized, however, that many details of these interesting pathophysiologic responses still need to be clarified.

Antithrombogenic Features of the Endothelium

In the physiological state, a truely impressive number of properties of the endothelial surface antagonize platelet aggregation, inhibit blood coagulation, and promote fibrinolysis.

Antiplatelet Actions

Three factors exhibit antiplatelet actions: PGI_2, EDRF, and adenosine. The endothelial formation of PGI_2 from arachidonic acid and its release at the luminal surface is a well-established phenomenon. This ability seems to be almost unimpaired in patients receiving low-dose aspirin treatment [24].

The antiplatelet effect of the EDRF nitric oxide was discovered only about 2 years ago [7, 25]. In Fig. 1 the production and the different actions of EDRF are schematically indicated. A great number of vasoactive substances, including acetylcholine, bradykinin, histamine, thrombin, ATP, and ADP, are known to bind to receptors at the luminal surface, initiating a Ca^{2+}-dependent formation of EDRF (NO) from the precursor substance L-arginine [32, 39]. The precise mechanisms involved in the generation of NO, however, are not yet fully understood. Interestingly, NO is released from the endothelial cells at the basal and also at the luminal side [2]. Through stimulation of the soluble guanylate cyclase and the resulting increase in cGMP levels relaxation of the

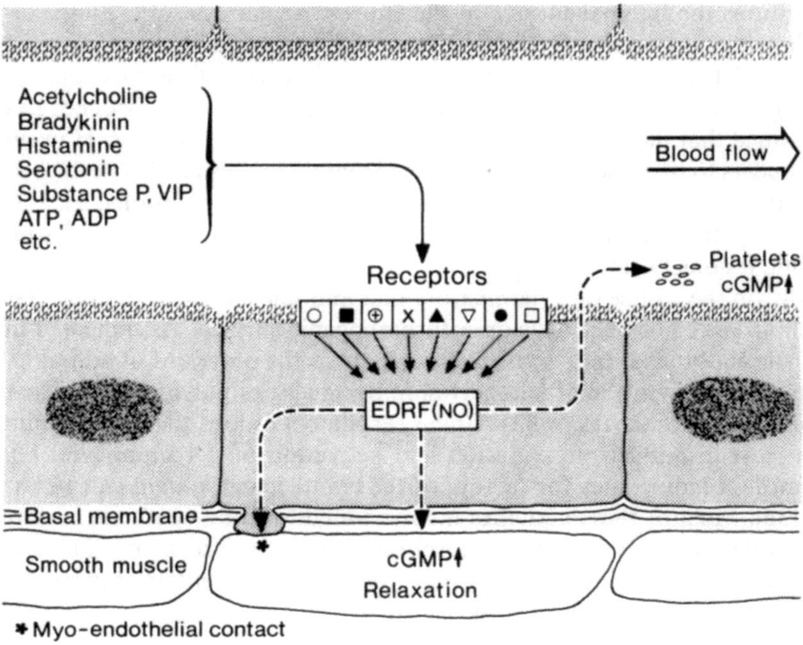

Fig. 1. Schematic illustration of steps involved in the production and action of the endothelium-derived relaxing factor (EDRF) nitric oxide (NO). Various vasoactive substances, when present intravascularly, bind to endothelial surface receptors, thereby inducing a Ca^{2+}-dependent luminal and abluminal release of NO. This causes an increase in cGMP levels in vascular smooth muscle cells, leading to relaxation, and in platelets, increasing their antiaggregatory potential (for further details, see text)

smooth muscle cells and thus vasodilatation is brought about. EDRF released into the vascular space similarly activates guanylate cyclase in platelets, and here the elevation of cGMP is a powerful antiaggregatory signal. Owing to the short half-life of the EDRF, which is in the order of seconds in blood, the antiplatelet action of EDRF is obviously restricted in vivo to the close vicinity of the endothelial production site (for details of EDRF actions, see reviews [1, 21]).

A localized action is also expected for the nucleoside adenosine, a strong inhibitor of platelet aggregation [4], which we have shown to be continuously formed and released by the endothelium, and which can be additionally generated at the vessel wall through dephosphorylation of adenine nucleotides by means of endothelial ectonucleotidases [18, 19, 26]. However, as mentioned above in the context of the metabolic barrier function, adenosine is also avidly taken up and metabolized by endothelial cells. This seemingly discrepant capability of endothelial cells for both uptake and release of adenosine raises the intriguing question of which process prevails.

Since under physiological conditions the adenosine concentration is known to be almost identical in the arterial and venous blood [40], the regulatory mechanisms outlined in Fig. 2 appear important. In the upper part of Fig. 2 the normal steady-state situation is shown. As indicated by the arrows, adenosine must be continuously released from the endothelium in excess of the amount that is taken up because also red blood cells incorporate adenosine. As a consequence of these dynamic processes a concentration gradient of adenosine is presumably established across the vessel lumen, the highest concentration existing close to the endothelial surface. Thus, it is mainly in this border zone where, already under normal conditions, adenosine can augment the antiplatelet actions of EDRF and PGI_2.

As depicted in the lower part of Fig. 2, the adenosine concentration can be locally enhanced when adenine nucleotides become stepwise dephosphorylated at the endothelial surface through the ectonucleotidase cascade, which consists of an ATPase, ADPase, and 5′-nucleotidase [18, 33]. Such a condition actually exists close downstream from a vascular lesion, where adenine nucleotides are liberated from injured cells and from aggregating platelets. It is easy to appreciate that the increased adenosine concentration must result in a much stronger antiplatelet action, thus preventing a spreading of platelet aggregation beyond the primary lesion. In this context it is important that the ecto-ADPase is thus not only involved in the extracellular formation of antiaggregatory adenosine but also in the rapid removal of the potent aggregatory stimulant ADP.

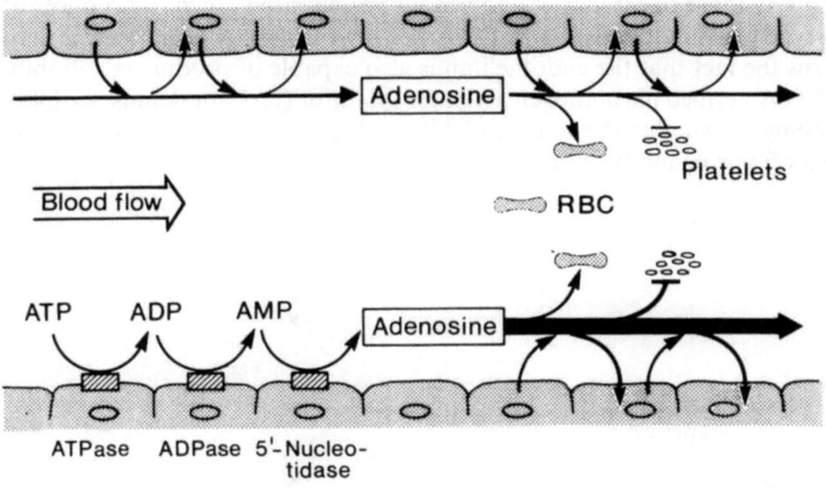

Fig. 2. Adenosine homeostasis in streaming blood under normal conditions (*above*) and after release of adenine nucleotides from damaged tissue or from platelets (*below*). Normally, formation and release of adenosine prevails over uptake by endothelial cells and red blood cells (*RBC*), thus establishing an antiaggregatory adenosine concentration in the plasma layer adjacent to the endothelium. This condition becomes greatly enhanced if adenine nucleotides occur intravascularly and become degraded by the ectonucleotidases (*thick arrow*)

Anticoagulant and Fibrinolytic Properties

The anticoagulant properties of the endothelium comprise two distinct mechanisms, both of which involve thrombin, the key enzyme of the coagulation cascade. One concerns heparan sulfate-rich membrane structures of the luminal surface, to which the natural clotting inhibitor antithrombin III (AT III) can bind [34]. This binding process causes an activation of AT III similar to that brought about by heparin. AT III was formerly shown to originate partly in the endothelium [8], however recent findings indicate that endothelial cells internalize plasma-borne AT III [46]. Apparently, most if not all circulating AT III is produced by the liver [23].

The second mechanism centers around a membrane receptor protein named thrombomodulin [15], and furthermore involves the endothelium-derived protein S [16, 42]. Interestingly, synthesis and binding of protein S seem to be modified by an α_1-receptor mediated process, with noradrenaline causing inhibition [6]. Both, thrombomodulin and protein S, are essential for establishing the so-called protein C pathway [14, 35], details of which are depicted in Fig. 3. It is well established that thrombin binds with high affinity to thrombomodulin, thereby losing its substrate specificity for fibrinogen, but obtaining a high specificity for protein C. This plasma factor, synthesized vitamin K-dependently in the liver, becomes activated (protein Ca). In cooperation with protein S, protein Ca exerts two antithrombogenic effects, namely an anticoagulant action and a fibrinolytic action (see below).

In addition to the anticoagulant mechanisms, the endothelium is also essentially involved in the regulation of fibrinolytic activity. Endothelial cells, particularly those of capillaries and venous vessels, are known to produce the tissue-type plasminogen activator (TPA; see review [44]). A rather new insight concerns the fact that the endothelium is also capable of producing an inhibitor of TPA, termed plasminogen activator inhibitor (PAI; for details, see [38]). Depending on whether the activity of TPA or PAI predominates, the endothelium can favor or inhibit fibrinolysis.

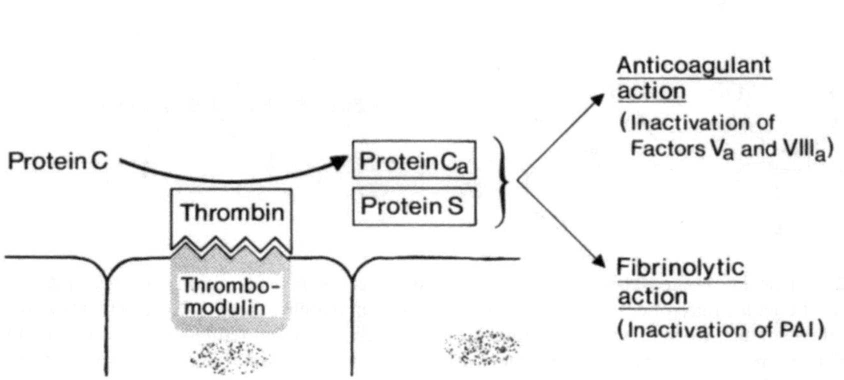

Fig. 3. Schematic illustration of the protein C pathway. (For details, see text)

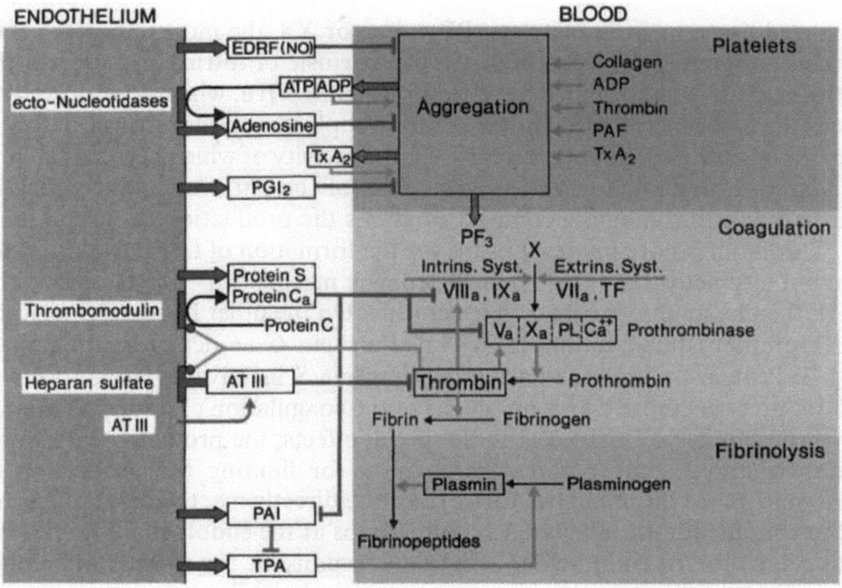

Fig. 4. Antithrombogenic features of the vascular endothelium displayed at its luminal surface. The most important interactions with platelets, blood coagulation, and fibrinolysis are depicted. For a detailed discussion, see text. The release of AT III from the endothelium has recently been questioned [46]. *PF_3*, Platelet factor 3; *TF*, tissue factor; *PL*, phospholipid; *PAI*, plasminogen activator inhibitor; *TPA*, tissue plasminogen activator

Synopsis of Antithrombogenic Features

Figure 4 summarizes the interactions of endothelial mechanisms with platelet aggregation, coagulatory processes, and fibrinolysis. As shown in the upper part of this scheme, platelet aggregation can be initiated by collagen, ADP, thrombin, platelet-activating factor (PAF), and thromboxane (TxA_2). During the aggregation process platelets release various substances, such as ATP, ADP, TxA_2, and platelet factor 3 (PF_3). Liberated ADP and TxA_2 promote additional aggregation. However, at the endothelial surface these effects are strongly counteracted by EDRF (NO), adenosine, and PGI_2. Furthermore, the endothelial ectonucleotidases not only enhance the level of antiaggregatory adenosine but also rapidly reduce the concentration of proaggregatory ADP. Because of these interactions, platelet aggregation normally does not occur at the surface of an intact endothelium.

In the middle section of Fig. 4 the multiple interactions with the coagulation cascade are outlined. In order to facilitate understanding of the details, some major aspects of the coagulation processes need briefly to be reviewed. The main effector of the coagulation system is known to be the prothrombinase complex, consisting of the activated factors Va and Xa in conjunction with phospholipids and Ca^{2+}. The phospholipids are derived either from damaged tissue or from platelets (PF_3). Factor Xa, the most important constituent, originates from factor X via the extrinsic or intrinsic system. In the extrinsic pathway the immediate effector is factor VII a, which for full activity needs the tissue factor, also known as thromboplastin. In the intrinsic pathway the responsible participant is factor IX a, the activity of which becomes greatly enhanced through factor VIII a. Regardless of the pathway involved, factor Xa in the prothrombinase complex catalyzes the production of thrombin.

Thrombin is not only responsible for the formation of fibrin from fibrinogen but also activates – in a kind of feedback mechanism – the factors V and VIII, thereby amplifying its own generation. On the other hand, after binding to thrombomodulin, thrombin activates protein C as depicted in detail in Fig. 3. Protein Ca in combination with protein S inactivates factors Va and VIII a, precisely those two components of the coagulation cascade potentiated by thrombin itself. Because of these special effects, the protein C pathway is today regarded a most potent mechanism for limiting the production of thrombin. Since thrombin can furthermore be directly inactivated through AT III in conjunction with heparan sulfate groups at the endothelial surface [34], it appears that the endothelium is actually responsible for control and limitation of coagulation.

As is depicted in the lower part of Fig. 4, the protein C system also influences fibrinolysis. It was only recently discovered that protein Ca neutralizes the plasminogen activator inhibitor of endothelial origin [37, 38]. Thus, the activity of TPA becomes predominant and results in an augmented formation of plasmin, the enzyme responsible for removing fibrin.

From all the hemostatic interactions outlined in Fig. 4 one may understand that the antithrombogenicity of the luminal vessel surface requires an intact endothelial lining. Vascular lesions with damage to the endothelial surface must induce platelet aggregation and coagulation solely at the site of damage, since spreading of both processes beyond the lesion is effectively counteracted by the antithrombogenic properties of the adjacent intact endothelium.

Thrombogenic Features of Perturbed Endothelium

Antithrombogenicity is not an unchangeable characteristic of the endothelium. It is a rather new insight that endothelial cells can develop certain thrombogenic properties, mainly in the course of inflammatory processes and immune reactions. Table 2 lists the most important thrombogenic reactions which can be induced when endothelial cells are stimulated or perturbed by various mediator substances. These mediators include endotoxin, i.e., lipopolysaccharides, and substances originating primarily in macrophages, lymphocytes, and endothelial cells themselves, such as interleukin-1 (IL-1), tumor necrosis factor (TNF), and PAF, as well as thrombin and histamine (see reviews [5, 9, 35]). Most of these substances can induce synthesis of tissue factor (thromboplastin) and its expression on the endothelial surface. As men-

Table 2. Induction of thrombogenic features in the vascular endothelium

Mediators	
	Endotoxin
	Interleukin 1
	Tumor necrosis factor
	Platelet activating factor
	Thrombin
	Histamine
Reactions of endothelial cells	
	Synthesis and expression of tissue factor
	Synthesis and activation of factor V
	Binding of factors Va, IXa, and Xa
	Reduced expression of thrombomodulin
	Enhanced synthesis of PAI
	Reduced synthesis of TPA
	Synthesis of PAF and IL-1

tioned above, tissue factor and factor VIIa act in concert to activate factor X in the extrinsic system (Figs. 4, 5). Other processes involve endothelial synthesis and activation of factor V and the binding of factors Va, IXa, and Xa to specific membrane receptor sites [41, 43]. As is apparent from Fig. 5, all these reactions lead to the formation of the prothrombinase complex, now adhering to the surface of a perturbed endothelium. In this way, generation of thrombin and, consequently, of fibrin becomes accentuated at the vessel wall.

It should also be mentioned that these pro-coagulatory events can be further enhanced because several mediators, such as endotoxin, IL-1, and TNF, simultaneously reduce the endothelial expression of thrombomodulin

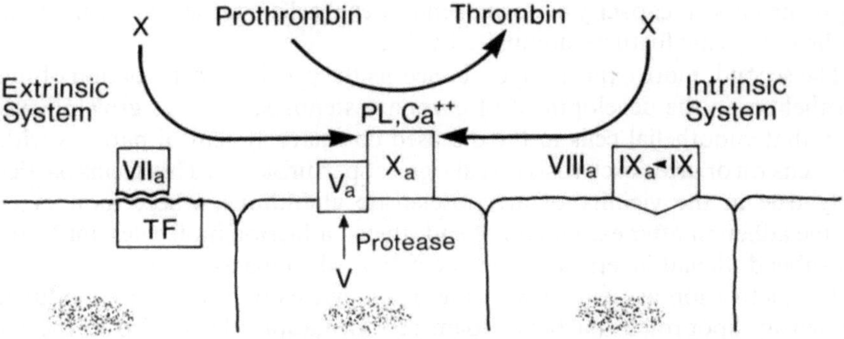

Fig. 5. Illustration of the prothrombogenic mechanisms induced through the action of various mediators at the surface of a perturbed endothelium. Most importantly, the prothrombinase complex originates at the endothelial surface via the extrinsic or intrinsic system, causing an accentuated formation of thrombin at the surface of irritated endothelial cells. These events occur in conjunction with inflammatory and immune reactions as well as during the development of arteriosclerosis of the vessel wall

[14, 35]. As a consequence, activation of protein C becomes impaired so that neutralization of PAI and down-regulation of thrombin formation are attenuated (see Fig. 4). Thus, more fibrin can be deposited at the surface of a perturbed endothelium. In addition, the persisting levels of thrombin and the endothelium-derived PAF provide strong proaggregatory stimuli for the platelets.

Endotoxin, IL-1, and thrombin can directly enhance the synthesis of PAI while reducing synthesis of TPA [35]. The net result is, obviously, a further reduction of fibrinolytic activity, which strongly favors the maintenance of the deposited fibrin network on the perturbed endothelial cells.

The last phenomenon listed in Table 2 relates to the surprising capability of endothelial cells to synthesize PAF and IL-1 themselves. Production of PAF can be induced, for instance, by IL-1, thrombin, and histamine; production of IL-1 is caused by IL-1 itself and by endotoxin and TNF [5, 35]. It is immediately apparent that, regardless of the respective mechanisms, endothelial formation of PAF and IL-1 strongly amplifies the thrombogenic properties of a once perturbed endothelium.

Additional Aspects

Any description of the antithrombogenic properties of the normal endothelium and of the thrombogenic features of a perturbed endothelium would be incomplete if two further aspects are not briefly addressed. One concerns observations that certain prothrombotic responses can not only be induced but are detectable even under normal conditions [35]. This applies, for instance, to the synthesis of factor V and the binding of factor Va (see Fig. 5) as well as to the endothelial formation and secretion of von Willebrand factor [22], known to be essential for the adhesion of platelets. There is, however, no doubt that the prothrombotic capacity of normal endothelial cells is rather small, and that antithrombogenic features dominate by far.

The second, more clinical aspect concerns the possible participation of the endothelium in the development of coronary stenoses. There is growing evidence that endothelial cells in the diseased coronary system of patients with hypertension or arteriosclerosis reveal signs of perturbation. This seems particularly true in the vicinity of arteriosclerotic alterations, where monocytes become adherent after expression of endothelial adhesion molecules, infiltrate into subendothelial layers, and become activated to macrophages.

This activation associated with the phagocytosis of oxidatively modified low-density lipoprotein particles (foam cell formation), leads also to the release of mediators (IL-1, PAF, TNF) which then cause or intensify the expression of thrombogenic features on the endothelial surface. As a result, local thrombin formation increases, giving rise to an accelerated platelet aggregation. In addition, the formation and deposition of fibrin becomes locally enhanced because fibrinolytic activity decreases due to an overall preponderance of PAI [20]. The extent of these processes, the concomitant proliferation of the vessel wall augmented by growth factors (PDGF) derived from platelets and endothelial cells [17], and the reduced formation of EDRF in such altered vessel segments or their attenuated response to EDRF [1], together, finally determine when blood flow becomes critically impaired.

The outlined concept reflects a rather qualitative view, and there is no doubt that many details require further experimental clarification and quantification. However, it must be accepted that in patients with a diseased coronary system pathophysiological consequences do result already from a perturbed and not yet destroyed endothelium. They involve, besides morphological and functional disturbances of the vessel wall, all three components of hemostasis: platelets, coagulation, and fibrinolysis.

References

1. Angus JA, Cocks TM (1989) Endothelium-derived relaxing factor. Pharmacol Ther 41:303–351
2. Bassenge E, Busse R, Pohl U (1987) Abluminal release and asymmetrical response of the rabbit arterial wall to endothelium-derived relaxing factor. Circ Res 61 [Suppl II]:II-68–II-73
3. Bevilacqua MP, Gimbrone MA (1987) Inducible endothelial functions in inflammation and coagulation. Semin Thromb Hemost 13:425–433
4. Born GVR, Cross MJ (1963) The aggregation of blood platelets. J Physiol (Lond) 168:178–195
5. Braquet P, Paubert-Braquet M, Koltai M, Bourgain R, Bussolino F, Hosford D (1989) Is there a case for PAF antagonists in the treatment of ischemic states? TIPS 10:23–31
6. Brett JG, Steinberg SF, deGroot PhG, Nawroth PP, Stern DM (1988) Norepinephrine down-regulates the activity of protein S on endothelial cells. J Cell Biol 106:2109–2118
7. Busse R, Lückhoff A, Bassenge E (1987) Endothelium-derived relaxant factor inhibits platelet activation. Naunyn-Schmiedeberg's Arch Pharmacol 336:566–571
8. Chan TK, Chan V (1981) Antithrombin III, the major modulator of intravascular coagulation, is synthesized by human endothelial cells. Thromb Haemost 46:504–506
9. Cotran RS (1987) New roles for the endothelium in inflammation and immunity. Am J Pathol 129:407–413
10. Cryer A (1983) Scale and diversity of interactions at the vascular endothelium. In: Cryer A (ed) Biochemical interactions at the endothelium. Elsevier, Amsterdam, pp 1–3
11. DiCorleto PE, Chisolm GM (1986) Participation of the endothelium in the development of the atherosclerotic plaque. Prog Lipid Res 25:365–374
12. Eckel RH (1989) Lipoprotein lipase: a multifunctional enzyme relevant to common metabolic diseases. N Engl J Med 320:1060–1068
13. Engelberg H (1989) Endothelium in health and disease. Semin Thromb Hemost 15:178–183
14. Esmon CT (1987) The regulation of natural anticoagulant pathways. Science 235:1348–1352
15. Esmon CT, Owen WG (1981) Identification of an endothelial cell cofactor for thrombin-catalyzed activation of protein C. Proc Natl Acad Sci USA 78:2249–2252
16. Fair DS, Marlar RA, Levin EG (1986) Human endothelial cells synthesize protein S. Blood 67:1168–1171
17. Gajdusek C, Carbon S, Ross R, Nawroth P, Stern D (1986) Activation of coagulation releases endothelial cell mitogens. J Cell Biol 103:419–428
18. Gerlach E, Nees S, Becker BF (1985) The vascular endothelium: a survey of some newly evolving biochemical and physiological features. Basic Res Cardiol 80:459–474
19. Gerlach E, Becker BF, Nees S (1987) Formation of adenosine by vascular endothelium: a homeostatic and antithrombogenic mechanism? In: Gerlach E, Becker BF (eds) Topics and perspectives in adenosine research. Springer, Berlin Heidelberg New York, pp 309–320

20. Grulich-Henn J, Müller-Berghaus G (1989) The role of vascular endothelial cells in the regulation of fibrinolysis. Z Kardiol 78 [Suppl 6]:25–29
21. Ignarro LJ (1989) Biological actions and properties of endothelium-derived nitric oxide formed and released from artery and vein. Circ Res 65:1–21
22. Jaffe EA (1984) Synthesis of factor VIII by endothelial cells. In: Jaffe EA (ed) Biology of endothelial cells. Nijhoff, Boston, pp 209–214
23. Léon M, Aiach M, Coezy E, Guennec J-Y, Fiesinger J-N (1983) Antithrombin III synthesis in rat liver parenchymal cells. Thromb Res 30:369–375
24. Lorenz R, Boehlig B, Üdelhofen W, Weber PC (1989) Superior antiplatelet action of alternate day pulsed dosing over split dose administration of aspirin. Am J Cardiol 64:1185–1188
25. Moncada S, Radomski MW, Palmer RMJ (1988) Endothelium-derived relaxing factor. Identification as nitric oxide and role in the control of vascular tone and platelet function. Biochem Pharmacol 37:2495–2501
26. Nees S, Gerlach E (1983) Adenine nucleotide and adenosine metabolism in cultured coronary endothelial cells: formation and release of adenine compounds and possible functional implications. In: Berne RM, Rall TW, Rubio R (eds) Regulatory function of adenosine. Nijhoff, Boston, pp 347–360
27. Nees S, Böck M, Herzog V, Becker BF, Des Rosiers C, Gerlach E (1985) The adenine nucleotide metabolism of the coronary endothelium: implications for the regulation of coronary flow by adenosine. In: Stefanovich V, Rudolphi K, Schubert P (eds) Adenosine: receptors and modulation of cell function. IRL, Oxford, pp 419–436
28. Nees S, Herzog V, Becker BF, Böck M, Des Rosiers C, Gerlach E (1985) The coronary endothelium: a highly active metabolic barrier for adenosine. Basic Res Cardiol 80:515–529
29. Nees S, Des Rosiers C, Böck M (1987) Adenosine receptors at the coronary endothelium: functional implications. In: Gerlach E, Becker BF (eds) Topics and perspectives in adenosine research. Springer, Berlin Heidelberg New York, pp 454–469
30. Newman WH, Becker BF, Heier M, Nees S, Gerlach E (1988) Endothelium-mediated coronary dilatation by adenosine does not depend on endothelial adenylate cyclase activation: studies in isolated guinea pig hearts. Pflügers Arch 413:1–7
31. Palmer RMJ, Ferrige AG, Moncada S (1987) Nitric oxide release accounts for the biological activity of endothelium-derived relaxing factor. Nature 327:524–526
32. Palmer RMJ, Ashton DS, Moncada S (1988) Vascular endothelial cells synthesize nitric oxide from L-arginine. Nature 333:664–666
33. Pearson JD, Carleton JS, Hutchings A, Gordon JL (1980) Metabolism of adenine nucleotides by ectoenzymes of vascular endothelial and smooth muscle cells in culture. Biochem J 190:421–429
34. Preissner KT (1988) Anticoagulant potential of endothelial cell membrane components. Haemostasis 18:271–306
35. Rogers GM (1988) Hemostatic properties of normal and perturbed vascular cells. FASEB J 2:116–123
36. Ryan US (1986) The endothelial surface and responses to injury. Fed Proc 45:101–108
37. Sakata Y, Curriden S, Lawrence D, Griffin JH, Loskutoff DJ (1985) Activated protein C stimulates the fibrinolytic activity of cultured endothelial cells and decreases antiactivator activity. Proc Natl Acad Sci USA 82:1121–1125
38. Schleef RR, Loskutoff DJ (1988) Fibrinolytic system of vascular endothelial cells. Role of plasminogen activator inhibitors. Haemostasis 18:328–341
39. Schmidt HHHW, Klein MM, Niroomand F, Böhme E (1988) Is arginine a physiological precursor of endothelium-derived nitric oxide? Eur J Pharmacol 148:293–295
40. Sollevi A, Torssell L, Öwall A, Edlund A, Lagerkranser M (1987) Levels and cardiovascular effects of adenosine in humans. In: Gerlach E, Becker BF (eds) Topics and perspectives in adenosine research. Springer, Berlin Heidelberg New York, pp 599–613
41. Stern D, Nawroth P, Handley D, Kisiel W (1985) An endothelial cell-dependent pathway of coagulation. Proc Natl Acad Sci USA 82:2523–2527
42. Stern D, Brett J, Harris K, Nawroth P (1986) Participation of endothelial cells in the protein C–protein S anticoagulant pathway: the synthesis and release of protein S. J Cell Biol 102:1971–1978

43. Stern DM, Kaiser E, Nawroth PP (1988) Regulation of the coagulation system by vascular endothelial cells. Haemostasis 18:202–214
44. van Hinsbergh VWM (1988) Regulation of the synthesis and secretion of plasminogen activators by endothelial cells. Haemostasis 18:307–327
45. Vanhoutte PM, Katusic ZS (1988) Endothelium-derived contracting factor: endothelin and/or superoxide anion. TIPS 9:229–230
46. van Iwaarden F, Acton DS, Sixma JJ, Meijers JCM, de Groot PhG, Bouma BN (1989) Internalization of antithrombin III by cultured human endothelial cells and its subcellular localization. J Lab Clin Med 113:717–726
47. Wolinsky H (1980) A proposal linking clearance of circulating lipoproteins to tissue metabolic activity as a basis for understanding atherogenesis. Circ Res 47:301–311
48. Yanagisawa M, Kurihara H, Kimura S, Tomobe Y, Kobayashi M, Mitsui Y, Yazaki Y, Goto K, Masaki T (1988) A novel potent vasoconstrictor peptide produced by vascular endothelial cells. Nature 332:411–415

Synergetics of Fluid-Dynamic and Biochemical Catastrophe Reactions in Coronary Artery Thrombosis

H. Schmid-Schönbein [1]

Introduction: Toward an Understanding of the Synergetics of the Cardiovascular System

The cardiovascular system is an ensemble of dynamic elements (pumps, conduits, and feedback regulators) that offers a striking example of dynamic stability, adaptability, and efficacy in complex biological systems. The fundamental regularities of such cooperative systems have become the topic of a new scientific discipline, termed synergetics [1, 2] or chaos theory [3–7], dealing with the emanation of dynamic cooperativity in physical, chemical, and biological processes. Large-scale biological order is comprehensible as the cooperativity of many subsystems, i.e., as the result of joint efforts in dynamic systems; the latter must be construed as limited compartments in which there is a continuous flow of energy and matter. Provided that in such systems a steady state far from thermodynamic equilibrium is created, coherent behavior spontaneously sets in, i.e., an a priori unexpected, highly efficient, and stable cooperativity which is governed by universal physical and thermodynamic laws. In this context it is important to realize that synergetics is concerned with processes rather than with reactions; the consideration of forces is replaced by consideration of powers (in the classical sense of thermodynamics).

In the cardiovascular system the present paradigmatic system of transport reactions (as described by Poiseuille's law, Ohm's law) must be replaced by the analysis of dynamic and cooperative processes (e.g., those between the heart as a pulsatile pump, the compliant vascular network, and the blood as a multiphase fluid). Concepts for this approach can be taken from synergetics, a neologism coined by Haken [1, 2] to describe regularities responsible for the spontaneous creation of highly organized dissipative structures in dynamic multiphase systems and for their coherent behavior, which induces the transitions of random events at the microscopic level to macroscopic cooperativity whenever the systems are not in thermodynamic equilibrium. The application of synergetic concepts as developed by Haken [1, 2] for various physical systems by Prigogine and Stengers [3], Schuster [4], and Hess and Markus [5] for autocatalytically amplified chemical systems and by Ruelle and Takens [6] and Mandelbrot [7] for the development of turbulent flow can help not only to

[1] Abteilung Physiologie, Klinikum der RWTH, Pauwelsstrasse, 5100 Aachen, West Germany

W. Bleifeld et al. (Eds.)
Unstable Angina

provide insight into the intricate cooperativity [8] of the components of the cardiovascular system but also proves to be extremely helpful in understanding catastrophic reactions in vascular pathology.

The chaos theory was developed in the study of nonbiological multiphase systems; its application in cardiology has led to a better understanding of arrhythmias [9]. The transfer of chaos concepts to biology and medicine, however, tends to produce semantic confusion [2]; the original and still generally accepted understanding of the term chaos refers to systems that are not subject to law, but in which reactions occur by chance. More specifically, chaos was and still is understood colloquially to describe a confused, unorganized, and unpredictable state of primordial matter before the creation of distinct and orderly forms.

The present review starts from the assumption (detailed in [8]) that the intact circulatory system of blood constituents (macrocirculation, microcirculation, extravascular percolation due to the process of filtration and reabsorption) can be interpreted as a large ensemble of simple dynamic systems that are coherent in behavior. Mechanical coherence (in the synergetic sense) in a system of connected conduits follows from the simple laws of communicating tubes; however there is also chemical coherence of the processes in which the blood constituents take part.

Since not only the intravascular, but also the interstitial convective transport processes are powered by the rectified flow of energy, the stability of flow is also exerting control over the stability of chemical reactions in these two compartments. Moreover, by keeping the environment (i.e. the milieu exterieur of the cells) in stable order, stable perfusion of the interstitial space therefore helps to maintain intracellular integrity. The cooperativity and coherence of rectified flow in the entire systemic circulation therefore stabilizes (a) the directionality of vascular perfusion and interstitial percolation, (b) the distribution of flows (ordered attendance of blood constituents to individual vessel segments and to the interstitial spaces), and (c) the biochemical processes taking place in the different parts of the large interstitial compartment by strongly favoring stable or linear catalyzed reactions and by effectively inhibiting unstable or non-linear catalyzed reactions.

The Concept of Coherent Rectified Flow and Its Disturbances as a Cause of Cardiovascular Pathology

The input of energy and matter into the proximal aorta and the large arteries is highly pulsatile; for this reason the system is powered phasically. Fluid-dy-

[2] The concepts and semantics of synergetics and of chaos theory are new; they have not yet penetrated biomedical thinking and are therefore often misunderstood. In the attempt to provide the reader of the present review with an everyday model of the behavior of a dynamic model, the behavior of windsleeves is explained in the didactic appendix, to which those readers who are here confronted for the first time with synergetics are referred before continuing the present text.

namic rectification occurs in a conduit network, itself optimalized geometrically [10]. Due to the great frictional energy dissipation associated with the perfusion of microscopic tubes, the energy is lost as the blood moves through the terminal vessels. A small – but by no means negligible – remainder of the systolic cardiac energy is normally conserved to do work in filling the right ventricle. The concept of rectified flow can be generalized to include all those processes that normally guarantee stable laminar flow. The results of passive rectification processes reduce the degrees of freedom of the constituents of the cardiovascular system; despite the presence of influences of kinetic energy, gravitational effects, and the prima vista complex conduits that tend to destabilize the blood flow, the process of blood motion is highly robust toward external and internal disturbances, adaptable and stable. Speaking in synergetic terms, this process in the systemic circulatory system can be said to be under the influence of one strong-attractor process (the powered flow of energy and matter from the arterial energy reservoir to the right venticle in diastole). If – for sake of argument – we neglect the pulmonary system for a moment, we can state that the contractile process in the contracting myocardium replenishes the power – the product of flow rate (m^3/s) and pressure ($N/m^2 = Nm/s$) – to the moving blood. This results, then, in the periodic boosting of the Windkessel vessels; from these the motion of the highly complex fluid blood through a complicated system of conduits proceeds under pulsatile input of energy and matter from one to the next segment. Rectification is based on damping processes in the vessel walls, impedance matching of the resistance vessels to the large conduits (see "Stabilizing Mechanisms"), dynamic fluidization of red cell plasma mixtures, and electrostatic repulsion processes between the glycocalices of blood cells and endothelial cells (see [24]). All cooperate in minimizing deviating motions and thus frictional energy losses in the moving blood. It goes without saying that this greatly enhances the efficacy of transport processes in the cardiovascular system.

In discussing the synergetics of blood circulation, one must also keep in mind that there are multiple biological functions of the cardiovascular system beyond those related to transport of blood gases and metabolites. For example, constituents of the blood must fulfill pivotal influences in all catalyzed (immunologic, hemostatic) reactions taking place in response to injury. For these aims, the rectified and cooperative flow must become separated. As detailed in the section "Stabilizing Mechanisms", strictly unidirectional Poiseuille flow completely inhibits the occurrence of self-amplifying biochemical reactions between plasmatic and cellular components of blood for three clear reasons (Fig. 1): (a) the steady laminar flow leads to automatic dilution of activated enzymes; (b) activated enzymes (e.g., serin proteases) are immediately bound by inhibitor principles (e.g., thrombin by antithrombin III, AT_{III}); and (c) the association of activated proteases with plasmatic protease inhibitor proteins links the reaction site to an infinite reservoir of inhibitor principles (e.g., antithrombin, α_2-macroglobulin) and connects every part of the vascular system to an infinite sink of scavenger mechanisms that remove the reaction product (e.g., the FIIa-AT_{III} complex).

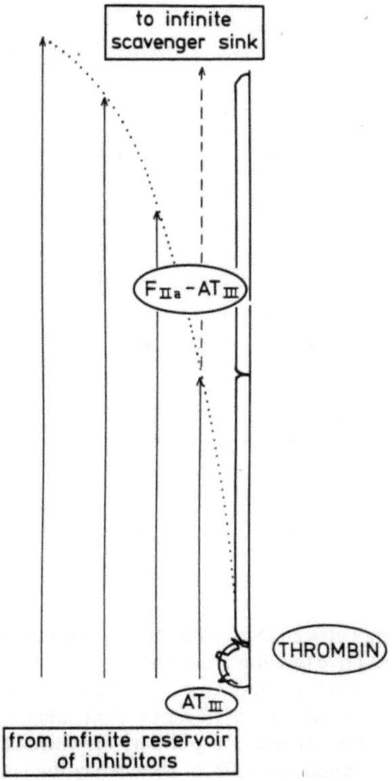

Fig. 1. Schematic representation of the functional coherence of laminar flow and biochemical reactions in the flowing blood (as examplified in the linear reaction between an activated enzyme (here thrombin) and its inhibitor (here antithrombin III, AT_{III})). Strictly linear convective motion guarantees that reaction product (here the complex of antithrombin III – factor IIa, F_{IIa}) is removed, coupling the reaction to an infinite sink for scavenger mechanisms. Similar linear scavenging reactions take place between all other activated proteases and protein inhibitor molecules (e.g., α_2-macroglobulin), plasmin and antiplasmin, arachidonic acid, and albumin; between released serotonin and passing thrombocytes; and between oxygen radicals and flowing radical scavengers (e.g., the glutathione of the passing RBC)

Conversely, noncoherent or disturbed flow (e.g., vortex or eddy movements, local stagnation phenomena) facilitates all catalyzed reactions in the blood vessels. We can regard the occurrence of (mechanical) flow separation as both the cause and the consequence of chemical divergence phenomena [1–5] or of phase transitions, which in turn cooperate in destabilizing blood flow [8]. As we will see below, the transition from laminar to incoherent flow becomes an order parameter controlling the manifestation of chemical reaction involving cellular and plasmatic blood components. We can regard separated flow as a divergence process with low fractal dimension [11], producing short-lived vortices that act as flow reactors. In these vortices networks of catalyzed, self-perpetuating, and self-amplifying chemical reactions (e.g., those of the coagulation system) can take place (Fig. 2).

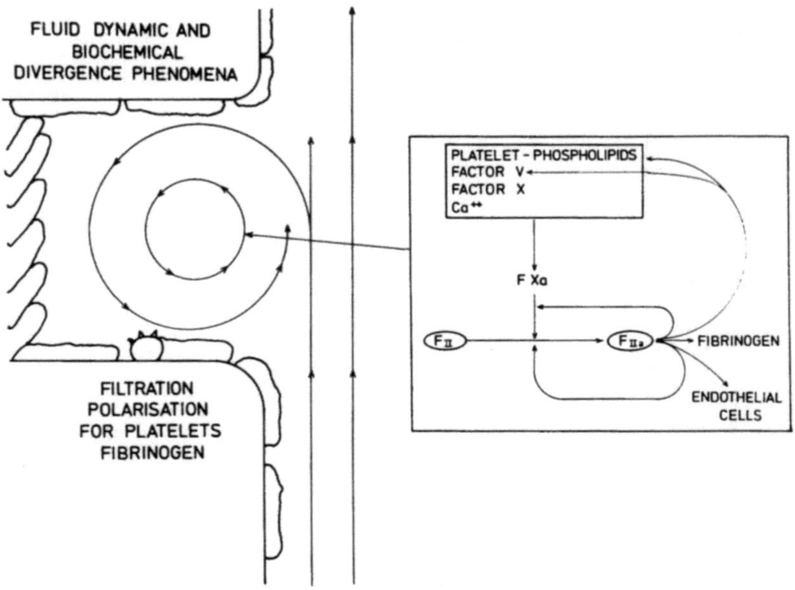

Fig. 2. Schematic representation of the functional coupling between incoherent blood flow and an enzymatically amplified reaction. Unless removed by convective dilution (and binding to its inhibitor), thrombin initiates a multitude of positive feed back reaction loops (e.g., that by activating platelets and factors V, X, and II). Also, it acts on endothelial cells by severing their integrity allowing local accumulation of fibrinogen and thrombocytes, as reaction partners for chemical reactions, and induces a fluid/solid phase transition (due to induction of fibrin polymerization and platelet aggregation). Similar reaction loops occur between the activated factor XII and the alternate pathway of the complement system, the kinin system, between platelet-derived activators and fresh platelets, and between them and the adjacent endothelial cells, the interstitium, and the smooth-muscle cells

It is the purpose of this communication to demonstrate the synergetics of fluid-dynamic, cytological, enzymatic, and hemorrheological aspects in a pathogenetic concept of circular causality for atherogenesis and thrombogenesis, and hence for unstable angina. It is proposed that (a) atherogenic reactions can be regarded as the consequences of long-term but low-grade divergence reactions caused by repetitive fluid-dynamic flow separation episodes which are associated with strictly localized traumatizing events injuring the wall in noncylindrical vascular segments, and that (b) thrombotic reactions in abnormally shaped macrovascular beds follow fundamental rules established for catastrophic or deterministic chaos reactions in other, related scientific fields and can be reduced to geometric, fluid-mechanical and enzymatic reasons generating a flow reactor in the classical sense of a dissipative structure [3] [3].

[3] The multitude of cytological [11], enzymological [12] reactions and their synergy (see [13] and [14]), but also the secondary rheological changes in platelets (see [15]) can thence be put into a common perspective.

Stabilizing Mechanisms in the Cardiovascular System and Their Breakdown in Aging and Disease

The synergetic interpretation of the mammalian cardiovascular system must start from the fundamental fact that the input of energy and matter (i.e., the mechanical work, $\Delta P \times Q$, associated with each systole) is generated in an extremely phasic fashion. The short systolic acceleration phase (0.1 s) in the systemic circulation, the complex geometry, and the multiphase nature of the blood are therefore endogenously unstable and hence susceptible to flow separation [16]. In fluid-dynamic terms, the motion of blood in the proximal arteries is associated with high Reynolds' numbers and pronounced pulsatility of Reynolds' numbers (see [16]).

There are numerous mechanisms to compensate for the input instability (Table 1). In the present context the storage of energy in the proximal elastic arteries (Windkessel vessels), the myogenic, metabolic, and nervous control of the small arterioles and the physiolocial adaptation of these two (impedance matching) tend to stabilize the motion of blood [17], i.e., attenuate Reynolds' number pulsatility. In fluid-mechanical terms, the Windkessel function can be reduced to the reduction of forward velocity in systole, increase in forward velocity in diastole, i.e., attenuation in flow pulsatility (but see "Fluid Dynamics"). The systolic dilatation of the aorta and the proximal arteries attenuates the ratio of kinetic energy over viscous energy by decreasing systolic peak flow in comparison to that occurring in nondistensible vessels when both are phasically powered [18]. Conversely, the elastic recoil (contraction) of the distended walls in diastole leads to maintained forward flow during the cardiac pause. Even at peak flow velocity, the ratio of kinetic energy over shear stress is kept relatively low, but, most importantly, the protosystolic acceleration is attenuated.

The action of the Windkessel vessel thereby helps to stabilize laminar flow in complex conduits. It follows from the same logic that the physiological changes taking place in the walls of arterial systems during aging produce an unavoidable loss of a major rectifying mechanism. It is generally known that the enhancement of peak systolic pressure and hence of pulse pressure is a sign of physiosclerosis during aging. More importantly, however, the flow pulsatility is greatly augmented, and therefore the pulsatility in Reynolds' number [16] is much more pronounced.

Another important change taking place during the process of physiological aging is the geometric deformation of arteries. The juvenile circulatory system is physiologically shaped in accordance to fluid-dynamic optimality principles [10]. Not only the taper of individual arterial segments but also the branching angles, the radii of curvature, and the ratio of cross-sectional areas of sequential segments are structured in such a fashion that flow is forced into the stable laminar shearing, the danger of flow separation being minimized by the progressive drop in the Reynolds' number from proximal to distal arteries [19–21]. This geometric order is lost as a quasiphysiological side effect of aging, so

Table 1. Rectifying mechanisms of the cardiovascular system to stabilize blood flow

1. Myocardium
   1.1. Frank-Starling mechanism of the right and left ventricles in complying to changes in preload and afterload (see 6.5)
   1.2. Rectification of flow directionality due to action of all cardiac valves
   1.3. Mediation of sympathetic and parasympathetic inotropic and chronotropic effects
   1.4. Active diastolic filling due to elastic and kinetic energies operating in A-V ring displacement mechanism (see 6.5)
2. Large arteries
   2.1. The Windkesselfunktion
   2.2. Impedance matching due to dilatation in physical exercise
   2.3. Site of sensor mechanisms for stability of boosted steady state, regular for cardiovascular depressor reflexes
3. Arterioles
   3.1. Matching in microvascular conductance and cell attendance to metabolic demands (input regulation)
   3.2. Matching of microvascular conductance to arterial steady state (myogenic and metabolic output autoregulation)
   3.3 Attenuation of pressure and flow pulsatility
4. Exchange capillaries
   4.1. Axial RBC alignment
   4.2. Marginal plasma lubrication
   4.3. Active control of cytological and plasmatic interactions: electrostatic repulsion between cellular glycocalices (endothelial cells, blood cells) and between cells and plasmatic colloids
   4.4 Maintenance of flow rate and directionality of reversed osmosis (concentration, performance of chemical work when Pcap > COP) and colloidal osmosis (performance of osmotic work when Pcap < COP; see 6.5.)
5. Interstitial tissue
   5.1. Directed percolation and irrigation of pericellular spaces for nutrient and mediator supply
   5.2. Obligatory link of scavenger input and output
6. Veins
   6.1. Venous valve mechanism
   6.2. Venous tone adaptation to adapt capacity
   6.3. Venous tone adaptation to adapt site of volume receptors to match blood volume to systemic capacitance
   6.4. Obligatory adaptation of cardiac filling (venous output) to microvascular perfusion (venous input)
   6.5 Obligatory setting of intravascular pressure to atmospheric pressure (zero transmural pressure, ensuring colloidal osmosis in exchange vessels)

that the gross enlargement of the proximal arterial bed, the meandering, and the loss of compliance cooperate in slowly changing the arterial bed into a system of enlarged and stiffened conduits no longer following the rules of optimality. The above-mentioned fluid-dynamic and the presently discussed geometric alterations in the vascular bed therefore pose a potentiated risk for flow destabilization (see [20] and [21]).

The arterioles – by their efficacy in matching impedance to net flow [22] – stabilize pressure and flow in arteries. In the microcirculation there are a host of mechanisms that exert rectifying effects on the blood flow at the level of the exchange vessels (to be discussed elsewhere [23]). In the present context the sequence of filtration and reabsorption (reversed osmosis at the arteriolar and osmosis at the venular end of microvessels) must be viewed as cooperative effects of a mechanism producing coherent tissue percolation. It is of the utmost significance to appreciate that the tunica intima of the large arteries (i.e., the subendothelial space) is a part of the extravascular compartment (in essence part of the interstitium). Its lack of proper irrigation in the course of the atherogenic process represents another form of incoherent flow (see [8], [24]).

The rectifying mechanisms in the low-pressure system (veins and right heart in diastole) are beyond the scope of the present communication. Suffice it to say that the action of the venous valves and the so-called Frank-Starling mechanism cooperate in rectifying flow and keep the highly unstable venous homestretch in an energized form [8]. In the present context it is important to know that myocardial insufficiency (by its interference with perfect matching of venous return and cardiac output) must be viewed as a destabilizing mechanism for blood flow.

Lastly, obliterating atherogenesis as well as essential hypertension (as the typical forms of vascular pathology associated with unstable angina) both interfere with the physiological rectifying mechanisms [23], albeit in an indirect fashion. The fundamental pathomechanisms of essential hypertension, namely elevated cardiac output and/or enhanced peripheral resistance, remove the arterial system from its dynamic optimality [10], i.e., predisposes to flow separation. Both hemodynamic abnormalities can cause the symptom of elevated blood pressure; however, they augment flow pulsatility much more than they enhance mean arterial pressure or diastolic pressure [16, 18]. Obliterating atheromatosis by the combination of enhanced pressure loss over the stenosis and compensatory arteriolar vasodilatation produces severe changes in the microvascular rectifying mechanism (described elsewhere). It goes without saying that the effects of hypertension and obliteration are more pronounced if superimposed upon an aged, less well stabilizing arterial vasculature.

Functional Haemostasiology: Thrombotic Process Occurring in Flow Reactors Rather than in Test Tubes

The conceptional advantage of physiological synergetics lies in its ability to relate apparently independent biological processes in a meaningful schema of causality. For this purpose the conventional fluid-dynamic approach as well as the conventional biochemical approach to biomedical problems, have to be extended, simply with the aim of bringing these two areas of experimental investigation into a common dimensional system, namely that of energy flow, of energy barriers and energy gradients, of flow of matter, and of the ratio of reaction rates and flow rates. As we try to understand unstable angina as a process related to (unphysiological yet normal hemostatic or prothrombotic) reactions occurring in abnormally shaped coronary arteries, we have to view the enzymatically driven reactions as processes in (more or less short-lived) flow reactors (see "Didactic Appendix").

For obvious reasons, the bioenergetic details of enzymatically controlled events occurring in rectified and coherent flow and those occurring in incoherent flow are beyond the scope of the present review; these will be dealt with, however, in a contribution to a symposium on blood coagulation [24]. Suffice it to say here that:

1. The conventional techniques for studying blood or blood components taken from their natural habitat (coherently flowing blood) detach the blood, as it were, from the infinite reservoir of scavengers and the infinite sink for activator-inhibitor complexes, as discussed in the section "The Concept of Coherent Rectified Flow."
2. Blood taken from its state of coherent flow and sequestered into any container of limited volume is turned into a dynamic system in its own right, i.e., it displays the enzymatic, proteolytic, and fibrinoplastic potentials of blood. The multitude of hemostasiological data on coagulation reactions in normal blood and in blood taken from patients have to be viewed as reaction potentials: they can, within limits, be extrapolated to reactions taking place in fully incoherent flow in vivo.
3. Fully incoherent flow, however, is the exception rather than the rule; therefore, if we accept the natural hemostatic reactions (physiological as well as pathological ones) as events in a flow reactor, the continuous through-put of energy and matter, the production of reaction products (activated proenzymes, activated monomers, activated platelets) and the phase transitions of activated reaction products (polymerization of fibrin-monomers into macromolecular fibers and fiber networks, aggregation of platelets, combination of polymerization and aggregation) have to be taken into account.
4. There are not just the well-known physicochemical differences between the walls of test tubes and those of blood vessels, but also between normal and pathological vessels. Clearly, the walls of containers for autocatalytically driven proteolytic reactions are – to a greater or lesser degree active – reaction partners for either coherent or incoherent biochemical events in a blood sample. The antithrombotic properties of endothelialized vascular segments again have to be seen from an energetic point of view (due to the barrier of hydration energy of the components of the glycocalix of endothelial cells) (Fig. 3). Conversely, the thrombogenic properties of acutely or chronically deendothelialized vascular segments are only in part related to the breakdown of the energy barrier just referred to. They are, however, related to an energetic sink from the high-pressure system into the interstitium [24].

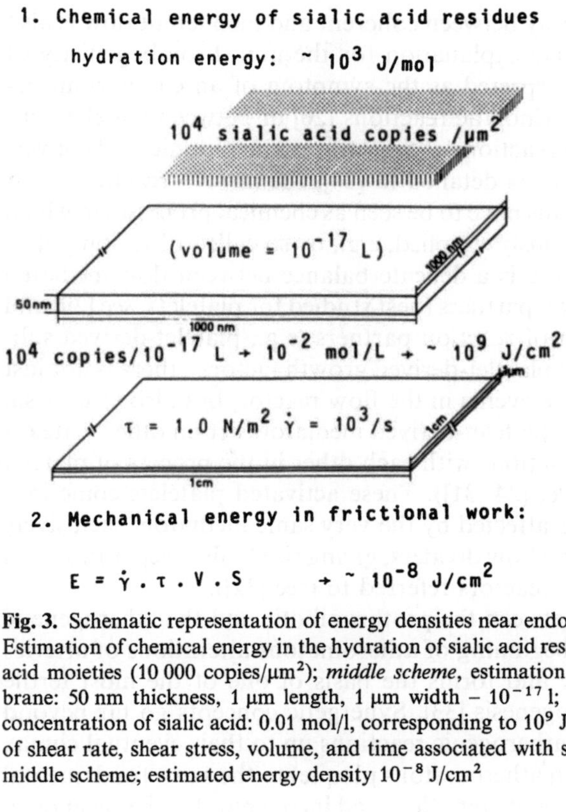

Fig. 3. Schematic representation of energy densities near endothelial surfaces and cell surfaces. *1*, Estimation of chemical energy in the hydration of sialic acid residues; *upper scheme*, density of sialic acid moieties (10 000 copies/μm^2); *middle scheme*, estimation of hydrophilic volume near membrane: 50 nm thickness, 1 µm length, 1 µm width – 10^{-17} l; *lower scheme*, estimation of molar concentration of sialic acid: 0.01 mol/l, corresponding to 10^9 J/cm^2. *2*, Mechanical work: product of shear rate, shear stress, volume, and time associated with shearing the volume depicted in the middle scheme; estimated energy density 10^{-8} J/cm^2

In summary then, we can hope to understand the synergy between the biochemical and the biophysical events leading to coronary atheromatosis, to coronary thrombosis, and to the sequelae of thrombotic events in perfused coronary artery only if we segregate ourselves without compromize from the current concept of isolated fluid-dynamic and chemical reactions. Contemporary hemorrheology, i.e., the study of physical properties of blood as a function of biochemical composition and of changes in these, has thus paved the way to the transition from what might be called test-tube biochemistry[4] of extracellular reactions to the flow reactor approach that has long been taken by workers such as Hess [25] for understanding control in intracellular biochemical chain reactions.

---

[4] The fundamental differences between test-tube reactions, in which several chemical reactants are brought together simultaneously and the flow reactor processes, into which reactants are continuously being fed and from which reaction products are continuously removed are beyond the scope of the present review; the reader is referred to Chapter 9 of [1].

The conceptional dichotomy between coherent and incoherent flow is also introduced as a comprehensive explanation for the non-thrombogenicity of blood in vivo, previously interpreted as the symptom of an equilibrium between thromboplastic and fibrinolytic reactions [26] or between platelet-activating and platelet-inhibiting reactions of the various arachidonic acid conversion reactions [27]. Moreover, as detailed in [24], the in vivo reactions near injured parts of the arterial walls have to be seen as chemical processes in which reaction partners are continuously supplied, e.g., by so called filtration polarization [28], and in which there is a delicate balance between flow-mediated supply and removal of reaction partners (best studied for platelets, see [29] and [30]). Since there is filtration of reaction partners (e.g., platelet-derived substances such as serotonin and platelet-derived growth factors), there is not just an influence of the wall on the events in the flow reactor, but also vice versa. In a strictly localized fashion, platelet-derived mediators act on other platelets and condition them for interactions with each other in the process of platelet aggregation (see, for example, [24, 31]). These activated platelets come into contact with endothelial cells affected by the very same mediators exclusively in the immediate vicinity of the flow dividers, giving rise to flow separation and hence the generation of flow reactors referred to (see [32]).

The very close relation between the prothrombotic and the atherogenetic reactions of platelets at the beginning of atheromatous alterations of arteries has been stressed repeatedly and forms the basis of one of the most fertile current hypotheses of atherogenesis [33]. Synergetic concepts go far beyond this. They relate all steps of atherogenic reactions up to their eventual climax (thrombosis on the basis of an atheromatous plaque) to the same fundamental functional abnormality, i.e., incoherent flow and incoherent biochemical reactions in the extracellular spaces (vascular lumen and the extracellular space in the macrovascular walls). Recent progress in the imaging of disturbed flow in human subjects (e.g., [34]) provide support for our earlier hypothesis (see [13, 14, 16, 18]) that arterial thrombosis occurs in areas of separated flow, a concept well supported by detailed fluid-dynamic studies (see [17, 19–21]) and capable of leading out of the deadlock between the low shear [35] and the high shear [36] controversy on the influence of fluid dynamics on atherogenesis and thrombosis (see also [18]).

Instability of Blood Motion: Separated Flow as Deterministic Chaos

In conventional fluid mechanical terms (uncritically transferred to hemodynamics) one differentiates between laminar and turbulent flow. Even advanced text books on biofluid mechanics leave their readers with the impression that there is one critical Reynold's number at which a sudden transition from laminar to turbulent flow occurs. As discussed repeatedly [13, 16, 18], one must divorce oneself decidedly from this misconception.

The fluid-dynamic conditions prevailing in the arterial system never allow full-fledged (stochastic) turbulence for the simple reason that high velocities prevail only for short intervals (in the range of 100–200 ms). We should therefore discontinue the use of the term altogether in biofluid dynamics and replace it by the term vortex-forming and -carrying laminar flow and conceive of it in synergetic terms as of a divergence phenomenon (see Figs. 2, 5).

To appreciate the physical basis for the generation of deterministic vortices as separated flow, we must first recapitulate the physics of stable laminar flow. The thermodynamics and synergetics of Poiseuille flow in the cardiovascular system (i.e., a branching network of tapering tubes) has not been fully worked out. We can calculate, however, the energetics of each vascular segment, which represents a conduit boosted by the flow of energy and matter through it. The energy content (Nm = joules) is equal to the sum of potential energy – product of pressure (N/m^2) and volume (m^3) and of kinetic energy ($0.5\ mv^2$). For each segment, the content reflects the difference between energy inflow – equal to a power (Nm/s or watts) pressure differential ($\Delta P\ N/m^2$) and volumetric flow rate (m^3/s) – and energy outflow. The systolic cardiac output of energy and matter (product of stroke volume, m^3, and aortic pressure, N/m^2) is equivalent to a phasic input of energy, the kinetic energy of which is in part conserved as such, in part converted to potential energy (in actual fact the conformational energy of distended elastic elements in the walls of the Windkessel vessels); in part it is dissipated in performing frictional work associated with fluid element deformation (see [49]). For the sake of simplicity let us combine the potential and the kinetic energy as free energy of the system; this is mostly dissipated in performing frictional work in the peripheral vessels. However, a small part is conserved as kinetic energy of the venous blood, used to perform the work associated with distending the myocardium in diastole (the dynamic basis of the Frank-Starling mechanism). In terms of synergetics, we therefore come to the conclusion that the process of perfusing the individual vascular segments takes place (more or less) far from thermodynamic equilibrium, and that each segment represents a dynamic system (compartment) in a boosted steady state, a term explained in detail in [8].

It follows from the geometry and topology of the vascular network that the dynamics of the process of blood motion differs as it is displaced from arteries to exchange vessels to venules and veins. It follows from Poiseuille's law that the energy dissipation for any given volume displacement in unit time is markedly enhanced in smaller than in larger vessels. Likewise, it follows from continuity considerations that the kinetic energy is continuously reduced as that blood moves from larger (and more rapidly perfused) to smaller (and less rapidly perfused) vessels. Note, however, that even at the microscopic tubes there is a finite yet very small kinetic energy in each perfused microvessel. The venular and venous beds, characterized by continuously increasing hydraulic conductance (and hence progressively decreasing frictional losses; see [23]) are capable of funneling the sums of the kinetic energies contained in the microvessels to those in the two venae cavae, the two atria, and the two ventricles in diastole.

Before we proceed to separated flow, we must dwell briefly on the specific dynamics of the truly laminar (or Stokes' flow) as a dynamic process in cylindrical vessel when the fluid adheres to its walls (no slip condition). The fluid molecules cohere to each other, are in brownian motion, but can change places. What is felt as frictional energy dissipation is the result of multiple collisions (and exchange of impulses) when molecules traveling in spiraling trajectories [23] are involved in many more collisions than in the resting fluid. The energy dissipated in this process in unit time (work, equal to the product of power and time) can be calculated from the product of shear rate and shear stress, multiplied by the volume undergoing shear ($s^{-1} \cdot N \cdot m^{-2} \cdot m^3 = Nm/s$). As they are forced to collide when fluid lamellae glide past each other, a unique kinematic process is established: following a simple principle of minimum energy dissipation, the well-known three-dimensional parabolic velocity profile emanates. The reason is simple: frictional energy dissipation is largely restricted to the marginal layers; the axial portions far from the wall move without energy dissipation (because the velocity differences are lowest here); the remaining laminae glide past each other with equal velocity gradients (or shear stresses); and the linear distribution of velocity gradients produce the well-known parabolic distribution of absolute velocities.

In each boosted vascular segment (and especially the microscopic ones where the axial migration further stabilizes the motion [23]) this process induces large-scale cooperativity; it leads to the minimum possible energy expenditure and hence to the maximum possible conservation of kinetic energy. Whatever the absolute flow rates and dimensions are, the more rapidly moving axial fluid elements are displaced with least frictional energy dissipation and thus convey a maximum of kinetic energy to the respective downstream segment. Furthermore, since the absolute ratios of kinetic energy over frictional losses (as measured by Reynolds' numbers) decrease, the deformation process becomes more and more stable, the smaller the perfused vessels are.

In all processes of fluid motion, the ratio of kinetic energy can be described in a so-called order parameter, namely the Reynolds' number (ReN), a ratio of parameters (ϱ = density, r = radius, u = velocity, η = viscosity) conventionally written as

$$\mathrm{ReN} = \varrho\, r\, u / \eta$$

but reflecting the ratio of kinetic energy ($\varrho\, u^2$) over shear stress, ($\eta\, u/r$), as becomes evident if the equation is rewritten, and numerator and denominator are multiplied by u:

$$\mathrm{ReN} = \frac{\varrho\, u^2}{\eta \dfrac{u}{r}}; \quad \text{where} \quad \frac{\eta\, u}{r} \mathrel{\hat{=}} \tau\, [\mathrm{Nm}^{-2}]$$

As indicated above, the concept of one critical Reynolds' number for the transition from laminar (friction dominated) to turbulent (kinetic energy dominated) flow is without value for biofluid-dynamic consideration. Instead, we must appreciate that the flow can become separated if there is a sudden change

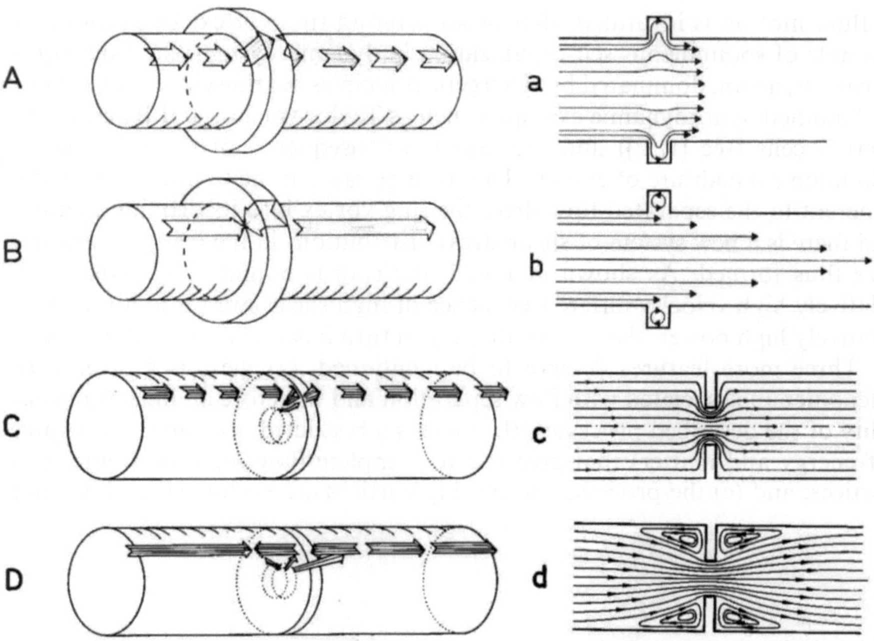

Fig. 4. Schematic representation of flow separation in the two most simple cases of geometric instability: expansion and stenosis of a cylindrical tube shown as en face view (**A–D**) and as cross-section (**a–d**). At very low Reynolds' numbers (**A**, **C**, **a**, **c**,) there is laminar, coherent flow following the contours of the conduit. At moderate Reynolds' numbers (**B**, **D**, **b**, **d**) flow becomes separated by formation of a ring vortex in the expansion as well as before and after the stenosis. In all cases of separation, backward flow occurs near the wall of expansion (see text for explanation). Also, boundary layers are formed between flow in the core and in the vortex (hence "incoherent flow")

in the conduit configuration simply because the kinetic energy of the fluid in motion is better conserved if the conduits suddenly become wider and, conversely, the shear stresses (and thus frictional energy dissipation) become larger if there is a sudden narrowing of the conduits. If, however, the narrowing is followed by a sudden widening, the kinetic energy is again better conserved, a fact again destabilizing flow (see Fig. 4).

These straightforward fluid dynamic considerations (detailed in the didactic appendix) will hopefully convince the biomedical community that any form of geometric abnormality in vascular conduits is associated with a sudden increase in the dispersion of local Reynolds' numbers. There is, in addition, a further instability, namely that in directionality, which can be reduced to the requirements of the law of continuity. For any given flow rate, the product of cross-sectional area and averaged velocity must be constant. Obviously, the average velocity is reduced (in proportion to the increase in cross-sectional area); hence if the axial velocities remain constant, continuity requirements can be met only if there are negative velocities, or in other words backward flow. Again following principles of least energy dissipation, a second process of fluid motion is instituted, that of an orbiting ring vortex. Its motion, an example of spontaneous self-organization in dynamic systems far from equilibrium is, again, dominated by synergetic principles bearing close similarity to well-studied hydrodynamic examples such as Taylor vortices and Benard convection cells (see [1, 3]) and are also the consequence of the principle of minimum expenditure of energy. The shear stresses at the boundary from the coherent to the separated flow drive the ring vortex into its orbiting motion, and there is a new system of shear stress distributions in the dissipative structure thus formed. As shown in Fig. 5, the ring is bounded by layers with relatively high velocity differences, hence of high shear stresses and therefore relatively high power; the core of the ring in turn has low velocity differences.

Three more features deserve to be mentioned: (a) there is a divergence phenomenon associated with flow separation and therefore an inherent instability of the described processes; (b) there is a restricted domain of flow rates (of energy and matter) that give rise to complete flow separation into ring vortices; and (c) the processes in the ring vortices are no longer in coherence

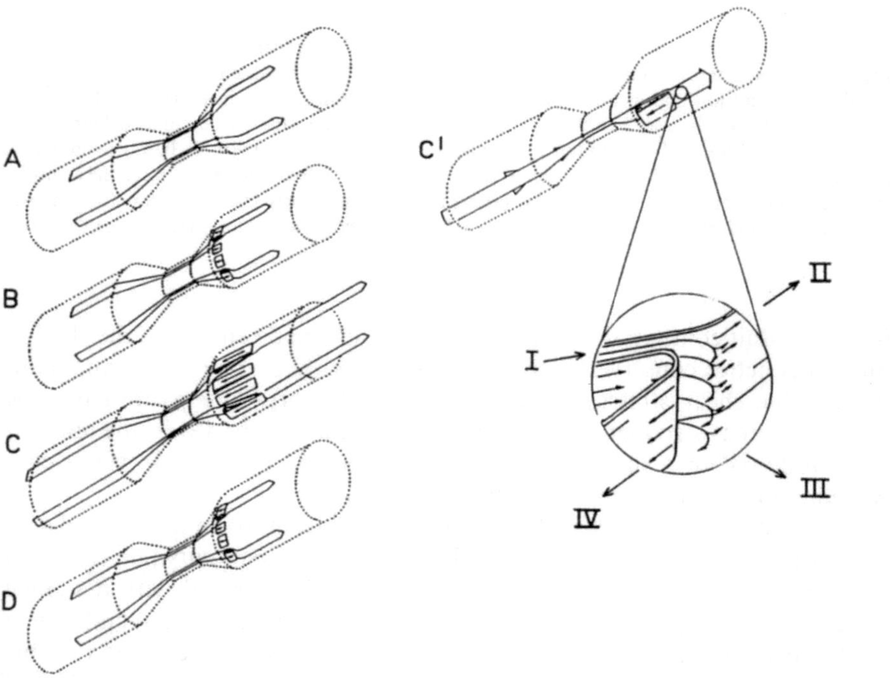

Fig. 5 A–D. Schematic representation of flow separation near stenosis in pulsatile flow. In diastole (**A**) the flow is fully laminar; in protodiastole (**B**) a ring vortex is developing, growing in size during peak systole (**C**) and followed by size reduction in late systole (**D**). *C'* Details in one segment of the so-called relaminarization point. The streamlines coming from the boundary layer (*I*) divide to feed into the laminar flow (*II*) and into the vortex (*IV*); some streamlines hit the wall (*III*), each one forming a stagnation point and their totality forming a showering jet washing the wall (see also Fig. 6). (Figure kindly supplied by Prof. Pertkold, University of Graz, Austria)

with Stokes' flow and are highly influenced by other processes to be discussed below (strange-attractor processes). We shall therefore refer to such fluid dynamic separation processes as incoherent flow (see "Didactic Appendix").

All types of secondary flow and/or vortices found in the vascular tree in segments with markedly noncylindrical configuration basically can be explained by the same straightforward fluid-dynamic considerations; the term vortex-generating and vortex-carrying laminar flow appears appropriate and must be differentiated both from coherent laminar and from stochastically turbulent flow. The shape and stability of vortices, the dynamics of their evolution and devolution in pulsatile flow, their longevity in pulsatile flow, and the events taking place in them, are, however, difficult to predict. We have earlier proposed to refer to the full spectrum of transport phenomena near a stenosis as "Alexander Naumann vortex transport", see [13] and [14]. However, sudden discontinuities in geometry, as well as sudden changes in flow velocity (or a combination of both) is bound to destabilize flow.

From a synergetic point of view, three important features of the whirl-generating laminar flow must be appreciated: (a) strictly locally, a satellite dissipative structure with its own cooperativity and coherence is formed, which is (b) stabilized to a certain extent as a new system of potential walls and potential sinks and hence traps certain blood elements (see "Instability of Blood Motion"), and which (c) creates a dynamic flow reactor which exhibits shearing motion without convective dilution and thence promotes autocatalytically enhanced proteolytic reactions (see "Instability of Blood Motion").

In this context, the classical notion of boundary layers between fully developed and separated flow must be extended. In the engineering sciences, the energy losses in flow separation and those necessary to form a boundary layer are of major concern. In the arterial system, however, the energy dissipated is only a small fraction of the total cardiovascular energy. Here, the energy associated with shearing the boundary layers is biologically important: shear stresses traumatic in magnitude act on the suspended particles of the blood, especially blood platelets and red blood cells (see [11, 15]). As flow separates and boundary layers develop, traumatizing streamlines are formed during the systolic peak flow; interestingly, the latter feed those directed toward the wall further down at the relaminarization zone. Here they divide, part of them moving downstream and the other part feeding into the vortex (Fig. 5).

According to the response-to-injury theory (see [33]), the response of the mural system to any kind of injury initiates, sustains, and complicates the atherogenic process. It is conceivable, therefore, that any atheromatous lesion, via the described sequence of events, perpetuates itself for fluid-mechanical and biochemical reasons. A further complication is related to the fact that endothelial discontinuities (abnormal transcellular or paracellular flux) are exposed to very high transmural pressures, thus leading to marked filtration of plasmatic constituents with very little reabsorption. Thus wall insudation – as a special form of separated mural flow – is created as a pathological dissipative structure: the biochemical and cytological events taking place there are commonly looked upon as the response to injury (see [33]).

For the case of T and Y bifurcations, experimental evidence using laser Doppler measurements in models of the vessels and mathematical modeling converge in the concept that the back-flow phenomenon occurs regularly at sites opposite to the vertex. A closely related phenomenon in the proximity of bifurcations of peripheral arteries in patients has been made probable by the method of aliasing monitoring in so-called color-coded ultrasound Doppler anemometers [34]. As has been explained in detail elsewhere [13], there is ample reason to believe that the phenomenon of flow separation is also responsible for low output of hot-film anemometers positioned at the walls of the areas adjacent to the vortices [35]. Based on results and concepts in the 1960s it was justified to refer to these areas as low-shear regions (Caro et al. [35]) and to associate atherogenesis with the transport processes immediately near the endothelial surface. At present, it appears more reasonable to associate these areas with whirl-generating flow rather than with laminar flow with low velocity gradients. Anyway, it is helpful to accept both the intramural event (intimal insudation) as a form of incoherent flow – or as deterministic chaos [1–8].

Synergetic Concepts of Cytological, Biochemical, and Hemorheological Reactions in Flow Reactors

As discussed in the section "The Concept of Coherent Rectified Flow", synergetics conceives a priori of biochemical reactions as processes, because (a) it is taken into account that biological processes do not take place in a closed but rather in an open compartment, and (b) most biochemical processes are kept far from their thermodynamic equilibrium.

This also holds true for catalyzed reactions in vortices. It is obvious that the efficacy of these short-lived flow reactors and the consequences of the biochemical reactions taking place there depend primarily on the life time of this type of deterministic chaos. Fluid-dynamically speaking, the simple question whether geometry and/or fluid-dynamics of the pulsatile flow allows the formation of closed vortices predicts whether the autocatalytic activation proceeds or not. Synergetically speaking, ideal Poiseuille flow in blood conduits links scavenging reactions to an infinite source of "scavengins" [37], hence enforcing stable chemical reactions or synergetic order. On the other hand, if the source of an activated species is within the closed compartment of a cell or of a short-lived vortex, it is bound to initiate a network of processes, all of which are far from equilibrium.

As can be seen, the fluid-mechanical details of the blood motion in the large arteries exert pivotal influences upon hematological functions. This applies especially to the network of proteolytic enzymes forming the coagulation cascade, which are amplified by the fact that hemostatic functions are, of course, associated with marked rheological phase transitions, e.g., formation of large platelet aggregates in the fluid, deposition of blood components onto the wall, and the polymerization of soluble fibrin into insoluble fibrin. These phase transitions alter the flow behavior, which in turn exerts marked fluid-dynamic influences. In the case of flow separation they tend to amplify, as it were, the effects of biochemical divergence phenomena.

For reasons of space, the cooperativity of the biochemical, cytological, and fluid-dynamic processes taking place in the vortices near the predilection sites for atheromatosis cannot be detailed here; the reader is referred to recent reviews ([13, 24, 37] and "Didactic Appendix"). Synergetic concepts help to explain the sparing of the flow dividers or arterial vertices and their protection from progressive forms of atheromatosis and hence provide a compromise between the proponents of the high-shear [36] and the low-shear [35] concept of atheroma localization (see also [16]).

Synergetics of Enzyme Reactions in Closed Vortices: Thrombus Formation as Symptom of Deterministic Chaos

Long-lived and, hence, closed vortices are the epitomy of incoherent flow; they come into existence whenever streamlines in separated flow close upon themselves. If they survive for many cardiac cycles, i.e., when fluid particles are carried not only on complicated helical pathways but on such trajectories that lead them onto orbits with more or less circular pathways (Figs. 2, 6) the fluid element is subjected to shear without dilution. Individual trajectories are rounded, hence fluid lamellae (the combination of all trajectories in closed vortex) assume the shape of more or less regular spheriods, ellipsoids, or rings, and the vortices themselves are in a continuous rotational motion (rotating vortex balls or ring vortices).

As discussed elsewhere [13, 16, 38], these closed trajectories create velocity differences between individual trajectories (or fluid lamellae), in other words, a strictly deterministic shearing process, producing repetitive collisions between fluid elements and dispersed phase particles. Since individual particles and especially small initial aggregates reach across fluid lamellae, any velocity gradient between closed trajectories gives rise to particle encounters by convective (rather than by thermal energy). These collisions follow from the simple fact that particles traveling on faster trajectories hit those on a slower one from behind, make contact, and form more or less permanent chemical bonds. This process is the equivalent to heating a flow reactor; the effect (aggregate formation) is equivalent to a phase transition forming a solid in a fluid. This causes (a) progressive growth of aggregate and, if free thrombin is available, (b) progressive stabilization of the platelet aggregate to a white thrombus.

The chemical bonds responsible for the process of adhesion depend upon the plasmatic environment (fibrinogen, fibronectin, von Willebrand Factor) determining the collision efficiency of particles. Fluid-dynamics determines the collision frequency: one collision in coherent laminar Poiseuille flow, repetitive particle collision in vortices. Since there is convective contact but no convective dilution, incoherent flow amplifies by several mechanisms a host of molecular,

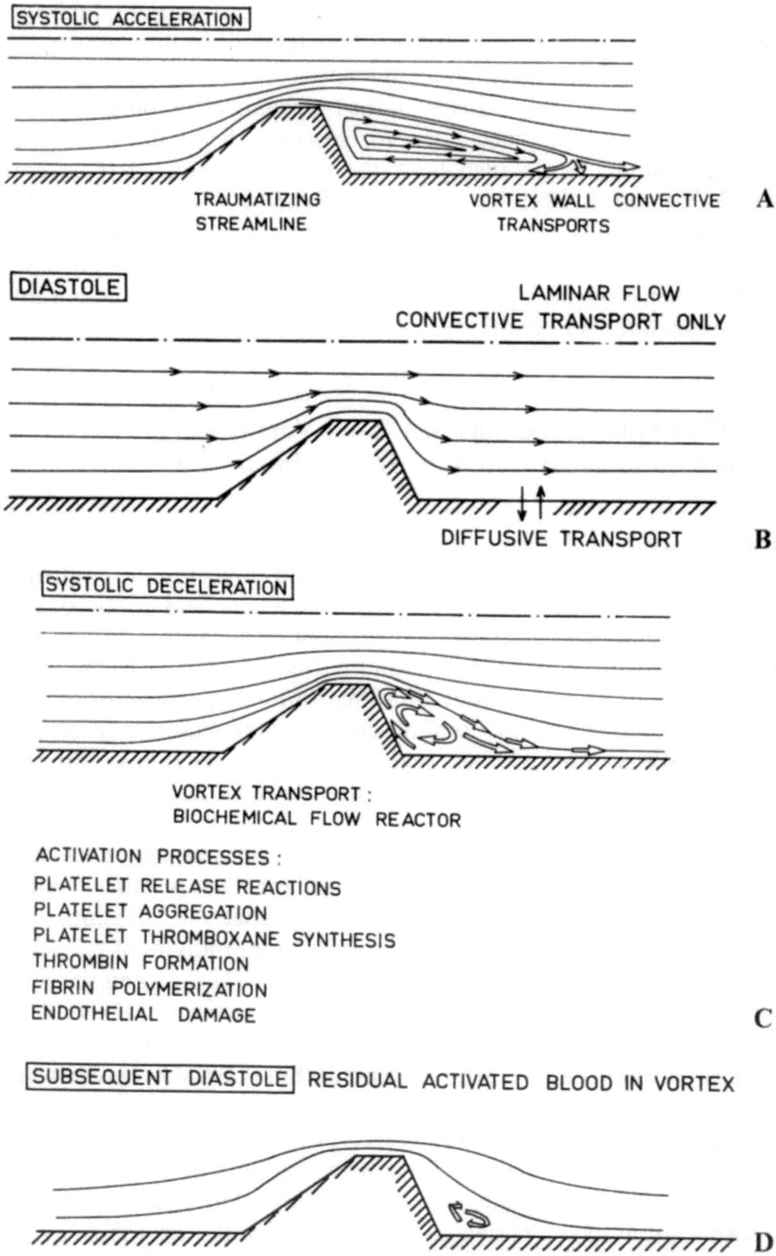

Fig. 6 A–D. Schematic representation of the evolution and devolution of vortices and the migrating stagnation points in pulsatile flow near an obstacle. **A** Laminar flow in diastole. **B** In peak systole there are high shear stresses near the surface of obstacle; the streamlines can become traumatizing to the blood, the material being partitioned to wall, vortex, and downstream conduit as schematically depicted in Fig. 5. **C** In the devolution of the vortex a short-lived biochemical flow reactor is formed, allowing various enzymatically amplified processes to take place. **D** In the subsequent diastole residua of the flow reactor remain trapped in the poststenotic area

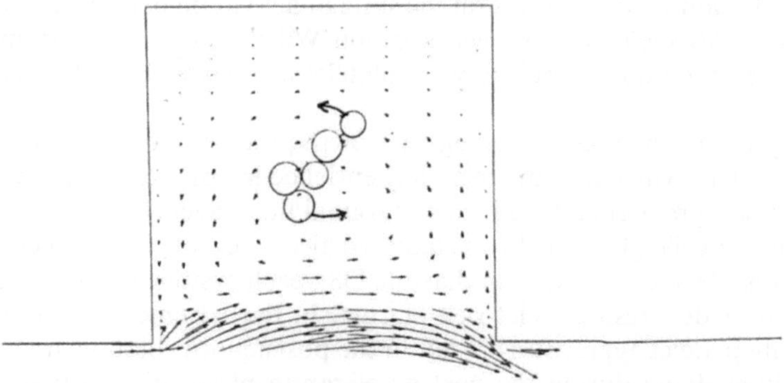

Synergetics of thrombus formation in closed vortices

1) Biophysics: Particle trapping in energetic trough

2) Cytological: Rarefication of RBC
   Platelet aggregation: sink for platelets

3) Biochemical: Accumulation of platelet activating mediators
   Flip-flop of procoagulant phospholipids in platelet membrane
   Autocatalytic amplification of coagulation proenzymes
   Fibrin polymerization

Fig. 7. Schematic representation of processes associated with separated and incoherent flow in a vortex. *Arrows* represent local velocity; *arrow density* represents shear rate. The high energy density in the boundary layer between separated flow and coherent flow prevents the particle from leaving the separated area. If the particle trapped in such an energetic trough is a platelet aggregate, it is subjected to continuous rotation, acting like a magnetic stirrer with catalytic surface

adhesive, and cellular interactions. Most importantly, autocatalytically amplified biochemical and cytological processes are made possible here – and only here. In short, coagulation can proceed despite the fact that the afflicted artery is still perfused.

At present, we have neither any detailed conception about the sequence of biochemical events that take place in such an element of fluid-dynamically separated blood, nor can we identify cause and effect relationships, temporal sequentiality, or hierarchies of cytological and enzymological processes. We can predict, nevertheless, that (a) the chemical processes are limited to the sites of vortices, and that (b) not only chemical processes amplify themselves there but also some pivotal rheological ones. Consequently, we have a dynamic system with positive feedback between physical and chemical events (see Fig. 7).

It is intuitively clear that the actual size of the aggregates is an important determinant of their fluid-dynamic behavior. They grow with time depending on (a) the particle supply, (b) adhesive properties of the components, and (c) the mixing rate (vortex rotation frequency). Platelet behavior is, of course, highly variable; adhesivity depends on the state of activation concentration of bridging molecules such as fibrinogen and von Willebrand factor and, most importantly, on the rapid stabilization of platelet aggregates by polymerized fibrin [39].

In energy terms, the platelet aggregate growth process can be regarded as a sink for platelets, which become relatively enriched in vortices [29] probably because these are preferentially fed from marginal fluid layers rich in platelets and poor in red cells [40, 41]. In unstable vortices, i.e., in those which are growing in systole and shrinking in diastole [38], each systolic evolution of a new vortex provides fresh platelet-rich plasma. In the extreme, when during standstill only platelet aggregates are left in the poststenotic dilation area, the vortex newly evolving during the next acceleration phase still contains the previously formed aggregates and receives fresh platelet-rich plasma, a phenomenon allowing a progressive aggregate growth. In short, any long-living vortex is linked to an almost infinite platelet reservoir.

Hemorheologists, when trying to decipher the role of fluid-dynamic factors in the various aspects of platelet function, approach thrombus formation as dynamic processes. The early results by Dintenfass [41] gave the clue that the direction of procoagulatory process, the extent of the process, and the resulting coagula are primarily a function of the incident shear conditions. The viscometric methods introduced by him are a very good model for the variable dynamics of vortices but are inadequate to model very short acting processes near stenoses and at boundaries of separated and coherent flow (see [13]). Our own group has since shown that the so-called shear activation of platelets in very rapid flow is based on overt mechanical platelet distruption (thrombocytorrhexis [14, 39]), and that secondary reactions in well-stirred compartments do take place within less than 1000 ms [14].

The synergetic interpretation given here for the stability of vortices containing aggregates or thrombi is borne out by experimental data from several laboratories. Our own studies of the flow behavior of blood element in idealized fluid-dynamic conditions (e.g., those in rotational viscometers [42]), at stagnation point flow [43], or in simple models of stenosis flow [44] have uncovered a number of such positive feedback hemostasiological events. Platelet aggregates, for example, have been shown to form preferentially in the center of closed vortices [13, 29].

The arterial wall at the site of vortex formation is directly affected by all these chaotic processes, the products of which are known to damage endothelial cells. It is known, of course, that the endothelial damage allows not only the penetration of blood cells (e.g., monocyte-macrophage [45]) but also the penetration of high molecular weight proteins without direct proteolytic activity, driven by a high filtration pressure. In the absence of a microvascular cleavage system (i.e., a system of vasa vasorum with capillaries and lymphatics), the monocytes, turning to resident macrophages in fulfilling their physiological scavenging reactions, proliferate locally. Lacking systems for reabsorption of transudated macromolecules, the repetitive charge of the intramural interstitial space of the arteries near bifurcations with low-density lipoproteins, fibrinogen, and platelet-derived growth factors is bound to induce an almost neoplastic hyperreaction of the local and the deposited cells.

Obviously, there is close functional relationship between the tumorlike proliferation of the intima (atheroma), the effect that it has on stability of flow, and hence the stability of biochemical reactions in the vortices subsequent to flow separation.

Fluid Dynamics of Arterial Flow in Normal and in Stenosed Coronary Arteries

The pulsatility of both pressure and flow in all parts of the proximal arterial system is uniquely accentuated in the coronary system (Fig. 8). Owing to the mechanical effect of the contracting myocardium on peripheral myocardial resistance there is strong protosystolic deceleration of arterial inflow, associated with marked backward flow and followed by very fast prodiastolic acceleration [46]. Exact details of this biphasic flow pulsatility and the interaction with pressure pulsatility are not presently known, but rapid progress has been achieved through the work of Kajiya et al. [47]. It can be hoped that the technological potential now available will soon provide us with information about this unique form of unstable flow in coronaries afflicted with atheromatous stenoses.

Even in the absence of detailed information we are safe in predicting that the bidirectionality of flow now established for proximal stenoses is more marked in the distal ones, especially in the vicinity of the transmural branches of the left descending coronary artery with their large mean volumetric flow rate and the pronounced systolic deceleration and flow reversal (Fig. 8).

Having appreciated that in the proximal arteries all phasic shifts in pressure, flow velocity, Reynolds' numbers, and hence spatial and temporal fluctuations in the ratio of kinetic energy to viscous energy dissipation predispose to flow separation, it is intuitively clear that the coronaries, especially when afflicted with obliterating atheromatosis, must have a very instable arterial flow. It is furthermore predictable that – for any degree of cross-sectional reduction of the lumen – asymmetric stenoses give rise to more pronounced, more unilateral vortex formation.

A stenosed coronary artery branch site represents a very marked deviation from cylindrical conduit configuration, giving rise to much more sudden local instability in Reynolds' numbers than would occur by the action of an obstacle encroaching the lumen more gradually. It is obvious that the additional hemodynamic load (extra hydraulic resistance) can in principle be compensated more or less perfectly by collaterals or by distal arteriolar relaxation.

There are no such mechanisms conceivable to counteract biochemical destabilization due to the deviation in blood motion (biomechanical destabilization of flow, platelet-based procoagulatory reactions). It may be mentioned that the presently popular hypothesis for explaining the anginal attack

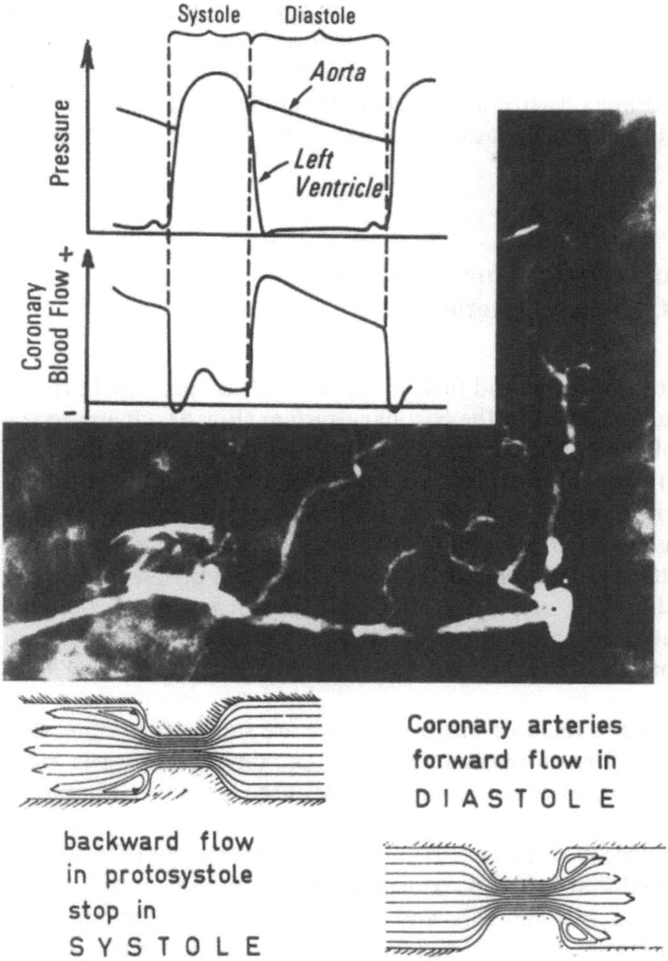

Fig. 8. Schematic representation of flow pulsatility in the coronary vascular bed. Due to physiological backward flow in the coronary arteries in protosystole, flow stop in systole, and forward flow in diastole, secondary flow and all its sequelae must be expected to occur both upstream and downstream of coronary stenosis

of the Prinzmetal type in assymmetric stenoses (contraction of the less afflicted segment of the coronary arteries [48]) can be included in this stability concept: the notion of an uncontrolled thromboxane-induced vasospasm adjacent to thrombotic reactions is in full agreement with the synergetic considerations presented here. It is not only logical to assume that a localized vasoconstrictor hyperresponse can be caused by localized release from reacting platelets, but one can likewise assume that the constriction enhances flow instability and hence incoherent flow with all its cytological and biochemical consequences.

It must be stressed, however, that there is a close relationship between the destabilization tendency of flow at a stenotic area and the presence or absence of arterio-arterial shunt vessels, simply because these limit flow destabilization in functional hyperemia. Any increase in flow rate, such as occurs subsequent to arteriolar relaxation in increasing the absolute local Reynolds' number as well as its fluctuations, obviously tends to accentuate flow separation. Relaxation in the most peripheral arterioles actively controlling proximal flow rate (run off), if accommodated by shunt vessels, reduces the hydrodynamical efficacy of the atheromatous obliteration. The influence of extra flow in functional hyperemia on the fractional proximal conductance [49] in generalized arteriolar relaxation depends linearly on the total flow rate over the stenosis. It is well known from detailed measurements in peripheral vascular obliteration that in uncompensated stenosis the arteriolar relaxation primarily causes a poststenotic pressure drop – during functional hyperemia – and hence a high pressure gradient across the stenosis. To summarize, we can say that the more effective the collaterals are, the lower the postexercise drop in distal arterial pressure, the more stable flow, and the less likely flow separation and its sequelae, namely thrombotic events.

The hemodynamic reason for this regularity is straightforward: collaterals in parallel to the stenosed segment (in elevating overall proximal conductance) reduce net energy dissipation for any given flow rate. Any stenosed vessel not adequately compensated during peak functional flow, in steepening the pressure gradient and hence the shear stresses, is likely to induce trauma to the flowing blood (and especially platelets) during functional hyperemia. This can be predicted to be proportional to the extra flow rate which the stenosed vessel must convey during functional hyperemia. Not only velocity is then more pulsatile but also the local Reynolds' number. This fluid-dynamic regularity is based on simple considerations of continuity; since coronary artery pulsatility is always so much more pronounced than that in any other bed, one is safe in predicting that uncompensated forms of obliteration will have far higher tendency to instability, in Reynolds' number and flow separation in functional hyperemia.

If associated with overt coronary thrombosis, the synergetic concepts presented here provide a stringent hypothesis relating thrombotic events to physical exertion. To summarize, the synergetics of hemodynamic events (flow pulsatility, lack of compensation), of fluid-dynamic events (unstable blood motion, flow separation), and of a state of hypercoagulability (local, generalized) makes the catastrophic event of a sudden coronary thrombosis a plausible reaction. It occurs by chance but it proceeds by necessity.

Functional Conclusions

Unstable angina, i.e., the often fatal consequence of pronounced coronary atheromatosis has been referred to as "the Friday afternoon disease" by cardiac surgeons (see Messmer, this volume), a term full of sardonic humor and deep insight into its fundamental unpredictability, which seems to exceed the tolerance of internists for risky situations. Synergetics and chaos theory provide an intellectual framework for explaining the fact that in the wide domain of synergetic order the various cardiovascular, hemostatic, and metabolic functions are funnelled down to the point where patient lives near the threshold of suprasynergetic chaos. The patient lives near watersheds (called bifurcations in chaos theory) where the progression of a delicately balanced steady state of procoagulatory and anticoagulatory (or fibrinolytic) processes (taking place near the atheromatous plaques) might suddenly get out of control and decide to divert and to go the lethal way. The patient's prognosis quoad vitam is linked to the unpredictable outcome of a strictly local event, since the potential sequelae of coronary thrombosis would have such severe consequences on the overall flow of energy and matter in his cardiovascular system that the organism as a whole is threatened by infrasynergetic chaos in case of pump failure and cardiogenic shock. The disease entity of unstable angina therefore offers itself as a paradigmatic example for an interpretation of disease processes as the consequence of disturbed cooperativity between the multiple dynamic systems.

Normally, many of these function as dissipative structures that form spontaneously as a kind of side effect of the continuous flow of matter and energy in the human organism as a consequence of highly cooperative systems forming one large, coherent dynamic system. The disease is then reducible to a fluid-dynamic, rheological, and chemical incoherence phenomenon. More specifically, the interpretation presented here lays out a platform for the comprehensive understanding of the multiple subsystem process abnormalities. In applying synergetics and chaos theory we come to a new dynamic understanding of risk factors. If we define risk to the stability of a system as something that creates (or is suggested to create) an adverse hazard for a contingent injury, risk factors are pathogenetic mechanisms that qualify as strange attractor processes in that they only act under a very special set of boundary conditions.

In the case of unstable angina, the obliterating atheromatosis, especially if asymmetrically placed, and when sparing arterial segments with conserved contractility, certainly poses the prime risk and the biggest hazard for destabilizing blood flow and for allowing the occurrence of positive feed-back cytological and biochemical reactions. As so often in dynamic systems, phenomena of circular causality can occur, for example, the potentiation of one abnormality (fully separated flow) by one or several others (platelet reactions forming a hemostatic plug, but also producing a potent vasoconstrictor, e.g., thromboxane). The destabilizing effect of coagulatory processes is self-evident, that of the vasoconstrictor principle slightly more involved. One may safely postulate that thromboxane is not formed in excess amounts if there is laminar flow. Once formed in separated flow, however, it can constrict the proximal segment in cases of asymmetric atheromatosis as well as all more distal arterioles. Consequently, there is overall flow retardation but still very marked pressure pulsation. This combination of effects aids in destabilizing the laminar flow by fundamental fluid-mechanical mechanisms, namely rapid acceleration (or rapid fluctuations in local Reynolds' numbers).

Interestingly, a rheological event appears to take over the role of a director of events in instituting strange-attractor processes. A platelet aggregate, even if loose in structure and without immediate hemodynamic consequence, effectively prevents the resumption of stable flow, while at the same time stabilizing the progression of thrombotic reactions. Particle aggregations of all kinds must be viewed as an isothermic phase transition by which the fluid-mechanical properties of the subsystems and the fluid-dynamic behavior of the whole system is changed. Since, on the other hand, the aggregated platelets are also biochemically activated, they act as the pivot of a series of highly nonlinear procoagulatory processes.

All processes taking place in dissipative structures, including the hemostatic process, are determined by chance and necessity. The necessity of the spontaneous generation of vortices as dissipative structures persisting in flow fields follows from the constraints of entropy production; their site is markedly influenced by geometric constraints (e.g., mountains in the case of weather, conformational abnormalities in that of blood vessels). There is a feature of necessity in the kind of processes determined by physicochemical reactions in cyclones (water content of the air, gradients of temperature, and barometric pressure). In thrombus-forming vortices, the genetically determined combination of reaction partners, their local accumulation, and the rate of diffusive and convective transport in vortices determine rate and extent of the phase transitions. In both systems there is the influence of chance, which determines both the time of the catastrophic reactions and the rate of cooperativity and hence of acceleration and the eventual extent and functional consequence of the physicochemical reactions.

Finally it should be noted that there is a notion of chance not only with respect to the acute event of the intracoronary catastrophe, but also in the formation of the atheromatous plaque. Flow separation as such, and especially the occurrence of traumatic forces in the streamlines passing an atheromatous arterial obliteration, are critically dependent upon the existence and/or nonexistence of arterio-arterial collaterals. When the atheromatous growth process is slow enough to allow the transformation of preexisting microvessels into patent collaterals, the stability of flow through the stenosed segment is far less in jeopardy. All processes that promote rapid proliferation of strictly localized atheromatous plaques are therefore much more likely to induce the kind of instability described, simple because – in the absence of collaterals – any increase in volumetric flow rate over a stenosed vessel leads to much higher local Reynolds' numbers and hence to much less stable flow.

Didactic Appendix: Propaedeutic Introduction to Synergetics and Biomedical Chaos Theory in Cardiovascular Physiology

In the past, the analysis of disease states such as those occurring in the atheromatous coronary arteries in patients afflicted with unstable angina were reduced to isolated anomalies, e.g., those of the morphology, of the hemostatic, fibrinolytic, and platelet reactions, and of the myocardial metabolism (see elsewhere in this volume). The fast progress of hemorheological research into the dynamics of thrombus formation has opened our eyes to the necessity to consider simultaneous changes in the hemodynamic and fluid-mechanic processes (and their dependency upon the chemical composition of the blood), the morphology of the vessels, and the speed of hemostatic and coagulatory reactions (see [24]). In short, dynamic processes rather than isolated reactions have to be analyzed. The physiology then can be comprehended as a stable order (synergetic cosmos, see [8]), and pathophysiological disturbances as a destabilization and deterministic chaos. The explanatory power of synergetic philosophies requires the reader's familiarity with presently new and extraneous semantics, for obvious reasons of space restraint this new terminology cannot be extensively covered in the present review. Readers are therefore referred to introductory texts cited in the bibliography [1–8].

The basic concepts for understanding such dynamic processes have been worked out in theoretical physics, for example by H. Haken for physical and by I. Prigogine [5] for physicochemical processes; one is safe in predicting, however, that there will be a significant impact of these new rational interactionist interpretations on interdependent biological functions. At present, however, semantics and philosophy of synergetics and chaos theory are so far removed from concepts customary in medicine that the vivid simplicity of a cartoon appears justified, showing the dynamic play of a windsleeve as an example of dissipative structuring. Its volatile yet stable pattern, reflecting a boosted steady state, emanates from the joint efforts of two phases (air, solids) in processes driven by several energies (gravitational, frictional, elastic).

It becomes structured, gains spontaneous cooperativity and stability exclusively when it transmits the flow of energy and matter. Since the latter is associated with finite frictional energy losses, it serves as a good example of the principle of dissipative structuring and the generation of synergetic order. Furthermore, the concept of a limited range of such dynamic order (synergetic cosmos, Fig. 9) can be illustrated, framed by two types of chaos.

If there is very little air flow, there is infrasynergetic (or indeterminate) chaos: The flow of energy is insufficient to rectify the sleeve, and thus the subsystems cannot cooperate. The motions are erratic, influenced by strange attractor processes, i.e., those related to the pressure acting on the outside of the sleeve and the folds there, as well as friction in the hinges and at the interface between sleeve ring and pole. The system can neither store nor amplify energy. As the wind power reaches a threshold (called the synergetic threshold), the dynamic cooperativity of subsystems emanates spontaneously, catalyzed, as it were, by the appropriate design of the subsystems. The taper of the sleeve is pivotal in ensuring controlled flow of energy:

[5] I. Prigogine gained the Nobel prize in Physics in 1977 for his pioneering work in non-equilibrium thermodynamics. There is a rapidly growing appreciation of his concepts in biology and medicine in Europe; he has also exerted pivotal impact upon pioneers in so-called chaos theory.

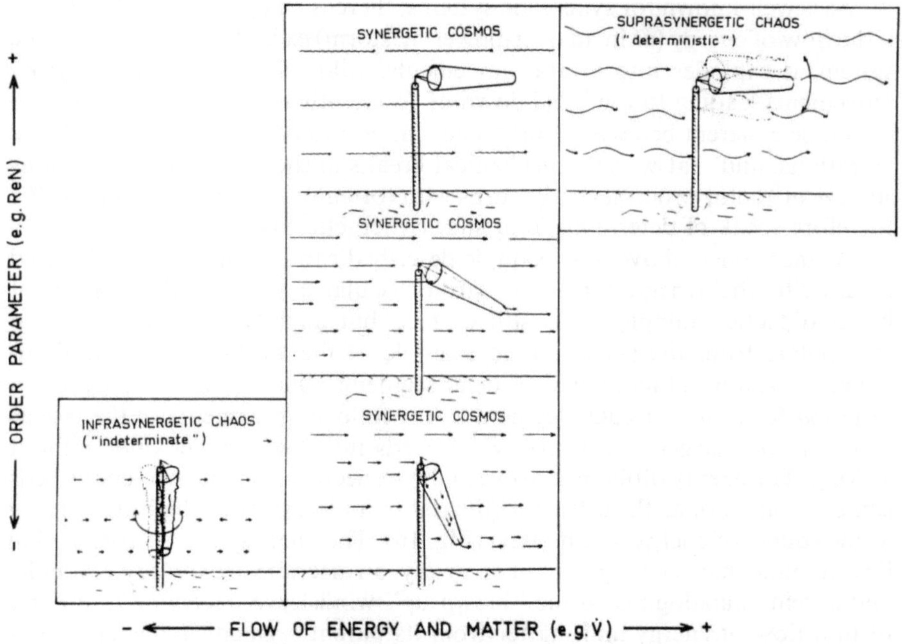

Fig. 9. Functional cooperativity of dynamic systems as exemplified by a "windsleeve". The continuous flow of energy and matter produces a wide range of synergetic order bounded by chaotic behavior if the system is not adequately boosted (infrasynergetic or indeterminate chaos), or when it is overpowered (suprasynergetic or deterministic chaos)

1. It creates an appropriate outflow impedance and hence allows the system to be boosted.
2. It rectifies the channel by placing the orifice so that it ensures maximum possible uptake of power.
3. When fully straightened out, it ensures strictly laminar flow, hence minimizing the frictional energy dissipation. It thereby concentrates the energy export and produces the apparent effect of an amplification.

For all these features, strictly passive processes are responsible, all following from principles of minimum energy expenditure, jointly producing spontaneous cooperativity, coherence, and stability. The reaction to the incident flow of energy is so reliable and the stability is so robust that such systems can be used to convey information (a typical feature of many, if not all synergetic systems). The example chosen also is a vivid description of the elementary fact that a "structuring" influence can be exerted by energy dissipation (hence the term "dissipative structure") to differentiate them from conventional "conservative structures" the shape of which is the result of energies "stored" in elastic elements.

As is well-known for synergetic systems, there is an upper limit of stability; if the flow of energy (as in an over-powering storm) exceeds the capacity of the system, it explodes into erratic movements, wild, unpredictable, and jerky movements leading to the breakdown of cooperativity, of amplification, and of course coherent behavior. Turbulency, intermittency of orientation, elastic vibrations, and – at worst – mechanical breaks in the sleeve (all classified as strange attractor processes) take turns with (often short) periods of order. We therefore speak of deterministic or suprasynergetic chaos.

As mentioned above, the example described can – within limits – be used to describe the synergetics of the cardiovascular system. In the absence of better didactic examples, it is still correct, but already comprehensible, to extrapolate from the aerodynamic example of the windsleeve to the fluid-dynamic example of individual vascular segments. One can picture the motion of blood from one vascular segment to the following segments of the tree as if it were one larger windsleeve which feeds into two smaller ones without leaking. The energy difference between the respective arterial and venous beds can be thought of as the attractor (the right and left sides of the heart serving as the source of energy and matter) (Fig. 10). The analogy used is permissible if we assume that each segment of an artery, an arteriole, a capillary, a venole, and a vein is analogous to the "blown up" windsleeve, receiving in orderly form a flow of energy and matter from its parent segment immediately upstream and conveying it loss free into the two daughter vessels immediately downstream. Despite a continuous dissipation of energy (as heat), each segment is kept in a boosted steady state (i.e., far from local thermodynamic equilibrium), conveying a finite amount of material as well as its kinetic energy to the parts of the vascular network lying downstream. Even though most of the kinetic energy supplied by the heart to the blood in the arteries is used up in frictional work, a characteristic residual part of the kinetic energy is conserved in the momentum of the blood in venous return. This energy is spent in working to expand the diastolic myocardium (or in supplying the energy for cardiac preload). It goes without saying that the stability of the motion in each segment, and hence that of the entire vascular system, depends on a number of factors; namely appropriate morphological design of the system, adequate filling, phasic input of sufficient energy, careful impedance matching, high fluidity of the perfusate, and lack of local viscidizing mechanisms.

The coherence between macrovascular and microvascular, between systemic and pulmonary, between intravascular and transmural, and between interstitial and lymph flow guarantees laminar one way traffic (see [8]) in each individual vessel segment and the establishment of a characteristic arrangement of motions; each part of the extracellular space behaves coherently with all others, making them into one cooperative dynamic system.

The role of laminar flow in synergetic order, in coherence between mechanical and chemical processes can also be illustrated by the model of the windsleeve (Fig. 11). Assuming the material of the sleeve to be soluble in an organic solvent, it is plausible that in the synergetic domain neither the addition of the solvent, nor that of glowing particles would have major consequences. Both

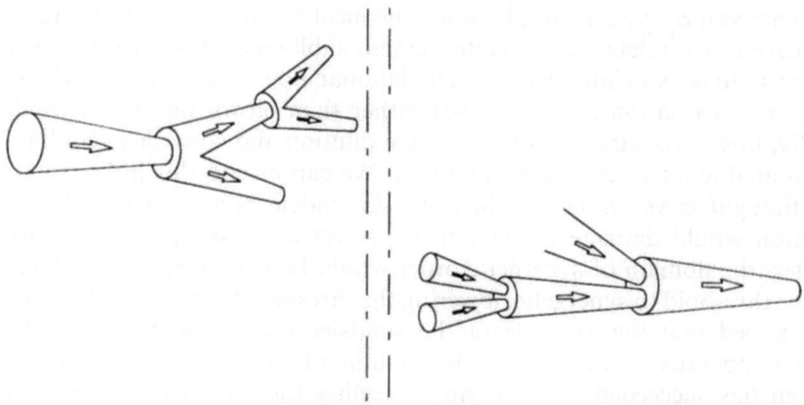

Fig. 10. Schematic representation of the synergetics of a highly simplified cardiovascular network by a system of "boosted windsleeves" (see Fig. 9). Assume that on the arterial side, each vascular segment conveys all its material and most of its initial energy (in the form of kinetic energy) into the two daughter vessels (the "branched windsleeve") immediately downstreams. By this process, while there is substantial dissipation of energy ("frictional losses"), each segment conveys a certain amount of the initial kinetic energy to the terminal branches. On the venular and venous side (*right of the two broken lines*) the kinetic energy is collected, as it were, so that under physiological conditions a small, but significant residuum of the kinetic energy of the blood supplied to it in the aorta is transferred to the vena cava and from there to the right atrium

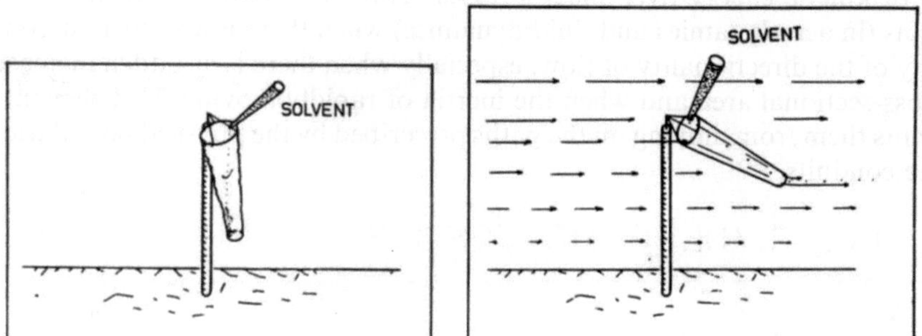

Fig. 11. Schematic representation of the interactions between physical and chemical processes in the windsleeve as dynamic system: if in infrasynergetic chaos, destructive reactions (dissolution of fabric by "solvent", oxidation by energy rich initiators, "glowing particles") can take place. Subsequent to the action of these processes, the system is less stable. Conversely, if in synergetic order, the reaction rates are suppressed by laminar flow: the reactions are "blown out" rather than "blown on", and the system can survive a temporal "crisis" largely undisturbed

potential activators, which would induce chemical reaction and or oxidation in the sleeve in its indeterminate state, remain subliminal. Provided that the synergetic state is associated with strictly laminar flow, the processes of dissolution or of oxidation are blown out rather than blown on by the wind. Physically, this is associated with convective dilution and convective cooling, a process analogous to chemical inhibition. We can extend this little experiment of thought as we assume that in a period of indeterminate chaos a chemical reaction would damage the system (i.e., destroyed its optimal design). Thereafter, the domain of synergetic order would be narrowed down (elevation of the threshold to synergetic, lowering the threshold to chaotic behavior).

It is hoped that the example of the windsleeve as an analogue of the coherent, cooperative, and stable mode of laminar blood motion in the vascular system has succeeded in conveying a feeling for the basic concepts of synergetics and that we can thus proceed to a description of their potential disturbances in the sense of flow destabilization. One can picture a local, unilateral impediment (encroaching like a dam into the entry of one segment): due to straightforward fluid-dynamic reasons detailed elsewhere [8, 13], the strictly laminar flow becomes locally de-stabilized by the generation of secondary flow or vortices (Fig. 12).

In order to understand the generation of these vortices, we come back to the concept of Reynolds' number instability, i.e., the sudden change in the ratio of kinetic energy over shear stresses. This ratio shifts in flowing fluid systems (in aerodynamics and fluid dynamics) when there is a sudden discontinuity of the directionality of flow, especially when there is a sudden increase in cross-sectional area and when the inertia of rapidly moving fluid elements prevents them from moving on the paths prescribed by the physical boundaries of the conduits.

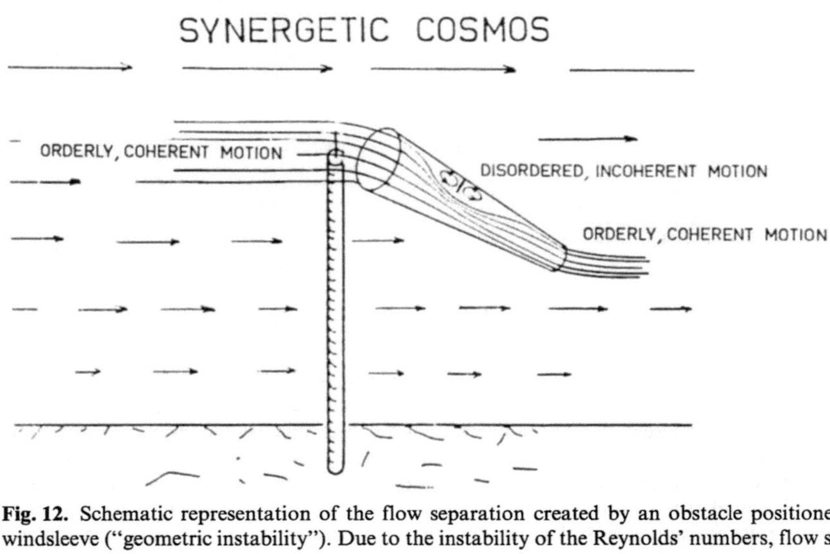

Fig. 12. Schematic representation of the flow separation created by an obstacle positioned in a windsleeve ("geometric instability"). Due to the instability of the Reynolds' numbers, flow separation occurs

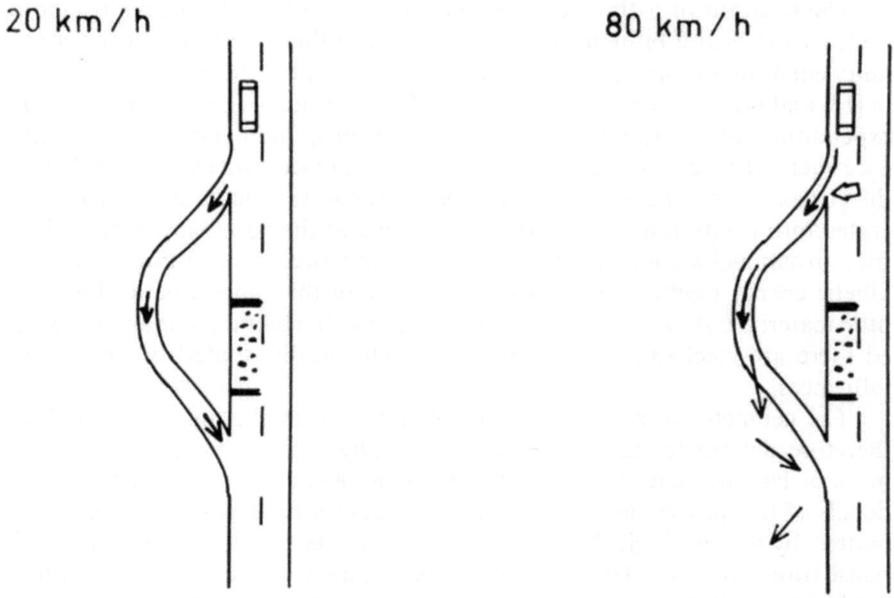

Fig. 13. Illustration of "incoherent motion" of an automobile forced to deviate from straight motion. If a curved path is taken at low velocity (20 km/h; *left*), the motion is "coherent" due to the predominance of frictional energy dissipation (between tire and road surface). If the speed (and hence the kinetic energy of the car) is too high (80 km/h; *right*) or the friction between road and tires is insufficient (icy surface, tires without traction) the automobile goes into "incoherent motion"

As will be understable from still another example of destabilized motion, a moving particle separates itself from the trajectories under the condition that the ratio of kinetic energy over viscous energy dissipation exceeds a critical level, the magnitude of which, however, depends on many factors. As illustrated in Fig. 13, the detour of an automobile forced onto a curved bypass around an obstacle on the road, is stable at low velocity and when there is high friction (e.g., when the car moves at 20 km/h along the bypass). The detour becomes unstable at 80 km/h, i.e., when the car moves with high kinetic energy and separates from the curvature of the road due to its inertia. As anyone knows, if there is an icy surface (or if the car's tires give poor friction), much lower velocities and therefore kinetic energies suffice to induce incoherent motion.

Leaving the descriptive example of the chaotic behavior of an individual particle (car, suspended individual cell) possessing high kinetic energy, we now return to the dynamics of a moving fluid. Here we are dealing with a dynamic system where all particles behave in a cohesive yet mobile fashion. Since all fluid particles cohere and hence interact with each other, the chaotic event at one site has long-range influences. Various physical laws (e.g., those of fluid incompressibility and cohesion, the requirements of conservation of mass, see [24]) are the reason for the remote influences that create to a greater or lesser extent vortices that are closed to a greater or lesser extent.

The creation of a three-dimensional structure of fluid vortices behind a stenosis and near a bifurcation closely related to the restrictions of the continuity equation (a topic beyond the present treatise, but dealt with extensively in [13] and [32]). Again being dominated by the principle of minimum energy expenditure, two independent flow regions form spontaneously, which influence each other, but which are no longer in coherence with each other. Hence the vortex is both chemically and physically separated, but is still being accelerated into rotation by the viscous drag acting at the boundary. Simple fluid friction assumes a dominating role as the driving force transmitting, as it were, kinetic energy (contained in particles moving in the main stream), but very little material is driven into the separated region; the blood components located there are mechanically mixed, but not chemically diluted by convective influences.

The geometry of a conduit, in combination with the pulsatility of flow, therefore determines the establishment of fully separated – in other words more or less incoherent – flow, by creating a new, dissipative structure. The details of this process are determined by geometry by the flow of energy and matter, by the rheological behavior of the contents and its changes following phase transitions. The latter determine the nature and velocity of the incoherent biochemical processes taking place there (as detailed in the sections "Stabilizing Mechanisms", "Instability of Blood Motion", and "Fluid Dynamics of Arterial Flow").

Hopefully, the reader will understand that all described phenomena have nothing whatsoever to do with turbulence, i.e., the stochastic motion of fluid elements. Obviously, each vortex formed is a highly deterministic system of laminar fluid motion, a kind of volatile structure and not a random chaos. A macroscopic element of fluid, bounded by nothing but steep gradients of energy flux, does not just form an innocent dissipative structure. Instead, as a dynamically separated piece of an explosive liquid in an orbiting three-dimensional vortex ball, it goes into chemical chaos. The high gain of the autocatalytically accelerated biochemical reactions taking place in this well-mixed liquid element warrant calling this dynamic system a flow reactor, located within a container structured by gradients of energy dissipation within a fluid.

One last everyday example is offered here to illustrate the cooperativity of physical and chemical incoherence. This is the example of a permanently orbiting system of vortices behind the pillar in a polluted river. One can visualize the notorious styrofoam bits bouncing around in circles, and take the rotten smell of organic material (which is also often trapped there) as an indicator of proteolytic degradation in an eddy of a liquid forced into mixing motion, but not diluted by the fluid moving past it (Fig. 14).

The details of this type vortex motion are highly complex, yet we can also refer to them as a deterministic chaos or as a suprasynergetic chaos, simply because it cannot be generated unless there is the transition through a phase of highly ordered motion (laminar flow with high kinetic energy). The proteolytic degeneration in this case is accelerated by another type of positive feed-back, namely that occurring when the presence of microorganisms and

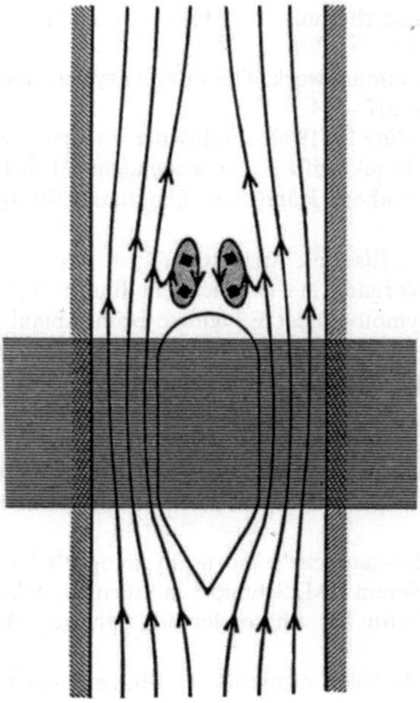

Fig. 14. Schematic representation of the influence of "separated flow" (behind the pillars of a bridge over a river). As can be readily seen, particles (e.g., pieces of styrofoam) are preferentially trapped there, and biochemical reactions (proteolysis of organic garbage) take place there. The vortices driven by the laminar flow are well mixed but not diluted (or "washed out") due to the high stability of the "incoherent flow"

that of breakdown products potentiate each other – a well-studied type of unstable reaction analyzed by chaos theoreticians [1–8].

References

1. Haken H (1978) Synergetics. An introduction – nonequilibrium phase transitions and self-organization in physics, chemistry and biology. Springer, Berlin Heidelberg New York
2. Haken H, Haken-Krell M (1989) Entstehung von biologischer Information und Ordnung. Wissenschaftliche Buchgesellschaft, Darmstadt
3. Prigogine I, Stengers I (1986) Dialog mit der Natur. Neue Wege naturwissenschaftlichen Denkens, 5th edn. Piper, Munich
4. Schuster HG (1981) Deterministic chaos: strange attractors and chaotic motions of dynamical systems. Rev Mod Phys 53:655–673
5. Hess B, Markus B (1984) Time pattern transitions in biochemical processes. In: Frehland E (ed) Synergetics – from microscopic to macroscopic order. Springer, Berlin Heidelberg New York
6. Ruelle D, Takens F (1971) On the nature of turbulence. Commun Math Phys 20:167–189
7. Mandelbrot BB (1982) The fractal geometry of nature, chap 10: geometry of turbulence intermittency. Freeman, New York, pp 97–124
8. Schmid-Schönbein H (1990) Synergetic order and chaotic malfunctions of the circulatory systems in "multiorgan failure": breakdown of cooperativity of hemodynamic functions as cause acute microvascular pathologies. In: Update in intensive care and emergency medicine, vol 11. Springer, Berlin Heidelberg New York

9. Glass L, Schrier A, Belair J (1986) Chaotic cardiac rhythms. In: Holden AV (ed) Chaos. Princeton University Press, New York, pp 237–264
10. Murray CD (1926) The physiological principle of minimum work. The vascular system and the cost of blood volume. Proc Natl Acad Sci USA 12:207–214
11. Schmid-Schönbein H, Böddeker L, Kiesewetter H, Pütz H (1980) Einfluß der Thrombozytenzahl auf die räumliche Ausbreitung der Gerinnung in rekalzifiziertem, stehendem Citrat-Plasma. In: Deutsch E, Lechner K (eds) Fibrinolyse, Thrombose, Hämostase. Schattauer, Stuttgart, pp 681–685
12. Zwaal RFA, Hemker HC (1986) Blood coagulation. Elsevier, Amsterdam
13. Schmid-Schönbein H (1988) Thrombose als ein Vorgang in "strömendem Blut": Wechselwirkung fluiddynamischer, rheologischer und enzymologischer Ereignisse beim Ablauf von Thrombozytenaggregation und Fibrinpolymerisation. Hämostasiologie 8:149–172
14. Schmid-Schönbein H, Wurzinger LJ (1986) Transport phenomena in pulsating post-stenotic vortex flow in arteries. An interactive concept of fluid-dynamic, haemorheological and biochemical processes in white thrombus formation. Nouv Rev Fr Hematol 28:257–267
15. Frojmovic MM, Panjwani R (1975) Blood cells structure-function studies: light transmission and attenuation coefficients of suspensions of blood cells and model particles at rest and with stirring. J Lab Clin Med 86:326–343
16. Naumann A, Schmid-Schönbein H (1983) A fluid-dynamicist's and a physiologist's look at arterial flow and arteriosclerosis. In: Schettler G, Nerem RM, Schmid-Schönbein H, Mörl H, Diehm C (eds) Fluid dynamics as a localizing factor for atherosclerosis. Springer, Berlin Heidelberg New York, p 9
17. Liepsch D (1987) Strömungsuntersuchungen an Modellen menschlicher Blutgefäß-Systeme. VDI, Düsseldorf (Fortschrittberichte VDI ser 7, Strömungstechnik no 13)
18. Schmid-Schönbein H, Naumann A (1984) Fluiddynamische, zellphysiologische und biochemische Aspekte der Atherogenese unter Strömungseinflüssen. Westdeutscher Verlag, Opladen, pp 6–38
19. Friedman MH, Deters OJ, Mark FF, Bargeron CB, Hutchins GM (1983) Geometric effects on the hemodynamic environment of the arterial wall: a basis for geometric risk factors? In: Schettler G, Nerem RM, Schmid-Schönbein H, Mörl H, Diehm C (eds) Fluid dynamics as a localizing factor for atherosclerosis. Springer, Berlin Heidelberg New York, pp 71–78
20. Karino T, Goldsmith HL (1979) Aggregation of human platelets in an annular vortex distal to a tubular expansion. Microvasc Res 17:217–237
21. Karino T, Goldsmith HL (1979) Adhesion of human platelets to collagen on the walls distal to a tubular expansion. Microvasc Res 17:238–262
22. Kenner TH, Busse R (1980) Cardiovascular system in dynamic. Plenum, New York
23. Schmid-Schönbein H (1990) Synergetics of normal and pathological blood movements in the cardiovascular system. In: Mosora F, Caro C, Baquey CH, Schmid-Schönbein H, Pelissier R, Krause E (eds) Biomechanical transport processes. Plenum, New York
24. Schmid-Schönbein H (1990) Synergetics of thrombus formation in flow: the concept of fluid-dynamic coherence and its breakdown. In: Schettler G, Heene DL, Harenberg J (eds) New trends in haemostasis. Springer, Berlin Heidelberg New York Tokyo (in press)
25. Höök M, Kjellen L, Johansson S, Robinson J (1984) Cell-surface glycosaminoglycans. Ann Rev Biochem 53:847–869
26. Lasch HG, Huth K, Heene DL, Müller-Berghaus G, Horder MH, Janzarik H, Mittermayer C, Sandritter W (1971) Die Klinik der Verbrauchskoagulopathie. Dtsch Med Wochenschr 96:715
27. Schrör K (1988) Eicosanoids and atherosclerosis. In: Hennerici M, Sitzer G, Weger HD (eds) Carotid artery plaques. Karger, Basel, pp 37–46
28. Forstrom RJ, Bartelt K, Blackshear PL et al. (1975) Formed element deposition onto filtering walls. Trans Am Soc Artif Intern Organs 21:602–608
29. Karino T, Goldsmith HL (1979) Adhesion of human platelets to collagen on the walls distal to a tubular expansion. Microvasc Res 17:238–262
30. Richardson PD (1973) Effect of blood flow velocity on growth rate of platelet thrombi. Nature 245:103–104
31. Booyse FM, Hoveke TP, Kisieleski D, Rafelson ME (1972) Mechanism and control of platelet-platelet interaction. 1. Effects of inducers and inhibitors of aggregation. Microvasc Res 4:179–198

32. Schmid-Schönbein H (1989) Hämostasiologie 9 (2)
33. Ross R (1986) The pathogenesis of atherosclerosis – an update. N Engl J Med 314:488–500
34. Zierler RE, Phillips DJ, Kirk WB, Primozich JF, Strandness DE (1987) Non-invasive assessment of normal carotid bifurcation hemodynamics with color flow ultrasound imaging. Ultrasound Med Biol 13:471–476
35. Caro CG, FitzGerald JM, Schroter RC (1971) Arterial wall shear. Observation, correlation and proposal of shear dependent mass transfer mechanisms for atherogenesis. Proc R Soc Lond [Biol] 177:109–159
36. Fry DL (1968) Acute vascular endothelial changes associated with increased blood velocity gradients. Circ Res 22:165–197
37. Beguin Y, Lindhout T, Hemker HC (1988) The mode of action of heparin in plasma. Thromb Haemost 60:457–460
38. Schmid-Schönbein H, Wurzinger LJ (1988) Vortex transport phenomena of the carotid trifurcation: interaction between fluid-dynamic transport phenomena and hemostatic reactions. In: Hennerici M, Sitzer G, Weger HD (eds) Carotid artery plaques. Karger, Basel, pp 64–91
39. Wurzinger LJ (1988) Thrombogenese und Hämodynamik. Hämostasiologie 8:173–182
40. Perkkiö J, Wurzinger LJ, Schmid-Schönbein H (1987) Plasma and platelet simming at t-junctions. Thromb Res 45:517–526
41. Dintenfass L (1964) Rheologic approach to thrombosis and atherosclerosis. Angiology 15:333–343
42. Schmid-Schönbein H (1977) Microrheology of erythrocytes and thrombocytes, blood viscosity and the distribution of blood flow in the microcirculation. In: Meessen H (ed) Microcirculation. Springer, Berlin Heidelberg New York, pp 289–384 (Handbuch der allgemeinen Pathologie, vol 3, pt 7)
43. Petschek HE, Adams D, Kantrowitz AR (1968) Stagnation flow thrombus formation. Trans Am Soc Artif Intern Organs 14:256–259
44. Herbst K (1989) Arterielle Thrombose trotz hochdosierter Antikoagulation mit Heparin. Dissertationsschrift, Medizinische Fakultät der RWTH Aachen
45. Hartung HP, Hennerici M (1988) Role of macrophages in atherosclerosis. In: Hennerici M, Sitzer G, Weger HD (eds) Carotid artery plaques. Karger, Basel, pp 47–63
46. Gregg DE (1944) Changes in right and left coronary artery inflow with cardiac nerve stimulation. Am J Physiol 141:382–384
47. Kajiya F, Tomonaga G, Tsujioka K, Ogasawara Y (1985) Evaluation of local blood flow velocity in proximal and distal coronary arteries by Laser Doppler Method. J Biomech Eng 107:10–15
48. Rafflenbeul W, Lichtlen PR (1983) Quantitative coronary angiography: evidence of a sustained increase in vascular smooth muscle tone in coronary artery stenoses. Z Kardiol 72 [Suppl 3]:87–91
49. Schmid-Schönbein H (1990) Blood rheology and oxygen conductance from the alveoli to the mitochondria. In: Fleming JS (ed) Drugs and the delivery of oxygen to tissues. CRC, Boca Raton, pp 15–86

Coronary Morphology in Unstable Angina

A. E. Becker [1]

Introduction

The term unstable angina was introduced by Fowler in 1971 [1]. The condition is characterized by a rather varied clinical profile, such as angina pectoris of new onset and initiated by minimal exercise, a change in the "angina characteristics" in a patient who had already suffered from stable exercise-induced angina, or the occurrence of angina at rest or with minimal exertion. It is generally acknowledged that a discrepancy between myocardial oxygen demand and supply is the final mechanism involved. In other words, the basic principle is the same as that encountered in patients with classical effort-induced angina.

This concept is further strengthened by the observation that 10%–15% of patients with unstable angina develop acute myocardial infarction or sudden cardiac death [2]. The mortality rate within 1 year among patients with severe refractory angina at rest associated with electrocardiographic repolarization abnormalities has been estimated as close to 40% [3]. Patients who present with progressive angina or a change in the pattern of chronic angina carry a much lower annual mortality risk, although still in the range of 2%–5% [4, 5]. Obviously, the natural history of unstable angina is determined to a large extend by the precise definition of the condition, but this should not obscure the fact that unstable angina presages serious ischemic cardiac events.

All in all, unstable angina should be seen as a condition with myocardial ischemia as the leading pathogenetic mechanism but with a clinical profile intermediate between stable angina and myocardial infarction. The "in-between" state of the clinical condition is also reflected in the pathology encountered within the coronary arteries.

Coronary Atherosclerosis

The classical atherosclerotic plaque is composed of a central core of fatty debris embedded within dense collagen tissue, often further complicated by

[1] Vakgroep Pathologie, Academisch Medisch Centrum, Universiteit van Amsterdam, Meibergdreef 9, 1105 AZ Amsterdam Zuidoost, The Netherlands

W. Bleifeld et al. (Eds.)
Unstable Angina

extensive calcifications. It is presently well accepted that this composition describes an end stage of a dynamic disease process that has evolved over many years. Such lesions usually underlie chronic stable angina. The fixed stenosis sets the limitation for myocardial perfusion and thus becomes the critical lesion in case of an increase in myocardial energy demand.

Over the past decade, however, it has been shown clearly that marked variability occurs with respect to the component make-up of the atherosclerotic lesions [6]. In keeping with the current concept of atherogenesis [7], the lesions may vary from those dominated by cellular constituents, particularly proliferating vascular smooth-muscle cells, to those exhibiting the classical, almost acellular features [8]. Indeed, an immune-mediated response, encompassing activated lymphocytes and macrophages, within the affected intima may be one of the processes involved [9]. The wide variety in histopathologic expressions of atherosclerotic lesions has long been neglected, but its significance is presently widely acknowledged. Differences in component make-up of the atherosclerotic lesions may be crucial for successful coronary angioplasty [10] but may also be considered an important factor in evaluating intravascular ultrasound imaging [11]. Above all, however, instability of the atherosclerotic plaque is accepted as one of the most important pathologic features that correlates with different clinical expressions of myocardial ischemia.

Stable Versus Unstable Atherosclerotic Plaques

The variability in component make-up of atherosclerotic plaques dictates that some lesions show a small central core of atheromatous debris with a thick fibrous cap separating the atheroma from the lumen (Fig. 1), while other lesions show an extensive atheroma with an almost totally attenuated fibrous cap (Fig. 2). In some instances a fibrous cap may be absent and replaced by lipid-laden macrophages. The fibrous type of atherosclerotic lesion is considered a stable plaque and on that basis as "safe." There is general consent that this is the lesion that is present in patients with chronic stable angina. On the other hand, the lesion with little in the way of a fibrous cap is considered an unstable lesion, prone to further complications, and therefore "unsafe" [12, 13].

In the setting of an unstable atherosclerotic lesion two major types of complications are recognized. First, superficial intimal injury, characterized by denudation of the endothelial layer and localized platelet aggregation (Fig. 3). The process of endothelial cell injury and adhesion of monocytes and platelets could represent an intrinsic phenomenon inherent to the atherosclerotic lesion [14, 15].

Reconstruction of the intimal structure at sites of coronary thrombi has revealed that up to 25% of major intraluminal thrombotic episodes represent thrombosis that has developed at the site of a superficial intimal injury [16]. The superficial changes that affect endothelial cells, moreover, may represent

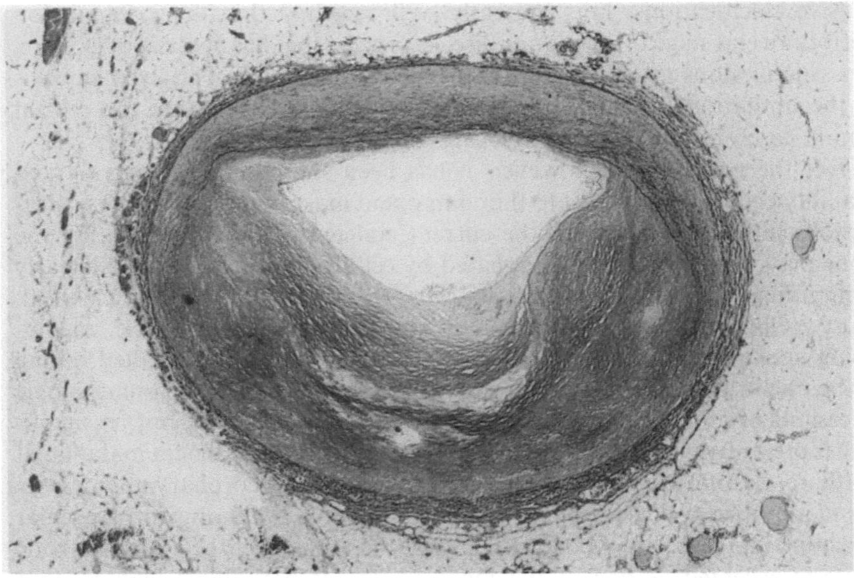

Fig. 1. Cross-section through a coronary artery with an eccentric atherosclerotic lesion. There is a small, almost slitlike central core of atheromatous debris, covered by a thick fibrous cap. This type of lesion is usually considered as "stable" and "safe." (Elastic tissue stain)

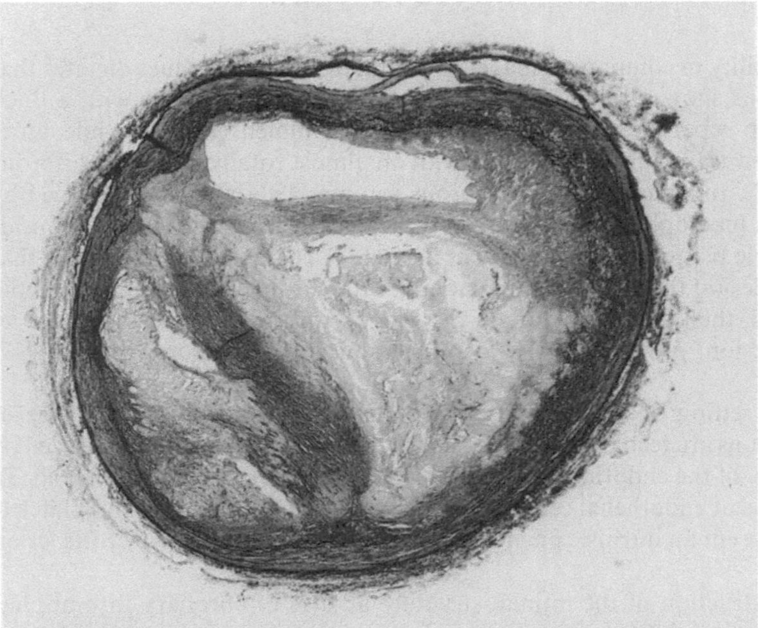

Fig. 2. Cross-section through a coronary artery showing an extensive atheroma with a markedly attenuated fibrous cap. This type of atherosclerotic lesion represents an unstable plaque and is widely considered "unsafe." (Elastic tissue stain)

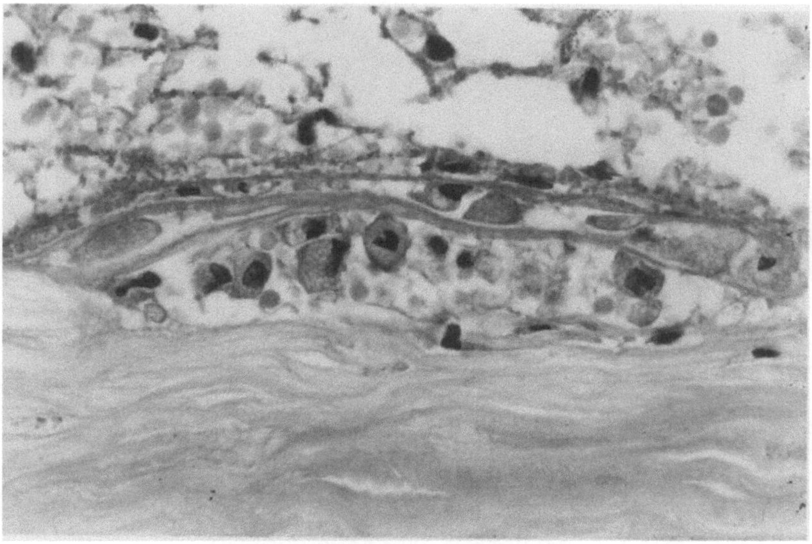

Fig. 3. Micrograph showing in detail the surface area of a fibrous cap. There is denudation of the endothelial cell layer with mural fibrin platelet aggregation. (Hematoxylin and eosin stain)

the morphologic expression of a functional cellular abnormality. Such endothelial cell dysfunction could affect the release of endothelial cell derived relaxation factor, as has been shown for regenerating endothelial cells [17]. This is a significant observation in view of the fact that human atherosclerotic coronary arteries show an abnormal reaction in vasomotor tone when acetylcholine is injected. Vasoconstriction occurs – rather than vasodilation, as expected [18]. Similary in vitro experiments with human coronary arterial segments obtained at cardiac transplantation have revealed that the response to endothelial cell derived relaxation factor was attenuated in atherosclerotic segments [19]. Hence, superficial intimal injury may have a much more profound effect on coronary artery dynamics than initially thought when seen through the microscope. From this perspective these "innocent" lesions may well play a role in the pathogenesis of unstable angina.

The second form of intimal complication to be considered is the so-called deep intimal injury. Such lesions are defined as tears or fissures that extend from the lumen into the plaque substance itself. The vast majority of instances in which coronary arterial thrombosis has occurred reveal an underlying plaque fissure as the immediate pathologic substrate (Fig. 4). The fibrous cap is torn, and blood has entered the lipid pool of the plaque, with thrombus formation as an immediate result. Occasionally, plaque fissuring may be complicated by wash-out of the intraintimal substances, leaving a crater partially covered with thrombus. Distal embolization, rather than thrombotic occlusion, is the consequence of this latter event.

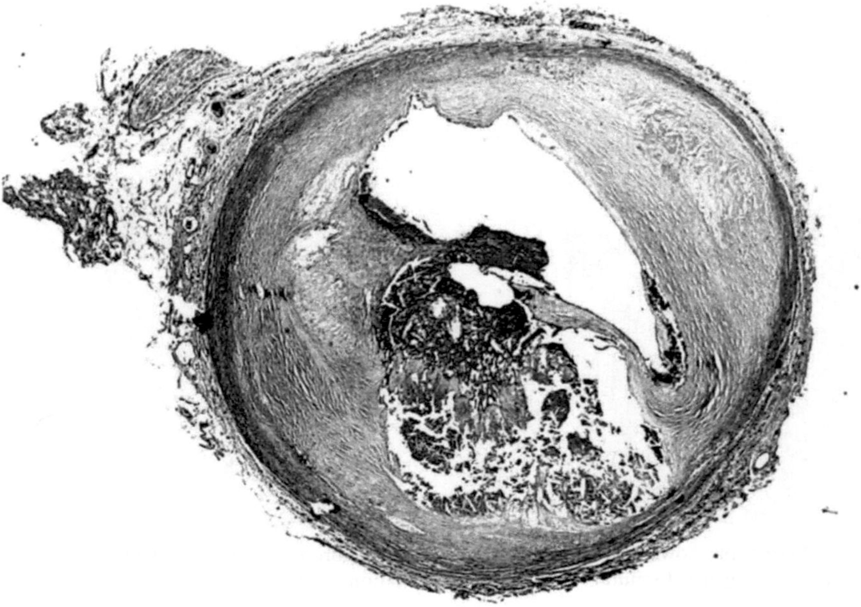

Fig. 4. Cross-section through a coronary artery showing a plaque fissure, characterized by a crack in the overlying fibrous cap with mural thrombosis and intraintimal hemorrhage. (Elastic tissue stain)

What is the clinical significance of a plaque fissure? First, the process of plaque fissuring with a predominantly intraintimal hemorrhage, not necessarily with thrombotic occlusion, is widely considered one of the mechanisms that accounts for a sudden increase in plaque size and, therefore, decrease in luminal diameter. This phenomenon contrasts with the slowly progressive increase in size of an atherosclerotic plaque under the conditions that have been set in motion as part of the atherosclerotic disease per se. It is important in this context that such sudden episodes leading to severe stenosis occur predominantly in arterial segments which were previously only minimally diseased [20]. The significance of a sudden plaque fissure is also suggested by the observation that only 33% of patients with a recent Q-wave infarction presented an obstructive coronary arterial lesion of more than 75% on a prior angiogram [21]. Finally, postmortem studies of patients with sudden cardiac death have revealed a high incidence of acute events with occlusive thrombosis [22, 23].

The concept of the atherosclerotic lesion and, in particular, its functional implications has changed drastically within the past decade. It is obvious that a whole range of morphologic changes can be present which to some extent may reflect plaque composition. The concept of "simple" fixed stenosis has been molded into one with multiple consequences that include dynamic effects on the vessel wall and intraluminal changes resulting in localized thrombosis and thromboembolic events within the microcirculation of the heart. The coronary morphology in unstable angina should be considered within this context.

Coronary Artery Pathology in Unstable Angina

Pathologic data in patients who died following an attack of unstable angina are scant. The presence of widespread atherosclerotic disease is well acknowledged, but within this setting further refinements that relate to intimal changes and dynamic aspects remain speculative. Nevertheless, some hard data are available. Falk [12] reported an 81% incidence of plaque rupture at sites of coronary thrombi in a cohort of patients who died after unstable angina. These observations further emphasize the significance of plaque fissuring as an important complicating factor in patients with unstable angina. The question remains, of course, whether plaque fissuring was also the cause of the onset of unstable angina. However, further evidence has evolved over recent years that indicate that acute coronary events do occur in patients with unstable angina. Angiographic studies reported by Ambrose and associates [24] have revealed that over two-thirds of the ischemia-related arteries in patients with unstable angina show eccentric stenoses with irregular borders. These findings have also been endorsed by others [25, 26]. It thus appears that plaque fissuring is a common event in patients with unstable angina. On the other hand, total thrombotic occlusion appears to be an uncommon phenomenon. In a series of patients catheterized shortly after an attack of unstable angina revealed only a 9% incidence of total occlusion [27].

Recently, angioscopy at the time of bypass surgery has revealed mural thrombi in 87% of patients [28]. Furthermore, intimal surface irregularities were a common finding, in contrast to the observations made in patients with chronic stable angina. The angioscopic data therefore support a concept of acute coronary events as the underlying pathologic substrate in patients with unstable angina. In fact, it brings into the picture the wide variety of both superficial and deep intimal lesions, as previously discussed. Biochemical studies, moreover, support a concept of platelet activation, with fibrin formation or fibrin dissolution, during episodes of unstable angina [29].

All in all, the accumulated data thus far support a concept of heterogeneity of the atherosclerotic lesions in coronary arteries in patients with unstable angina.

Conclusions

Unstable angina reflects basically an episode of myocardial ischemia due to a discrepancy between oxygen supply and demand. The variability in clinical expression already suggests that the pathogenetic mechanism that causes myocardial ischemia is not simply that of fixed coronary artery stenosis. Unstable angina, moreover, is a condition that shows a high tendency towards progression, with acute myocardial infarction or sudden cardiac death as the ultimate consequence. It is on the basis of the variable expressions also that unstable angina is considered an intermediate between chronic stable angina and acute myocardial infarction.

With this clinical profile in mind it should not come as a surprise that the pathology of the coronary arteries reflects a similar scope of abnormalities. The major hallmark is atherosclerotic lesions, but the presentation of the lesion may vary from one segment to another, both within the same artery and within the same patient. The leading factor, nevertheless, is an unstable atherosclerotic lesion, characterized by an attenuated fibrous cap. The superimposed pathologic features are then surface irregularities, characterized by localized platelet aggregations, and plaque fissuring with intraintimal hemorrhages and/or surface thrombosis and with or without total luminal occlusion. In other words, the entire spectrum of complicating features may be encountered in the patient who presents a bout of unstable angina. Furthermore, there is sufficient scientific basis to include dynamic aspects as part of the pathogenetic mechanism of unstable angina. Changes in vasomotor tone may have a profound effect on luminal diameter, particularly in eccentric lesions, and may therefore cause a major impediment to adequate myocardial perfusion. The linkage of this dynamic process to the atherosclerotic disease remains as yet hypothetical, but there is nevertheless overwhelming circumstantial evidence that a connection exists.

In a patient who presents with an acute episode of unstable angina, an acute coronary event is the most likely underlying pathology, however, one should keep in mind that these patients usually show a wide variability in the make-up of the atherosclerotic lesions and associated complications.

References

1. Fowler NO (1971) "Preinfarction" angina. A need for an objective definition and for a controlled clinical trial of its management. Circulation 44:755–758
2. Mulcahy R, Al Awadhi AH, de Buiteleor M, Tobin G, Johnson H, Contoy R (1985) Natural history and prognosis of unstable angina. Am Heart J 109:753–758
3. Patterson DLM (1988) Management in unstable angina. Postgrad Med J 64:271–277
4. Victor MF, Likoff MJ, Mintz GS, Likoff W (1981) Unstable angina pectoris of new onset: a prospective clinical and arteriographic study of 75 patients. Am J Cardiol 47:228–232
5. De Servi S, Ghio S, Ardissino D, Collarini L, Ferrario C, Salerno J, Vigano M, Montemartini C, Specchia G (1985) Management of crescendo angina. Eur Heart J 6 [Suppl F]:83–86
6. Becker AE (1985) Atherosclerosis – a lesion in search of a definition. Int J Cardiol 8:375–377
7. Ross R (1986) The pathogenesis of atherosclerosis – an update. N Engl J Med 314:488–500
8. Gown AM, Tsukada T, Ross R (1986) Human atherosclerosis. II. Immunocytochemical analysis of the cellular composition of human atherosclerotic lesions. Am J Pathol 125:191–207

9. van der Wal AC, Das PK, Bentz van de Berg D, van der Loos CM, Becker AE (1989) Atherosclerotic lesions in humans. In situ immunophenotypic analysis suggesting an immune mediated response. Lab Invest 61:166–170
10. Potkin BN, Roberts WC (1988) Effects of percutaneous transluminal coronary angioplasty on atherosclerotic plaques and the relation of plaque composition and arterial size to outcome. Am J Cardiol 62:41–50
11. Becker AE (1989) Ultrasound imaging and atherosclerosis. Int J Cardiac Imaging 4:99–104
12. Falk E (1985) Unstable angina with fatal outcome: dynamic coronary thrombosis leading to infarction and/or sudden death. Autopsy evidence of recurrent mural thrombosis with peripheral embolization culminating in total vascular occlusion. Circulation 71:699–708
13. Davies MJ, Thomas AC, Knapman PA, Hangartner JR (1986) Intramyocardial platelet aggregation in patients with unstable angina suffering sudden ischemic cardiac death. Circulation 73:418–427
14. Kim DN, Scott RF, Schmee J, Thomas WA (1988) Endothelial cell denudation, labelling indices and monocyte attachment in advanced swine coronary artery lesions. Atherosclerosis 73:247–258
15. Davies MJ, Woolf N, Rowles PM, Pepper J (1988) Morphology of the endothelium over atherosclerotic plaques in human coronary arteries. Br Heart J 60:459–464
16. Davies MJ (1989) Thrombosis and coronary atherosclerosis. In: Julian D, Kübler W, Norris RM, Swan HJC, Collen D, Verstraete M (eds) Thrombolysis in cardiovascular disease. Dekker, New York, pp 25–43
17. Shimokawa H, Aarhus LL, Vanhoutte PM (1987) Porcine coronary arteries with regenerated endothelium have a reduced endothelium-dependent responsiveness to aggregating platelets and serotonin. Circ Res 61:256–270
18. Ludmer PL, Selwyn AP, Shook TL, Wayne RR, Mudge GH, Alexander RW, Ganz P (1986) Paradoxial vasoconstriction induced by acetylcholine in atherosclerotic coronary arteries. N Engl J Med 315:1046–1051
19. Förstermann U, Mügge A, Alheid U, Haverich A, Frölich JC (1988) Selective attenuation of endothelium-mediated vasodilation in atherosclerotic human coronary arteries. Circ Res 62:185–190
20. Haft JI, Haik BJ, Goldstein JE, Brodyn NE (1988) Development of significant coronary artery lesions in areas of minimal disease: a common mechanism for coronary disease progression. Chest 94:731–736
21. Ambrose JA, Tannenbaum MA, Alexopoulos D, Hjemdahl-Monsen CE, Leavy J, Weiss M, Borrico S, Gorlin R, Fuster V (1988) Angiographic progression of coronary artery disease and the development of myocardial infarction. J Am Coll Cardiol 12:56–62
22. Davies MJ, Thomas A (1984) Thrombosis and acute coronary arter lesions in sudden cardiac ischemic death. N Engl J Med 310:1137–1140
23. van Dantzig JM, Becker AE (1986) Sudden cardiac death and acute pathology of coronary arteries. Eur Heart J 7:987–991
24. Ambrose JA, Winters SL, Stern A, Eng A, Teichholz LE, Gorlin R, Fuster V (1985) Angiographic morphology and the pathogenesis of unstable angina pectoris. J Am Coll Cardiol 5:609–616
25. Kranjec I, Delaye J, Didier B, Delahaye F, Grand A (1987) Angiographic morphology and intraluminal coronary artery thrombus in patients with angina pectoris: clinical correlations. Eur Heart J 8:106–115
26. Haft JI, Goldstein JE, Niemiera ML (1987) Coronary arteriographic lesion of unstable angina. Chest 92:609–612
27. Ambrose JA, Hjemdahl-Monsen CE, Borrico S, Gorlin R, Fuster V (1988) Angiographic demonstration of a common link between unstable angina pectoris and non-Q wave acute myocardial infarction. Am J Cardiol 61:244–247
28. Forrester JS, Litvack F, Grundfest W, Hickey A (1987) A perspective study of coronary disease seen through the arteries of a living man. Circulation 75:505–513
29. Fitzgerald DL, Roy L, Catella F, Fitzgerald GA (1986) Platelet activation in unstable coronary disease. N Engl J Med 315:983–989

Evidence for Intracoronary Thrombosis in Patients with Unstable Angina Pectoris

P. J. COMMERFORD, B. K. W. GREEN, and R. E. KIRSCH [1]

Introduction

A major difficulty that arises when discussing any aspect of unstable angina is that no good, all-embracing definition is available that acceptably encompasses all of the clinical syndromes often included. The term is applied to symptoms of a wide range of severity, occurring in a heterogeneous group of patients with a variety of clinical presentations and having in common a picture of presumed myocardial ischaemia and characterised by an unpredictable clinical course [11]. Patients with new-onset exertional angina and those with a change in the pattern of frequency and severity of exertional angina are considered unstable, as are others with severe, prolonged pain at rest associated with electrocardiographic evidence of ischaemia who do not have enzymatic evidence of myocardial necrosis. Angina occurring early after myocardial infarction is similarly labelled as being unstable.

Inevitably the decision as to whether or not a certain patient can truly be classified as having unstable angina is subjective and clinical, influenced both by the patient's report of his symptoms and the clinician's interpretation of the report. The most difficult decisions always relate to patients at the two ends of the spectrum of clinical severity. How much must the pattern of chronic stable angina change before a patient can be classified as having unstable angina? Can patients who have prolonged pain at rest and persistent electrocardiographic evidence of ischaemia be classified as having unstable angina? Some authors have chosen to regard such patients as having suffered a non-Q-wave infarct even in the absence of a detected enzyme rise.

It is not surprising given the heterogeneity of patients and the wide range of symptoms which are encompassed by the term unstable angina that there is still controversy about the pathogenetic mechanisms involved. Coronary spasm and abnormal vasomotion have been invoked, as have abnormal platelet reactivity and rapid progression of atherosclerotic plaques. Possible mechanisms have recently been reviewed in detail [50], and many are discussed elsewhere in this volume. Any and all of these may contribute, and at present it is fair to say that the final answer is not known.

[1] Cardiac Clinic and MRC Liver Research Centre, Department of Medicine, University of Cape Town and Groote Schuur Hospital, Observatory 7925, South Africa

W. Bleifeld et al. (Eds.)
Unstable Angina

Therapeutic trials of agents which inhibit thrombosis or alter platelet function [8, 30, 42, 45] have provided persuasive evidence that intracoronary thrombi may be important. Angioscopy [41], post-mortem angiography, and histological studies support this view [29].

In this chapter we reexamine the angiographic evidence for intracoronary thrombosis and biochemical evidence of activation of the fibrinogen-fibrin cascade in patients with unstable angina pectoris.

Angiographic Evidence of Intracoronary Thrombus in Patients with Unstable Angina

The reported prevalence of angiographically detected intracoronary thrombus ranges widely – from as low as 1% to as high as 58% (Table 1). Many factors may be responsible for the marked variability in reported prevalence of angiographically detected thrombus in these series; these include:

1. Differences in the clinical characteristics of the patients studied. Unstable angina is a term which describes a clinical syndrome. Variations in interpretation inevitably result in inclusion of a heterogeneous group of patients.
2. The decision as to what angiographic appearances truly represent thrombus is subjective.
3. The resolution of X-ray imaging systems varies, and small thrombi may not always be detected.
4. Layered, mural thrombi may not distort the contrast column and hence not be identified.
5. The time which elapsed between onset of symptoms, presentation and angiography was very different in different studies.
6. If thrombi are truly important, they may well be evanescent and altered by spontaneous endogenous fibrinolysis and therapy with anticoagulants and anti-platelet agents. Such therapy is by no means standard and not always reported in detail.

In 1981 Holmes and others [24] reported the clinical course, coronary artery anatomy and ventricular function of 16 patients in whom coronary artery thrombus was detected at the time of coronary angiography. The index cases were identified over a 3-year period in a total of 3553 patients undergoing angiography because they were suspected of having coronary artery disease. Intracoronary thrombus was diagnosed on the basis of a central filling defect (free of calcification) surrounded by contrast material. During the period in which these patients were identified 1202 underwent angiography for evaluation of an unstable course, defined as progressive escalation in the frequency and severity of angina pectoris in a 3-month period before catheterization despite conventional medical treatment. The 16 patients identified represented 1.3% of the patients with unstable symptoms. Three patterns of coronary artery thrombus were identified. In addition to thrombus immediately proximal and distal to high-grade coronary stenoses they identified thrombus in five

Table 1. Angiographic demonstration of coronary thrombi

Reference	Number of patients	Thrombus demonstrated	Time elapsed between symptoms and angiography	Pattern of angina
Holmes et al. [24]	1202	16 (1%)	<12 weeks	13 of 16 had pain at rest
Vetrovec et al. [48]	129	8 (6%)	< 4 weeks	Prolonged pain, ST, T wave changes
Zack et al. [52]	42	5 (12%)	<12 weeks	Prolonged pain at rest
	41	5 (12%)		Crescendo angina
Capone et al. [9]	44	23 (52%)	<24 h	Pain at rest
	75	21 (28%)	<14 days	Pain at rest
Bresnahan et al. [7]	67	24 (35%)	–	Pain at rest, crescendo angina Postinfarction angina
Williams et al. [51]	34	(29%)	5 days	Crescendo angina, rest pain <20 min
	59	(27%)	5 days	Acute coronary insufficiency, rest pain >20 min
Cowley et al. [10]	69	40 (58%)	1 h–5 days	Prolonged pain >15–20 min, pain at rest or marked increase in frequency of angina

patients in segments of the coronary arterial tree in which there was no high-grade coronary artery stenosis. Pathological confirmation of the coronary artery thrombus was obtained in three patients: in two at the time of surgery and in one at post mortem.

In a review of the coronary angiograms of 129 patients who underwent angiography within 1 month of the onset of unstable angina (defined as recent onset of increased frequency or severity or rest pain) and the intermediate coronary syndrome (prolonged pain of greater than 20-min duration with ST, T changes and no or minimal evidence of myocardial necrosis) Vetrovec and co-workers [47] found evidence consistent with intracoronary thrombus in 8 (6.2%). Filling defects consistent with thrombus were defined as partially occluding, non-opacified or hazy intracoronary filling defects outlined by contrast medium in at least two well-opacified views. All defects were found just distal to severe stenoses in vessels supplying a myocardial segment referable to the electrocardiographically defined area of ischaemia. Repeat angiography within 7 days showed enlargement of the filling defects in three and embolisation of fragments in two. Six of the eight patients had experienced prolonged pain, and all had resting ST segment and T wave changes on the electrocardiogram.

No evidence of intracoronary thrombus was found in 37 patients with chronic stable angina by Zack et al. [52]. In contrast, 10 of 83 (12%) of patients with unstable angina demonstrated intracoronary filling defects, intraluminal staining or total coronary occlusion with a convex dye outline, all of which were interpreted as compatible with intracoronary thrombus. Unstable angina was defined as either an episode of prolonged chest pain at rest leading to hospitalisation (42 patients) or an increase in the frequency and severity of chest pain (41 patients). There was no difference in the incidence of thrombi in the two groups, and contrary to the authors' expectations prolonged pain did not seem to be a useful marker for the presence of intracoronary thrombus.

The temporal relationship between angiographically demonstrated thrombus and symptoms of unstable angina was examined in studies of 119 patients with rest pain within 14 days of angiography [9]. Thrombi were considered to be present if spherical, ovoid or irregular intraluminal filling defects surrounded on three sides by contrast medium were seen just distal to or within a coronary stenosis. Intraluminal filling defects were found in 44 (37%) of the 119 patients with rest pain; none was found in a smaller control group of 35 patients with stable angina. Intraluminal filling defects were more frequently seen in 23 (52%) of the 44 patients who had experienced rest pain within 24 h before angiography than in those in whom angiography was delayed for 1–14 days, in whom they were only detected in 28%. The authors concluded that intracoronary thrombus is common in patients with unstable angina when symptoms occur at rest and plays an aetiologic role in the syndrome. The evanescent nature of the thrombi means that they may not be visualised after the clinical course has stabilized.

A prospective review for the presence of coronary thrombus of the angiograms of 268 patients without valvular heart disease identified 29 (11%)

with arteriographic criteria, which included contrast medium staining at the site of abrupt vessel occlusion and filling defects surrounded by contrast [7]. A total of 67 patients were identified as having unstable angina on the basis of angina at rest or a substantially new pattern of chest pain that had begun during the preceding 2 months. Thrombi were found in 24 (35%) of these patients. Thrombi were also identified in 5 (2.5%) of 201 patients with stable angina. All five had had a transmural myocardial infarction 3–18 months before angiography. The temporal relationship of the angiography to unstable symptoms is not clear.

The angiographic presence of intracoronary thrombus may be associated with a higher incidence of in-hospital cardiac events, including revascularisation, myocardial infarction or death when it is demonstrated in patients with acute coronary insufficiency or crescendo angina [51]. Filling defects, luminal staining at the site of high-grade stenoses and convexity at the site of total occlusion without vessel tapering were found in 29% of 34 patients with rapid acceleration of a previously established anginal syndrome which included rest pain of less than 20-min duration. The frequency of such appearances was much the same, occurring in 27% of the 59 patients with acute coronary insufficiency in whom infarction was excluded by absence of an enzyme rise at the time of admission. Thrombi were identified in seven of eight patients initially thought to have acute coronary insufficiency, but who subsequently were diagnosed as having acute myocardial infarction on the basis of an enzyme rise. The mean time to angiography was 5 days. Thrombus was identified more commonly (50%) in a small subset of patients studied within 48 h of presentation because of recurrent symptoms. Approximately 50% of patients had an in-hospital event, usually revascularisation, prompted by recurrent symptoms. Quantitative angiographic findings and identification of complex morphology and intracoronary thrombus identified patients at greatest risk of an event. These findings were most influential in the group with acute coronary insufficiency.

The same authors expanded their observation in a further report of 78 consecutive patients with unstable angina randomised to coronary angiography performed either on the day of presentation or later during the hospital admission [16]. There was no significant difference in the frequency with which thrombi were identified in the two groups. Coronary thrombi were found in 43% of patients undergoing early angiography and 38% of those investigated later. Twelve patients randomised to late angiography required urgent investigation because of recurrence of chest pain despite medical therapy (which did not include heparin and aspirin). Nine of these patients (75%) had angiographic evidence of intracoronary thrombus. The hypothesis that thrombus occurs more frequently in patients with early angiography was not confirmed, but, importantly, it was shown that thrombus had an important temporal link to the occurrence of chest pain at rest.

A recent report on patients studied very soon after episodes of chest pain found angiographic appearances compatible with intracoronary thrombi in a high percentage [10]. Sixty-nine patients with severe unstable angina defined as a prolonged episode of pain (> 15- to 20-min duration), pain at rest or marked increase in frequency of pain underwent coronary angiography within 5 days of admission. The mean time from onset of unstable symptoms to angiography was 9.4 days, and the mean time from last symptoms to angiography was 24 h, with a range extending from less than 1 h to 5 days. Intraluminal filling defects were found in 31 (45%) of 69 patients, and 9 additional patients (14%) had angiographic evidence of thrombus at a site of total occlusion with well-developed collaterals supplying the occluded vessel. Thus intracoronary thrombus was present in 40 of 69 patients (58%) with unstable angina.

These authors and others found, in addition to evidence of intracoronary thrombosis, that patients with unstable angina were more likely to have complex lesions. These are variously described as having hazy, ill-defined margins, irregular borders, luminal inhomogeneity and overhanging edges. Ambrose and others [2] described the frequent occurrence of their type II eccentric lesions in patients with unstable angina. The type II eccentric lesion was the most common morphologic feature of disease progression in patients with unstable angina [4]. They postulated that these asymmetric stenoses – in the form of a convex intraluminal obstruction with a narrow base or neck due to one or more overhanging edges or borders that were irregular or scalloped – could represent atherosclerotic plaques, partially occlusive thrombi or both and referred to post-mortem angiographic and pathologic correlations [29]. They further drew attention to the fact that similar lesions were seen in patients with acute infarction whose vessels were not totally occluded or were reopened with thrombolytic therapy [3]. Similar lesions were described by the same authors in non-Q-wave infarction [6], leading them to postulate a similar pathogenesis for the two conditions. In this study non-Q wave infarction was defined as follows: (a) all patients had prolonged rest pain and (b) new and persistent ST and T wave changes (lasting over 48 h) without new Q waves or (c) total creatine kinase level twice normal. Of 33 patients considered to have non-Q wave infarction 30 had persistent electrocardiographic changes with or without elevation of creatine phosphokinase. Such patients with prolonged pain, persistent ST, T changes without enzyme elevation might be classified by some as an extreme form of unstable angina or acute coronary insufficiency rather than non-Q wave infarction.

Several reports have thus documented specific coronary arteriographic appearances in patients with unstable angina. At least some of the described abnormalities are highly suggestive of intracoronary thrombi. Such appearances have been found most frequently when sought in close temporal relationship to unstable symptoms and in patients with prolonged pain at rest in association with resting ST, T wave electrocardiographic abnormalities. There is suggestive evidence that angiographic detection of appearances compatible with intracoronary thrombus identifies a subset of patients at increased risk of in-hospital complications.

Fibrinolytic Therapy for Unstable Angina

If intracoronary thrombus is important in the aetiology of unstable angina, then it is reasonable to assume that it should be possible to demonstrate clinical or angiographic benefit after administration of a thrombolytic agent. A number of studies have addressed this issue (Table 2). The studies have served to confirm the angiographic appearances of intracoronary thrombi when patients are investigated in close temporal relationship to symptoms of unstable angina and have shown that these thrombi may be altered by thrombolytic therapy; however, as yet striking clinical benefit has not been shown.

In the first such study [28] 40 patients with marked progression of symptoms within 6 weeks prior to evaluation were randomly assigned to an infusion of streptokinase (250000 units as a loading dose followed by 100000 units intravenously every hour) for 24 h followed by warfarin anticoagulation or to warfarin anticoagulation alone. Coronary angiography was not performed. During a 6-month follow-up period there were eight cardiovascular events (four myocardial infarctions and four sudden deaths) in the 20 treated with warfarin alone. There was only one event (sudden death) in the 20 patients treated with streptokinase. Despite the very favourable clinical outcome the authors emphasized the need for caution in drawing firm conclusions from a small series and suggested that it pointed to the need for exploration on a wider scale. The fact that it has not been tested on a wider scale, as suggested, can probably be attributed to the fact that larger studies of other agents that inhibit thrombosis or alter platelet function have shown dramatic benefit in patients with unstable angina [8, 30, 42, 45]. Studies with heparin and aspirin have had such dramatic benefit and have reduced the incidence of adverse effects to such a degree that it is unlikely that thrombolytic agents will be able to demonstrate substantial benefit. They are of interest however insofar as they shed light on the pathophysiologic role of intracoronary thrombus.

Intracoronary streptokinase infused into the ischaemia-related artery successfully reopened completely obstructed vessels or increased the diameter at the site of subtotal lesions in 22 of 29 patients with acute myocardial infarction, but no angiographically demonstrable change in luminal diameter occurred in the subtotal obstruction in five patients with unstable angina [38]. The clinical and electrocardiographic characteristics of the two groups of patients were similar. All had chest pain at rest lasting longer than 20 min, and the majority had electrocardiographic changes compatible with acute myocardial ischaemia. The diagnosis of unstable angina was based on an absence of a diagnostic enzyme rise. The authors concluded that narrowing of the ischaemia-related artery in these five patients was not due to fresh thrombotic material.

A study utilizing qualitative coronary angiographic techniques with vessel magnification and quantitative analysis with digital subtraction similarly failed to demonstrate overall benefit in 36 consecutive patients catheterised after an acute episode of unstable angina or recent non-Q wave infarction [5].

Table 2. Thrombolytic therapy in unstable angina pectoris

Reference	Number of patients	Thrombus demonstrated	Time elapsed between symptoms and angiography	Pattern of angina	Benefit
Lawrence et al. [28]	20	–	–	Progression of symptoms	Reduction in cardiovascular events during follow-up
Rentrop et al. [38]	5	–	<15 h	Prolonged pain	No angiographic benefit
Ambrose et al. [5]	36	24 (67%)	2.5 weeks	Prolonged pain, non-Q wave infarction	No benefit
Vetrovec et al. [48]	12	11	<5 days	Prolonged pain Abnormal ECG	Partial lysis in ten patients Improvement in symptoms
Mandelkorn et al. [31]	9	4 (44%)	<24 h	Prolonged pain	Angiographic improvement
Gotoh et al. [23]	37	21 (57%)	During spontaneous attacks	Prolonged chest pain >30 mins	Angiographic benefit; symptoms relieved
de Zwaan et al. [11]	41	28 (68%)	2–69 h (mean 19)	Recent onset, sudden worsening	Angiographic benefit
Gold et al. [21]	rt-PA 11 Placebo 11	0 8	Angiography performed after thrombolysis	Chest pain at rest with ST deviation	Improvement in symptoms, angiographic benefit
Nicklas et al. [34] Topol et al. [46]	40	16	<7 days	Chest pain at rest ECG evidence of ischaemia during pacing	Improved pacing threshold Facilitated safety of PTCA

Patients with totally occluded coronary arteries were excluded, as were those with lesions of less than 70% diameter stenosis. The percentage of diameter stenosis and percentage of area stenosis in all ischaemia-producing arteries were unchanged by intracoronary infusion of up to 300000 units of streptokinase over 30–40 min. The majority of patients (29) had unstable angina. The median length of time from onset of instability to angiography was 2.5 weeks but varied widely, and only 17 had angina within 24 h of catheterisation. The authors concluded that intracoronary streptokinase may be of limited utility in unstable angina but noted that patients in whom a significant improvement in the percentage of stenosis occurred after intravenous streptokinase infusion tended to have had more recent episodes of chest pain relative to catheterisation than did patients without improvement. Of the patients 50% had been treated with heparin before streptokinase, and this may have facilitated spontaneous fibrinolysis.

In contrast, a similar dose of intracoronary streptokinase produced angiographic evidence of partial or complete lysis in 10 of 13 (77%) ischaemia-related vessels in 12 patients treated within 5 days of recent prolonged angina or pre-infarction angina [48]. Importantly, 6 of the 13 vessels were vein grafts in patients who had previously undergone coronary bypass surgery. Angiographic benefit was associated with clinical improvement in that there was an improvement in symptomatic status and a decrease in rest angina after thrombolysis. One may question the relevance of the observations in postoperative patients to the usual patient presenting with unstable angina due to lesions in native coronary vessels. Nonetheless it could be concluded from this retrospective study that intracoronary streptokinase is successful in lysing angiographically demonstrated thrombi in at least some patients with unstable angina or pre-infarction angina.

Angiographic appearances compatible with intracoronary thrombi were identified in four (44%) of nine patients who underwent angiography within 24 h of an episode of rest pain [31]. Intracoronary streptokinase increased the stenotic diameter in two patients and completely dissolved filling defects in a further two. Two patients initially responding to streptokinase showed further anatomic change on restudy after 1 week of anticoagulation with heparin with further increase in luminal diameter and complete disappearance of a large intraluminal filling defect. Interestingly, thrombolysis was not demonstrated in any patient who was studied longer than 1 week after the onset of the rest pain syndrome. This is consistent with the postulate of Ambrose et al. [5] that thrombus in coronary arteries responsible for producing unstable symptoms may become organized and layered, as shown pathologically [14, 15], and may be resistant to thrombolytic agents.

Perhaps the most convincing evidence for the role of intracoronary thrombosis in unstable angina is presented in a very unusual study of 37 patients who underwent coronary angiography during spontaneous anginal attacks [23]. All patients had unstable angina with recurrent, prolonged (30–60 min) episodes of angina within 3 weeks, and none had suffered a recent myocardial infarct. Symptoms were refractory to conventional medical therapy, and the episode of pain during angiography was similar in duration and intensity to previous episodes and accompanied by similar electrocardiographic changes. Myocardial infarction did not follow the spontaneous pain at the time of angiography. Angiography during pain revealed that 21 (57%) of the 37 patients had intracoronary thrombus in major coronary arteries, 14 (38%) had fixed narrowings without angiographic evidence of thrombus, and 2 had coronary spasm. Intracoronary administration of urokinase in a dose of 24000 units per minute for 10–40 min resulted in improvement in 20 patients. Obstructed arteries were reopened or narrowings attenuated with relief of symptoms. Recurrent symptoms were more common in patients with intracoronary thrombus despite apparently successful thrombolytic therapy, and myocardial infarction within 4 weeks of catheterisation was observed more frequently in those with intracoronary thrombus than in those without. This study is particularly interesting in that it suggests that very different intracoronary pathological changes may be present in patients who are apparently clinically similar. Dynamic occlusion with intracoronary thrombus is obviously present in some, whereas others have severe stable narrowings. The short-term clinical outcome in the two groups may be very different.

Despite apparent angiographic benefit following thrombolysis clinical benefit was not shown in another group of patients in whom thrombolytic therapy was administered later, at a mean of 19 h, after symptoms of chest pain [11]. Coronary angiography was performed within 24 h of admission to hospital and between 2 and 69 h after the most recent episode of pain in 41 patients with unstable angina. Fifteen patients had a prior history of stable angina, half had rest angina of new onset, and 21 experienced episodes of chest pain of long duration. Electrocardiographic changes compatible with ischaemia at rest were present in all but two patients. Thrombolytic therapy was either intracoronary streptokinase (250000 units) or 100 mg intravenous single-chain recombinant tissue-type plasminogen activator (rt-PA) over 3 h. Angiography was repeated 1 day later. Of the 41 patients, 28 (68%) had angiographic evidence of intracoronary thrombus before and 16 after thrombolytic treatment.

Eleven of 21 patients treated with streptokinase, and 11 of 20 treated with rt-PA showed a decrease in severity of the coronary stenosis on repeat angiography 1 day later. Ischaemic symptoms and the need for coronary bypass grafting or angioplasty were not different in patients with or without a reduction in coronary stenosis after fibrinolytic therapy. Twenty-six patients had a decline in symptoms during observation over 10 days in hospital. The improvement in functional class did not correlate with the reduction in coronary stenosis. When clinical benefit was noted, it was often only temporary, and recurrent pain led to coronary angioplasty in 6 patients and bypass grafting in 13 during the 3-month follow-up. Noting the discrepancy and apparent dissociation between angiographic results and clinical benefit, the authors suggested that randomised, blinded, placebo-controlled studies would be necessary to establish whether fibrinolytic therapy was of value in patients with unstable angina.

A randomised, blinded, placebo-controlled trial of rt-PA was performed in a small group of 24 patients with unstable angina [21]. Patients entered all had chest pain at rest associated with reversible electrocardiographic changes of S-T elevation or depression within the previous week. Those with recent (2 weeks) myocardial infarction were excluded. Prior to randomisation patients received standardised therapy including nitrates, beta-blockers and calcium channel blockers. All received heparin anticoagulation treatment for 12–24 h before randomisation to placebo or a 12-h intravenous infusion of rt-PA at 1.75 mg/kg. Angiography was performed 1–3 days after completion of the infusion, and observations continued during a follow-up period of approximately 1 week.

Unstable angina pectoris persisted after completion of the infusion in 6 of the 11 patients receiving placebo and only 1 of 12 treated with rt-PA. Coronary angiography after completion of infusion demonstrated subocclusive thrombus in 8 of 11 patients receiving placebo but in none of 11 treated with rt-PA. There was a significant correlation between persistence of angina and the presence of intracoronary thrombus. Revascularisation procedures (angioplasty and coronary bypass grafting) occurred with similar frequency in the two groups. In the placebo group the interventions were necessary to control recurrent ischaemia whereas they were usually performed electively in patients treated with rt-PA. The authors concluded that the infusion of rt-PA stabilised patients presumably by removing intracoronary thrombus allowing definitive intervention to be performed during a stable phase of the disease.

Two other reports [34, 46] which appear to describe very similar if not identical patients fail to confirm this reduction in need for urgent revascularisation. Forty patients with chest pain at rest in the preceding 7 days, with angiographically significant coronary disease and provokable ischaemia on right ventricular pacing were randomised to receive either 150 mg rt-PA intravenously over 8 h or placebo. All patients were pretreated with aspirin, heparin, beta-blockers and calcium channel blockers. Angiography and right ventricular pacing was repeated 24 h later. There were no significant differences with regard to baseline characteristics between the two groups. Approximately equal numbers had angiographic evidence of intracoronary thrombus. The pacing threshold increased significantly for patients receiving rt-PA after therapy and did not change in the placebo group.

The greatest benefit was seen in patients with angiographically defined thrombus. Three patients treated with rt-PA and none in the placebo group had conversion of angiographic appearances to that of an insignificant residual stenosis (<60%). There was no difference between the two groups in overall rate of revascularisation by coronary artery bypass grafting or angioplasty. When angioplasty was necessary, it seemed safer in patients receiving rt-PA as the procedure was less likely to be complicated by abrupt closure. These reports support the contention that intracoronary thrombus is present in some patients with unstable angina. Fibrinolytic therapy may serve as complete treatment in a small number of such patients and promote the safety of angioplasty beyond maximal medical therapy including heparin. Benefit appears to be maximal in patients with angiographic evidence of intracoronary thrombus.

Fibrinopeptide A

Fibrinopeptide A (FPA) is a small 16 amino acid peptide released from the N-terminal of the α-chain of fibrinogen by the specific action of thrombin (Fig. 1). Liberation of FPA and another 14 amino acid peptide, fibrinopeptide B, uncovers the E domain of fibrinogen. The residual protein, fibrin monomer, polymerises to form fibrin clot [35]. Normal blood levels of FPA are low and become elevated during thrombotic and prethrombotic states before other markers of thrombosis.

Elevated levels of FPA reported in patients with acute myocardial infarction [12, 19, 33] are in keeping with the current understanding of the pathophysiologic role of intracoronary thrombosis in this condition. Values are highest in patients with transmural infarction in whom samples are obtained soon after the onset of symptoms, and sequential measurement shows that the values decline consistently over a 24-h sampling period [12]. Heparin administration reduces but does not normalise the elevated levels [19, 33]. Consistently elevated levels of FPA after fibrinolytic therapy for acute infarction or levels that increase despite adequate anticoagulation indicate ongoing fibrin generation and may be a marker for an increased risk of reocclusion [37].

If unstable angina and acute myocardial infarction have some pathophysiologic similarity, one might expect similar elevations of FPA in patients with unstable angina. Serneri and others [39, 40] reported on FPA levels in 98 patients with ischaemic heart disease. Fifty-three had suffered remote myocardial infarction 3–12 months previously. Fibrinopeptide A was higher in patients with remote infarction, spontaneous angina and effort angina than in controls. Levels were highest in those with "active disease" defined as at least one anginal attack per day. Gallino et al. [18] investigated FPA concentrations in urine and plasma in 19 patients with acute myocardial infarction and 17

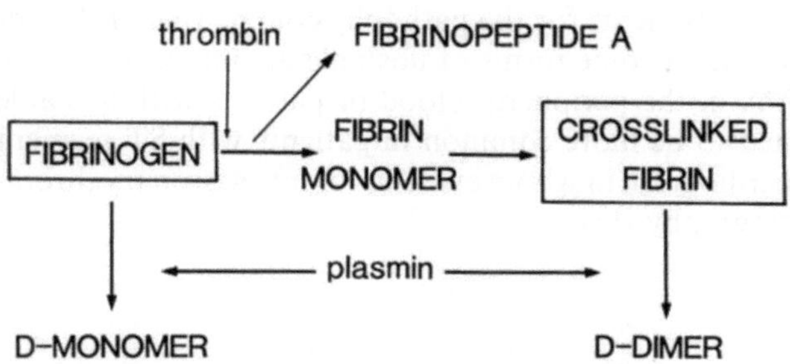

Fig. 1. A very simplified schematic diagram of the fibrinogen-fibrin cascade which illustrates the position of fibrinopeptide A and the antigens measured in our study. (Modified from [26])

with severe angina pectoris who had not had a recent (3 months) myocardial infarction. Nine of the 17 patients with angina pectoris were characterised as having unstable angina on the basis of a recent increase in frequency and severity of chest pain, frequent pain at rest and progressive decrease in exercise tolerance during the preceding 3 months. Levels of FPA in patients with unstable angina were similar to those measured in patients with acute myocardial infarction and were significantly higher than corresponding levels in patients with stable angina and normal control subjects.

Further convincing biochemical evidence for the pathophysiologic role of intracoronary thrombosis comes from a detailed study of 16 consecutive patients admitted to a coronary care unit with unstable angina [44]. Twelve patients had a crescendo pattern of chest pain, including pain at rest, and four had prolonged pain poorly relieved by nitroglycerin. All patients had transient ST segment depression or T wave inversion. Acute myocardial infarction was excluded by the usual electrocardiographic and enzymatic observations. Blood samples were obtained on the morning after admission, a mean of 18 h after the last episode of pain. Fifteen age- and sex-matched patients with stable exertional angina pectoris served as controls. Coronary angiographic characteristics, while not matched, were similar in the two groups. Mean plasma levels of FPA were considerably higher in patients with unstable angina compared to those in patients with stable angina. There was a wide range of the values obtained in those with unstable angina. The highest value was obtained in a sample collected shortly (1 h) after an episode of chest pain.

Blood tests were repeated in patients with unstable angina 5–8 days after admission and before coronary angiography. The mean level decreased significantly, but individual patients had varied responses. In 11 patients the individual values decreased and clinically the unstable pattern of angina was controlled in all these patients who showed a decrease in FPA; angina was still clinically unstable in two of three with increasing values and in one of three with unchanged levels. The half-life of FPA is very short (5 min), and the study was not prospectively designed to obtain blood samples in close temporal relationship to episodes of pain. However, the results which showed overall elevation of FPA in patients with unstable angina, fortuitously detected high levels in close relationship to pain, a decline in the levels in the majority of patients and persistent or rising levels associated with persistence of the unstable state are persuasive arguments for the pathophysiologic role of thrombosis in the aetiology of at least some forms of unstable angina pectoris [43].

Elevated levels of FPA in the peripheral blood of patients with unstable angina have been reported to be more common in patients with ST segment deviation on the electrocardiogram in whom evidence of intracoronary thrombus was detected at angiography [13].

Fibrin and Fibrinogen-Related Antigens in Unstable Angina

If intracoronary thrombus is important in unstable angina, and if it is one of the common pathophysiologic links in the syndromes of acute coronary ischaemia [17, 22, 49], then one might expect similar elevation of the intermediary fragments produced during fibrin formation or the specific breakdown fragments of these proteins in patients with unstable angina and acute myocardial infarction. We investigated patients with acute myocardial infarction, unstable angina and chronic stable angina using radioimmunoassay and antigen capture techniques for the measurement of these fragments [26]. Patients with acute non-cardiac pain and healthy volunteers served as controls. Unstable angina was defined as chest pain of at least 15-min duration occurring at rest in the absence of an increase in the MB fraction of creatine kinase in patients with objective evidence of coronary artery disease based on the angiographic demonstration of disease or diagnostic electrocardiographic changes during pain. Patients with chronic stable angina all had angiographic evidence of coronary artery disease, and none had had chest pain at rest within 14 days of blood sample collection. Patients with acute myocardial infarction and unstable angina were included only if they had had pain within 1 h of blood-sample collection.

Figure 1 is a simplified schematic diagram of the positions in the fibrinogen-fibrin cascade of the antigens measured in the study. To limit in vitro fibrinolysis, blood samples were collected in cold polystyrene tubes containing 3.8% sodium citrate and 0.025 *M* aminocaproic acid. All samples were taken with a 20-gauge needle, and no tourniquet was used. The initial 3 ml blood was used for other diagnostic tests. Blood samples were centrifuged immediately, and the plasma was stored at –70 °C until required. Serum was prepared by clotting the plasma in a mixture containing thrombin and soybean trypsin inhibitor for 4 h at 0 °C, as recommended by Merskey et al. [32]. Total serum fibrin and fibrinogen-related antigen was measured by radioimmunoassay with fibrin-derived D-dimer used as the competitive antigen and panspecific rabbit anti-human fibrinogen as the antiserum [36]. D-dimer, purified as described previously, was labelled with ^{125}I using the chloramine-T method [25].

Fibrin-related antigens (FRAs) were extracted from serum with the use of anti-human fibrinogen IgG covalently bound to activated aminophenylthioether paper disks [27]. After elution from the disk probes, the extracted antigens were subjected to 4%–11% gradient polyacrylamide gel electrophoresis. The gels were fixed and stained in a solution containing 33% methanol, 10% trichloro-acetic acid and Coomassie brilliant blue and then destained in an aqueous solution of 25% ethanol and 8% acetic acid. The proportions of the various FRAs were determined by densitometric analysis with the use of a Beckman Appraise densitometer, which automatically integrated the area under each curve. The presence of fibrin monomers and small fibrin polymers was confirmed with the ethanol gelation test [20].

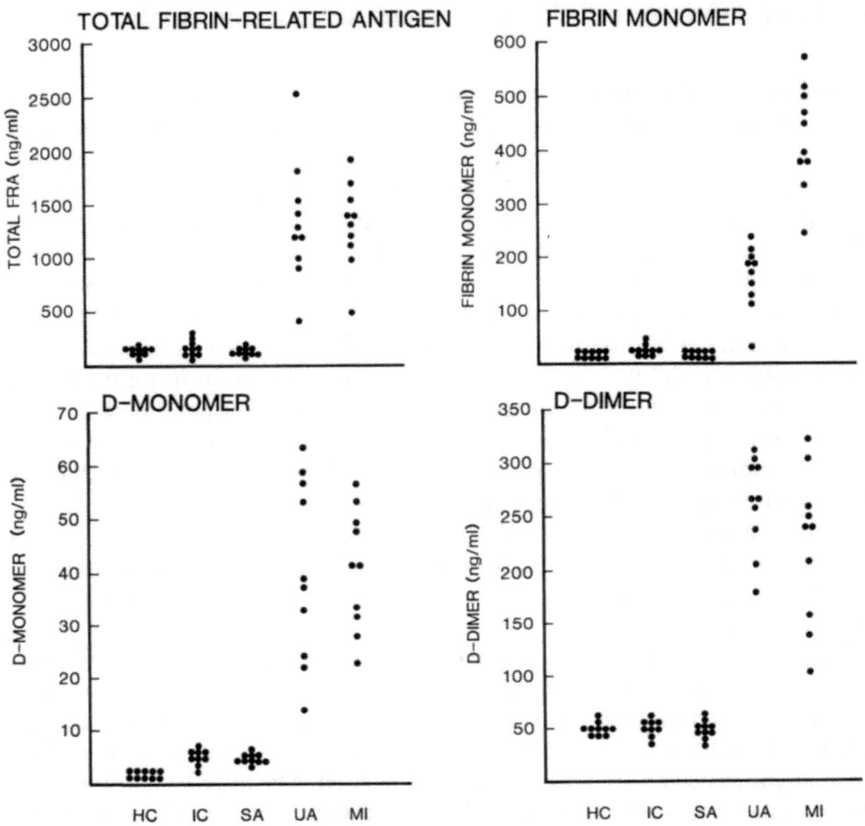

Fig. 2. Total concentrations of fibrin-related antigen, fibrin monomer, D-monomer and D-dimer in the serum of healthy controls (*HC*), controls with non-cardiac pain (*IC*), and in patients with stable angina (*SA*), unstable angina (*UA*), and acute myocardial infarction (*MI*). (Modified from [26] with permission)

Total FRA concentrations were normal in patients with chronic stable angina and those with non-cardiac pain but significantly elevated in patients with unstable angina and myocardial infarction (Fig. 2). The concentration of D-monomer, the terminal degradation fragment of fibrinogen used to distinguish fibrinogen from fibrin breakdown, was significantly higher in patients with unstable angina than controls or patients with stable angina and was in the same range as those with acute infarction. The concentration of D-dimer, which is the terminal degradation fragment of cross-linked fibrin present in serum during fibrinolysis, was in the normal range in patients with stable angina and non-cardiac acute pain but significantly elevated both in cases of unstable angina and acute infarction. Fibrin monomer is an intermediate product in the formation of cross-linked fibrin, and its presence indicates active fibrin formation. Concentrations were not elevated in patients with chronic stable angina. Patients with unstable angina had elevated concentrations of fibrin monomer, and patients with acute myocardial infarction had even higher levels (Fig. 2).

Other investigators have failed to confirm elevations of D-dimer in unstable angina and have reported that the levels were the same as in patients with stable angina pectoris [1]. They concluded that thrombus formation was important, but that the amount was too small to generate sufficient D-dimer to be detected in peripheral blood. The clinical characteristics of the patients studied may have differed from those of our patients, who all had prolonged pain at rest; samples were collected a median of 2.5 h after pain, and the assay used differed from ours. Their results differ also from those of others who have measured FPA.

Our original investigation led us to conclude that there was evidence of active thrombosis and thrombolysis in patients with unstable angina particularly when the clinical syndrome was defined as prolonged (> 15 min) pain at rest, usually associated with electrocardiographic changes, and when the observations were made within 1 h of the symptoms. The spectrum of patients considered to have unstable angina is, however, much broader than this and includes patients with typical exertional angina of recent onset and patients with a change in the severity and frequency of angina. Some patients present with a chest pain syndrome which may be angina pectoris, but in many of these clinical doubt exists, and diagnostic electrocardiographic features are not present.

Our original study showed a consistent and significant increase in total FRA concentration in patients with unstable angina. Unlike D-monomer, D-dimer and fibrin monomer, total FRA concentration can be assayed accurately and rapidly, with results being available in 5 h, using a four-layered enzyme-linked immunosorbant assay (ELISA). FRAs were captured using polyvalent goat anti-human fibrinogen IgG and measured using a monoclonal antibody, F11 (gift from EB Dowdle, Department of Clinical Science and Immunology, University of Cape Town) which recognises epitopes present on all FRAs containing the D domain of fibrinogen or fibrin. We have used the ELISA assay to measure total FRA concentration in a broader clinical spectrum of patients considered to have unstable angina.

All suitable patients admitted with a clinical diagnosis of unstable angina pectoris were treated with bed rest and soluble aspirin in a dose of 150 mg/day. None received heparin anticoagulation treatment. Nitrates, calcium channel blockers, and beta-blockers were prescribed at the discretion of the physician in charge of the patient. Blood samples were collected as soon as possible after admission and at 6-h intervals thereafter. The aim of this investigation was to confirm our earlier observations and to determine the behaviour over time of elevated FRA concentrations. Preliminary results in a small group of patients reveal two patterns. In the majority of patients (19) who presented with exercise-associated pain (either new onset or an exacerbation of a previously stable pattern) and without diagnostic changes of ischaemia on the resting electrocardiogram, the concentration of FRAs was usually well within the normal range or only slightly elevated (Fig. 3).

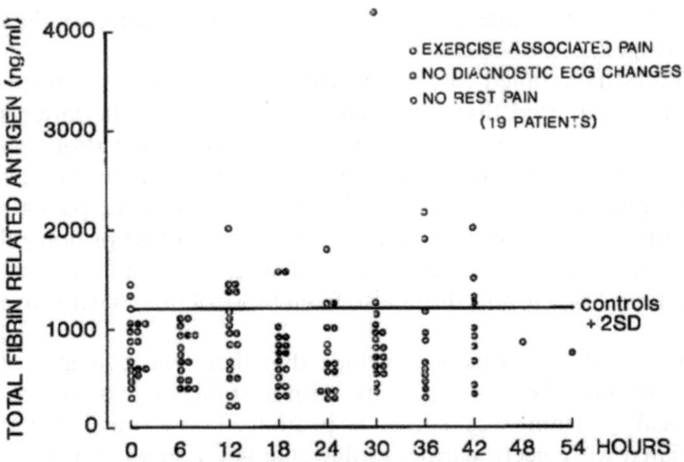

Fig. 3. Total fibrin-related antigen concentration in serum of patients with exercise-associated unstable angina. Serial samples collected 6 h after admission

Three patients who presented with chest pain considered to be angina pectoris and were subsequently shown to have angiographically normal coronary arteries had concentrations of FRAs which were within the normal range. In contrast, FRA concentrations in six patients who presented with prolonged pain at rest, or who had diagnostic ST segment and T wave changes of ischaemia were elevated at the time of admission or became elevated during the period of observation (Fig. 4).

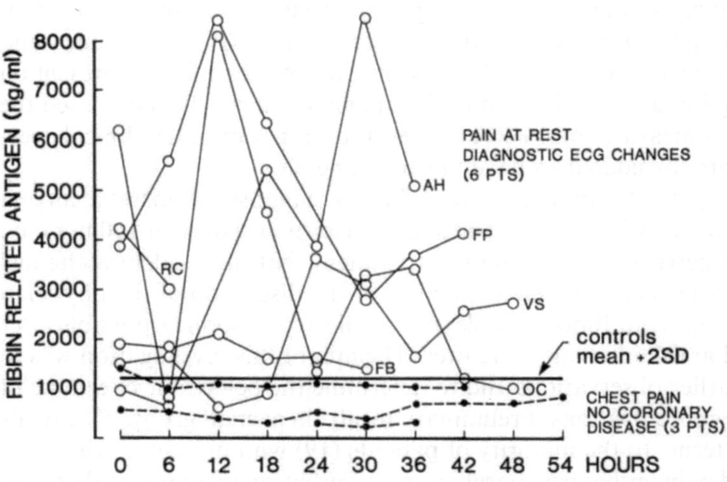

Fig. 4. Total fibrin-related antigen concentration in serum of patients with unstable angina and pain at rest with electrocardiographic changes of ischaemia (*open circles, continuous line*) and patients with chest pain and angiographically normal coronary arteries (*solid circles, broken line*). Serial samples collected 6 h after admission

These results confirm that in a subset of patients with unstable angina who have prolonged pain at rest and diagnostic electrocardiographic changes of ischaemia there is biochemical evidence of activation of the fibrinogen-fibrin cascade. While we cannot be certain that this activation is occurring specifically within the coronary circulation, such evidence has not been found in similar patients with non-cardiac chest pain and normal coronary arteries or in other patients with exercise-associated unstable angina who in all other respects have been managed identically. These results confirm our previous findings and are in accordance with those of Eisenberg et al. [13] who found the highest elevations of FPA in the subset of patients with unstable angina who had diagnostic ST segment changes at rest.

Conclusion

Coronary angiography reveals evidence of intracoronary thrombus in some patients with unstable angina pectoris, and such patients appear to be at increased risk of developing complications. There is suggestive evidence that thrombolytic therapy may be of some benefit in patients with unstable angina. The benefit at present seems small, and reports really only serve to confirm that intracoronary thrombus may have a pathophysiologic role. Biochemical studies confirm activation of the fibrinogen-fibrin cascade in a subset of patients with unstable angina. The most convincing evidence for the role of intracoronary thrombus in the pathogenesis of unstable angina comes from studies involving patients with prolonged pain at rest associated with electrocardiographic evidence of ischaemia. The evidence is most convincing when observations have been made in close temporal relationship to episodes of pain.

Given the broad clinical spectrum of unstable angina pectoris, it is hardly surprising that there is no unifying pathophysiologic explanation for the precipitation of the unstable state. At least in the subset of patients with prolonged pain at rest it seems as if intracoronary thrombus, superimposed on acutely altered coronary plaques may be responsible for abruptly reducing myocardial blood flow. If this is so, and if patients with intracoronary thrombi are at increased risk of in-hospital complications, then appropriate identification of such patients might influence the nature of therapy and the timing of interventions.

Assays such as those for FPA and for total FRA may serve non-invasively to identify patients with unstable angina in whom activation of the fibrinogen-fibrin cascade has commenced. Such identification may allow accurate pathophysiologic and clinical subclassification of the diverse syndrome of unstable angina contributing to improvements in therapy and appropriate timing of interventions.

References

1. Alexopoulos D, Stump D, Deshmukh P, Borrico S, Gorlin R, Fuster V, Ambrose JA (1989) Inability of thrombosis related markers to distinguish between unstable and stable angina pectoris. J Am Coll Cardiol 13:15A
2. Ambrose JA, Winters SL, Stern A, Eng A, Teichholz LE, Gorlin R, Fuster V (1985) Angiographic morphology and the pathogenesis of unstable angina pectoris. J Am Coll Cardiol 5:609–616
3. Ambrose JA, Winters SL, Arora RR, Haft JI, Goldstein J, Rentrop KP, Gorlin R, Fuster V (1985) Coronary angiographic morphology in myocardial infarction: a link between the pathogenesis of unstable angina and myocardial infarction. J Am Coll Cardiol 6:1233–1238
4. Ambrose JA, Winters SL, Arora RR, Eng A, Riccio A, Gorlin R, Fuster V (1986) Angiographic evolution of coronary artery morphology in unstable angina. J Am Coll Cardiol 7:472–478
5. Ambrose JA, Hjemdahl-Monsen CE, Borrico S, Sherman W, Cohen M, Gorlin R, Fuster V (1987) Quantitative and qualitative effects of intracoronary streptokinase in unstable angina and non-Q wave infarction. J Am Coll Cardiol 9:1156–1165
6. Ambrose JA, Hjemdahl-Monsen CE, Borrico S, Gorlin R, Fuster V (1988) Angiographic demonstration of a common link between unstable angina pectoris and non-Q wave acute myocardial infarction. Am J Cardiol 61:244–247
7. Bresnahan DR, Davis JL, Holmes DR, Smith HC (1985) Angiographic occurrence and clinical correlates of intraluminal coronary artery thrombus: role of unstable angina. J Am Coll Cardiol 6:285–289
8. Cairns JA, Gent M, Singer J, Finnie KJ, Froggatt GM, Holder DA, Jablonsky G, Kostuk WJ, Melendez LJ, Myers MG, Sackett DL, Sealey BJ, Tanser PH (1985) Aspirin, sulfinpyrazone, or both in unstable angina. N Engl J Med 313:1369–1375
9. Capone G, Wolf NM, Meyer B, Meister SG (1985) Frequency of intracoronary filling defects by angiography in angina pectoris at rest. Am J Cardiol 56:403–406
10. Cowley MJ, DiSciascio G, Rehr RB, Vetrovec GW (1989) Angiographic observations and relevance of coronary thrombus in unstable angina pectoris. Am J Cardiol 63:108E–113E
11. De Zwaan C, Bar FW, Janssen JHA, de Swart HB, Vermeer F, Wellens HJJ (1988) Effects of thrombolytic therapy in unstable angina: clinical and angiographic results. J Am Coll Cardiol 12:301–309
12. Eisenberg PR, Sherman LA, Schechtman K, Perez J, Sobel BE, Jaffe AS (1985) Fibrinopeptide A: a marker of acute coronary thrombosis. Circulation 71:912–918
13. Eisenberg PR, Kenzora JL, Schaab C, Jaffe AS (1989) Patients with ST segment deviation and unstable angina have consistent increases in thrombin activity. J Am Coll Cardiol 13:15A (Abstract)
14. Falk E (1985) Unstable angina with fatal outcome: dynamic coronary thrombosis leading to infarction and/or sudden death. Circulation 71:699–708
15. Falk E (1989) Morphologic features of unstable atherothrombotic plaques underlying acute coronary syndromes. Am J Cardiol 63:114E–120E
16. Freeman MR, Williams AE, Chisholm RJ, Armstrong PW (1989) Intracoronary thrombus and complex morphology in unstable angina. Relation to timing of angiography and in-hospital cardiac events. Circulation 80:17–23
17. Fuster V, Badimon L, Cohen M, Ambrose JA, Badimon JJ, Chesebro J (1988) Insights into the pathogenesis of acute ischemic syndromes. Circulation 77:1213–1220
18. Gallino A, Haeberli A, Baur HR, Straub PW (1985) Fibrin formation and platelet aggregation in patients with severe coronary artery disease: relationship with the degree of myocardial ischaemia. Circulation 72:27–30
19. Gallino A, Haeberli A, Hess T, Mombelli G, Straub PW (1986) Fibrin formation and platelet aggregation in patients with acute myocardial infarction: effects of intravenous and subcutaneous low-dose heparin. Am Heart J 112:285–290
20. Godal HC, Abildgaard U (1966) Gelation of soluble fibrin in plasma by ethanol. Scand J Haematol 3:342–350

21. Gold HK, Johns JA, Leinbach RC, Yasuda T, Grossbard E, Zusman R, Collen D (1987) A randomized, blinded, placebo-controlled trial of recombinant human tissue-type plasminogen activator in patients with unstable angina pectoris. Circulation 75:1192–1199
22. Gorlin R, Fuster V, Ambrose JA (1986) Anatomic-physiologic links between acute coronary syndromes. Circulation 74:6–9
23. Gotoh K, Minamino T, Katoh O, Hamano Y, Fukui S, Hori M, Kusuoka H, Mishima M, Inoue M, Kamada T (1988) The role of intracoronary thrombus in unstable angina: angiographic assessment and thrombolytic therapy during ongoing anginal attacks. Circulation 77:526–534
24. Holmes DR, Hartzler GO, Smith HC, Fuster V (1981) Coronary artery thrombosis in patients with unstable angina. Br Heart J 45:411–416
25. Hunter WM, Greenwood PC (1962) The preparation of iodine-131 labelled human growth hormone of high specific radioactivity. Nature 194:495–496
26. Kruskal JB, Commerford PJ, Franks JJ, Kirsch RE (1987) Fibrin and fibrinogen-related antigens in patients with stable and unstable coronary artery disease. N Engl J Med 17:1361–1365
27. Kruskal JB, Maeder DL, Purves LR, Franks JJ, Kirsch RE (1987) A diazophenylthio-ether-IgG probe for analysing fibrin- and fibrinogen-related antigens. S Afr Med J 71:211–217
28. Lawrence JR, Shepherd JT, Bone I, Rogen AS, Fulton WFM (1980) Fibrinolytic therapy in unstable angina pectoris. A controlled clinical trial. Thromb Res 17:767–777
29. Levin DC, Fallon JT (1982) Significance of the angiographic morphology of localized coronary stenoses. Circulation 66:316–320
30. Lewis HD, Davis JW, Archibald DG, Steinke WE, Smitherman TC, Doherty JE, Schnaper HW, LeWinter MM, Linares E, Pouget JM, Sabharwal SC, Chesler E, DeMots H (1983) Protective effects of aspirin against acute myocardial infarction and death in men with unstable angina. Results of a Veterans Administration cooperative study. N Engl J Med 309:396–403
31. Mandelkorn JB, Wolf NM, Singh S, Shechter JA, Kersh RI, Rodgers DM, Workman MB, Bentivoglio LG, LaPorte SM, Meister SG (1983) Intracoronary thrombus in nontransmural myocardial infarction and in unstable angina pectoris. Am J Cardiol 52:1–6
32. Merskey C, Johnson AJ, Lalezari P (1972) Increase in fibrinogen and fibrin-related antigen in human serum due to in vitro lysis of fibrin by thrombin. J Clin Invest 52:903–911
33. Mombelli G, Im Hof V, Haeberli A, Straub PW (1984) Effect of heparin on plasma fibrinopeptide A in patients with acute myocardial infarction. Circulation 69:684–689
34. Nicklas JM, Topol EJ, Kander N, O'Neill WW, Walton JA, Ellis SG, Gorman L, Pitt B (1989) Randomized, double-blind, placebo-controlled trial of tissue plasminogen activator in unstable angina. J Am Coll Cardiol 13:434–441
35. Nossel HL (1976) Radioimmunoassay of fibrinopeptides in relation to intravascular coagulation and thrombosis. N Engl J Med 295:428–432
36. Purves LR, Lindsey GG, Franks JJ (1980) Sites of D-domain interactions in fibrin derived D dimer. Biochemistry 19:4051–4058
37. Rapold HJ, Kuemmerli H, Weiss M, Baur H, Haeberli A (1989) Monitoring of fibrin generation during thrombolytic therapy of acute myocardial infarction with recombinant tissue-type plasminogen activator. Circulation 79:980–989
38. Rentrop P, Blanke H, Karsch KR, Kaiser H, Köstering H, Leitz K (1981) Selective intracoronary thrombolysis in acute myocardial infarction and unstable angina pectoris. Circulation 63:307–317
39. Serneri GGN, Gensini GF, Abbate R, Laureano R, Parodi O (1980) Is raised plasma fibrinopeptide A a marker of acute coronary insufficiency. Lancet ii:982–983
40. Serneri GGN, Gensini GF, Abbate R, Mugnaini C, Favilla S, Brunelli C, Chierchia S, Parodi O (1981) Increased fibrinopeptide A formation and thromboxane A_2 production in patients with ischemic heart disease: relationships to coronary pathoanatomy, risk factors, and clinical manifestations. Am Heart J 101:185–194
41. Sherman CT, Litvack F, Grundfest W, Lee M, Hickey A, Chaux A, Kass R, Blanche C, Matloff J, Morgenstern J, Ganz W, Swan HJC, Forrester J (1986) Coronary angioscopy in patients with unstable angina pectoris. N Engl J Med 315:913–919
42. Telford AM, Wilson C (1981) Trial of heparin versus atenolol in prevention of myocardial infarction in intermediate coronary syndrome. Lancet i:1225–1228

43. Théroux P (1987) A pathophysiologic basis for the clinical classification and management of unstable angina. Circulation 75 [Suppl V]: V103–V109
44. Théroux P, Latour J-G, Léger-Gauthier C, De Lara J (1987) Fibrinopeptide A and platelet factor levels in unstable angina pectoris. Circulation 75:156–162
45. Théroux P, Ouimet H, McCans J, Latour J-G, Joly P, Lévy G, Pelletier E, Juneau M, Stasiak J, DeGuise P, Pelletier GB, Rinzler D, Waters DD (1988) Aspirin, heparin, or both to treat acute unstable angina. N Engl J Med 319:1105–1111
46. Topol EJ, Nicklas JM, Kander NH, Walton JA, Ellis SG, Gorman L, Pitt B (1988) Coronary revascularization after intravenous tissue plasminogen activator for unstable angina pectoris: results of a randomized, double-blind, placebo-controlled trial. Am J Cardiol 62:368–371
47. Vetrovec GW, Cowley MJ, Overton H, Richardson DW (1981) Intracoronary thrombus in syndromes of unstable myocardial ischemia. Am Heart J 102:1202–1208
48. Vetrovec GW, Leinbach RC, Gold HK, Cowley MJ (1982) Intracoronary thrombolysis in syndromes of unstable ischemia: angiographic and clinical results. Am Heart J 109:946–952
49. Willerson JT, Hillis LD, Winniford MD, Buja LM (1986) Speculations regarding mechanisms responsible for acute ischaemic heart disease syndromes. J Am Coll Cardiol 8:245–250
50. Willerson JT, Golino P, Eidt J, Campbell WB, Buja LM (1989) Research on unstable coronary syndromes. Specific platelet mediators and unstable coronary artery lesions. Circulation 80:198–205
51. Williams AE, Freeman MR, Chisholm RJ, Patt NL, Armstrong PW (1988) Angiographic morphology in unstable angina pectoris. Am J Cardiol 62:1024–1027
52. Zack PM, Ischinger R, Aker UT, Dincer B, Kennedy HL (1984) The occurrence of angiographically detected intracoronary thrombus in patients with unstable angina pectoris. Am Heart J 108:1408–1412

Platelet Activation in Patients with Unstable Angina

C. W. Hamm, W. Terres, and W. Bleifeld [1]

Unstable angina has become accepted as a clinical entity of coronary heart disease associated with a high risk of myocardial infarction and sudden cardiac death [1–4]. In recent years the pathogenetic mechanisms of unstable angina have been intensively investigated with the aim of better characterizing this high-risk group of patients. Evidence is now accumulating that platelet activation plays a major role in a complex cascade of events originating in arteriosclerotic plaque rupture and resulting in occlusive thrombus formation.

Pathophysiology of Platelet Activation Following Plaque Rupture

Injury of the vascular endothelial cell monolayer is considered to be the underlying event in the initiation and progression of coronary atherosclerosis. The contact of circulating blood platelets with subendothelial collagen fibers results in adhesion of platelets to collagen and in reversible or irreversible aggregation of platelets with each other, if the proaggregatory stimulus is strong enough (Fig. 1). Irreversibly aggregated platelets release various active proteins [5–9]:

- Adenosine diphosphate (ADP) and thromboxane A_2, which activate other platelets. Thereby platelet activation is a self-perpetuating process
- Serotonin and thromboxane A_2, substances which contract vascular smooth muscle
- Platelet factor 3, which activates the intrinsic pathway of coagulation
- Platelet-derived growth factor, which stimulates the proliferation of vascular smooth-muscle cells and fibroblasts [10, 11]
- Other factors such as platelet factor 4 [12] and β-thromboglobulin [13], with up to now largely unknown physiological functions

Aggregation of platelets with each other results in the formation of the so-called primary thrombus which is still mechanically unstable. Primary thrombus formation is opposed by the intrinsic protective mechanisms of the

[1] Abteilung für Kardiologie, Medizinische Klinik, Universitätskrankenhaus Eppendorf, Martinistrasse 52, 2000 Hamburg 20, West Germany

W. Bleifeld et al. (Eds.)
Unstable Angina

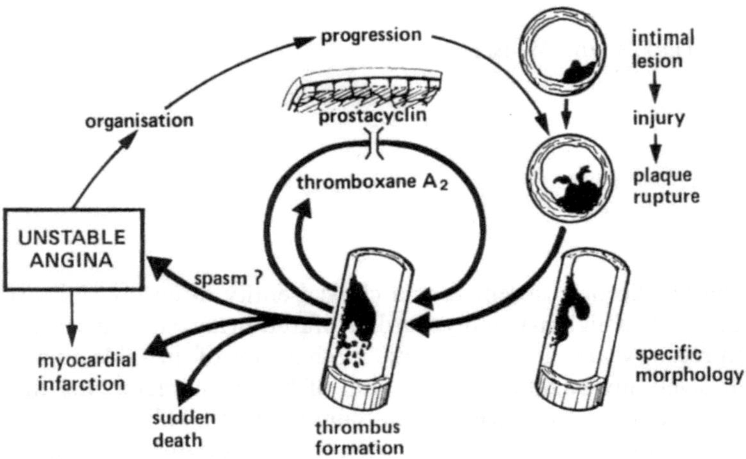

Fig. 1. Vicious circle in unstable angina

vessel wall. These mechanisms include the release of adenosine and prostacyclin from the endothelium. Prostacyclin and adenosine inhibit platelet aggregation [14], and prostacyclin was shown, in addition, to dissolve reversibly aggregated platelets [15]. They also act as vasodilators and thus may counteract the vasoconstrictive effect of the substances released from activated platelets.

While platelet activation occurs in only a few seconds, the simultaneous activation of the coagulation cascade is a process which takes some minutes. The result is the formation of thrombin, which stimulates the generation of fibrin from fibrinogen. Thrombin further promotes a close connection between aggregated platelets and fibrin by binding to platelet membrane receptors and by stimulating platelets [16]. The so-called secondary thrombus is formed by stabilization of the platelet thrombus by a fibrin network. Immigration of vascular smooth-muscle cells and fibroblasts into this secondary thrombus and their proliferation then result in persistent obstruction of the vascular lumen. Due to turbulent flow the probability of further endothelial injury is increased [17–19].

The link between coronary flow reduction and platelet deposition has been experimentally validated by Folts et al. [20]. Their observations could be confirmed in autopsies of patients with unstable angina suffering sudden cardiac ischemic death [21, 22]. Falk [21] and Davies et al. [22] found microscopic evidence of recurrent mural thrombus formation accompanied by intermittent thrombus fragmentation and embolization. According to autoptic and angiographic findings the thrombus superimposed on the ruptured plaque in myocardial infarction is most frequently occlusive [23], while in unstable angina a residual flow is usually preserved [24–27].

Although spontaneous plaque rupture is difficult to study in vivo, thrombus formation at the site of a fissured plaque (Fig. 1) generally follows the

Table 1. Platelet aggregation after induction with ADP and collagen in patients with angina pectoris at rest during the last 8 h prior to blood collection and in controls with stable exertional angina

		Angina at rest ($n = 18$)	Exertional angina ($n = 18$)
ADP	0.5 µmol/l		
	Rate of aggregation (%/min)	102±29	96±36
	Extent of aggregation (%)	44±18	37±15
	Number of irreversible aggregations	4 (22%)	2 (11%)
ADP	1 µmol/l		
	Rate of aggregation (%/min)	138±33	143±29
	Extent of aggregation (%)	65±14	60±19
	Number of irreversible aggregations	8 (44%)	9 (50%)
ADP	10 µmol/l		
	Rate of aggregation (%/min)	172±39	193±35
	Extent of aggregation (%)	82±10	82±8
	Number of irreversible aggregations	18 (100%)	18 (100%)
Collagen	1 µg/ml		
	Rate of aggregation (%/min)	100±46	118±60
	Extent of aggregation (%)	73±18	73±22
	Number of irreversible aggregations	15 (83%)	15 (83%)
Collagen	5 µg/ml		
	Rate of aggregation (%/min)	149±36	163±42
	Extent of aggregation (%)	85±10	84±7
	Number of irreversible aggregations	18 (100%)	18 (100%)

No significant differences between the groups.

same mechanisms as in experimental superficial endothelial injury. Plaque rupture results in an extended exposition of subendothelial structures such as collagen [28, 29]. This may lead to extensive activation of platelets and to the coagulation cascade. Concomitant with platelet activation local vasoconstriction occurs. Although no systemic enhancement of platelet aggregability was demonstrable in patients with unstable angina pectoris [30] (Table 1), it was suggested that the rapid formation of a large intracorconary thrombus should produce a measurable increase in the serum levels of platelet constituents or of their metabolites in urine [31].

Biochemical Markers of Platelet Activation

Considerable efforts have been made in recent years to find a biochemical marker of platelet activation in vivo. Such a marker could be very helpful to identify high-risk patients and to guide therapeutic decisions [32].

Thromboxane A_2 (TxA_2) is formed from arachidonic acid in activated platelets [33]. The estimated rate of thromboxane secretion into the circulation of normal subjects is extremely low [34]. After release in plasma there is rapid, nonenzymatic conversion of TxA_2 to thromboxane B_2 (TxB_2) which has only minor proaggregatory and vasoconstrictory effects [35, 36]. Therefore the measurement of immunoreactive TxB_2 in serum was considered to reflect in vivo TxA_2 biosynthesis [37]. However, all invasive sampling techniques were shown to be associated with considerable artificial ex vivo platelet activation [38]. This invalidates TxB_2 measurements in coronary sinus or peripheral blood samples [39–43]. Artifacts are minimized only when more stable, enzymatic metabolites of TxA_2, such as 11-dehydro-TxB_2, are determined [44, 45]. The alternative is to measure breakdown products of TxA_2 in urine. TxB_2 is found in urine but largely reflects renal TxA_2 generation under physiologic conditions [46]. In vivo platelet activation, however, is accurately estimated from the urinary excretion of 2,3-dinor TxB_2 (Tx-M) [47, 48].

Measurements of circulating platelet granule constituents, such as β-thromboglobulin and platelet factor 4, are subject to similar ex vivo platelet activation as arachidonic acid metabolites [13, 39, 40, 49–51]. The artifactual elevation of these substances has been shown [38, 52].

The natural antagonist to the effects of TxA_2 with respect to platelet aggregation and vasoconstriction is prostacyclin (PGI_2) which is released from endothelium [53–55]. The unstimulated excretion rate of PGI_2 into the circulation of human volunteers is extremely low [47]. In addition, PGI_2 is rapidly and nonenzymatically broken down to 6-keto-prostaglandin $F_{1\alpha}$, which is more stable than the parent compound [47]. Blood samples are commonly obtained by insertion of needles or catheters into vessels, a procedure that itself is most likely to traumatically stimulate PGI_2 synthesis [56]. Further artifacts may be induced by the use of radiocontrast medium [56]. To circumvent the problems of artifactual prostacyclin formation induced by blood sampling, the stable breakdown product 2,3-dinor-6-keto-prostaglandin $F_{1\alpha}$ (PGI-M) is measured in urine [57]. PGI-M excretion reflects accurately plasma levels of endogenous PGI_2 [58].

The analysis of arachidonic acid metabolites in urine has certain inherent limitations. The excretion of circulating prostanoids depends on intact renal function. Severe peripheral vascular disease such as in diabetes [59] or septicemia may stimulate prostanoid metabolism and thereby restrict measurements in myocardial ischemic syndromes. The use of nonsteroid anti-inflammatory drugs over a 2-week period also invalidates measurements due to cyclo-oxygenase inhibition [60, 61].

In conclusion, the measurement of urinary Tx-M and PGI-M represents a noninvasive and artifact-free approach to quantify endogenous PGI_2 and TxA_2 synthesis. Published data based on serum sampling have seriously been questioned [47]. The following evaluation therefore considers only results obtained in urinary samples.

Thromboxane and Prostacyclin Metabolites in Patients with Unstable Angina

Reliable evidence of platelet activation in patients with unstable angina was provided by studies of FitzGerald et al. [62] and Hamm et al. [63].

FitzGerald et al. measured the stable urinary metabolites Tx-M and PGI-M as well as serum 11-dehydro-TxB_2 in patients with various ischemic syndromes [62]. In patients with stable coronary artery disease the urinary levels of Tx-M and PGI-M were normal at rest and were not altered by exercise-induced myocardial ischemia. The largest increase of thromboxane synthesis was observed in 16 patients with unstable angina, in whom 84% of the episodes of chest pain were associated with phasic rises in the excretion of thromboxane metabolites. However, 50% of such increases occurred in the absence of chest pain, and 16% of the painful episodes were not associated with any alteration in the excretion of Tx-M. A rise in Tx-M excretion was frequently accompanied by a modest increase in PGI-M.

The study of Hamm et al. [63] confirmed and extended the biochemical studies using the same urinary metabolites in 24 patients with unstable angina

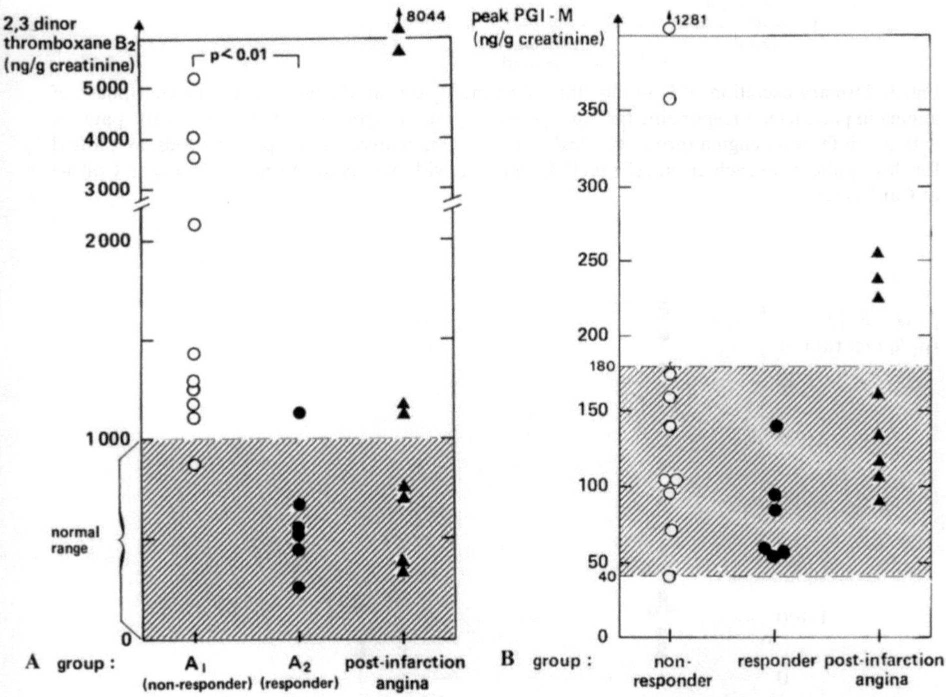

Fig. 2. Urinary excretion of 2,3-dinor-thromboxane B_2 (*TX-M*) (**A**) and 2,3-dinor-6-keto-prostaglandin $F_{1\alpha}$ (*PGI-M*) (**B**) in 16 patients with unstable angina resistant to medical treatment (group A_1) or responding to therapy (group A_2) and in 6 patients with sustained postinfarction angina (group B). Peaks of three consecutive 8-h sampling periods are plotted. (From [63] reprinted with permission from the American College of Cardiology)

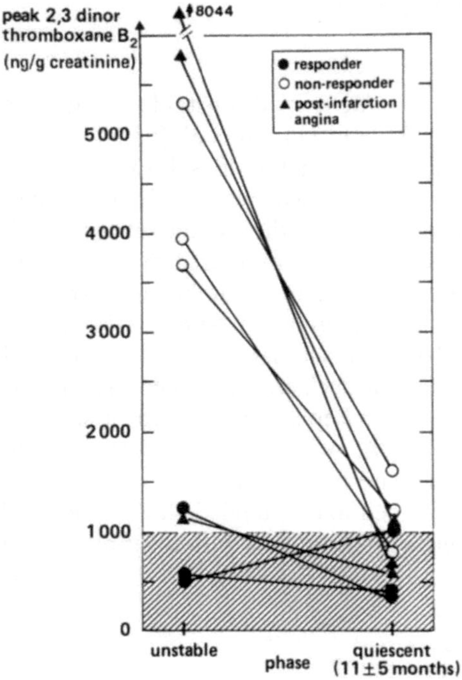

Fig. 3. Urinary excretion of 2,3-dinor-thromboxane B_2 during the acute and quiescent phase of angina in patients not responding (group A_1) and responding (group A_2) to treatment and patients with postinfarction angina (group B). Peaks of three consecutive 8-h sampling periods are plotted for three patients in each group. (From [63] reprinted with permission from the American College of Cardiology)

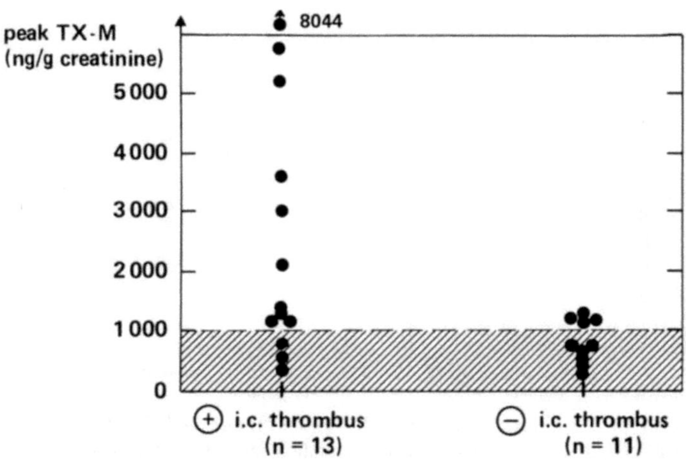

Fig. 4. Excretion of 2,3-dinor-thromboxane B_2 (*TX-M*) and angiographic evidence of intracoronary (*i.c.*) thrombus formation in 24 patients. (From [63] reprinted with permission from the American College of Cardiology)

who all underwent coronary angiography. Nine of ten patients whose condition could not be stabilized during therapy with heparin and antianginal agents including intravenous nitroglycerin for more than 48 h had elevated Tx-M levels compared with one of six patients who could be stabilized (Fig. 2). Elevated values were also found in four of eight patients with sustained postinfarction angina. Enhanced thromboxane synthesis was frequently associated with angiographic evidence of intracoronary thrombus formation (Fig. 3). Excretion of PGI-M (Fig. 2) was not depressed in any patient but correlated weakly with Tx-M ($r = 0.41$). When nine patients were restudied in a stable phase after 11 ± 5 months, Tx-M excretion had returned to normal or high normal levels (Fig. 4).

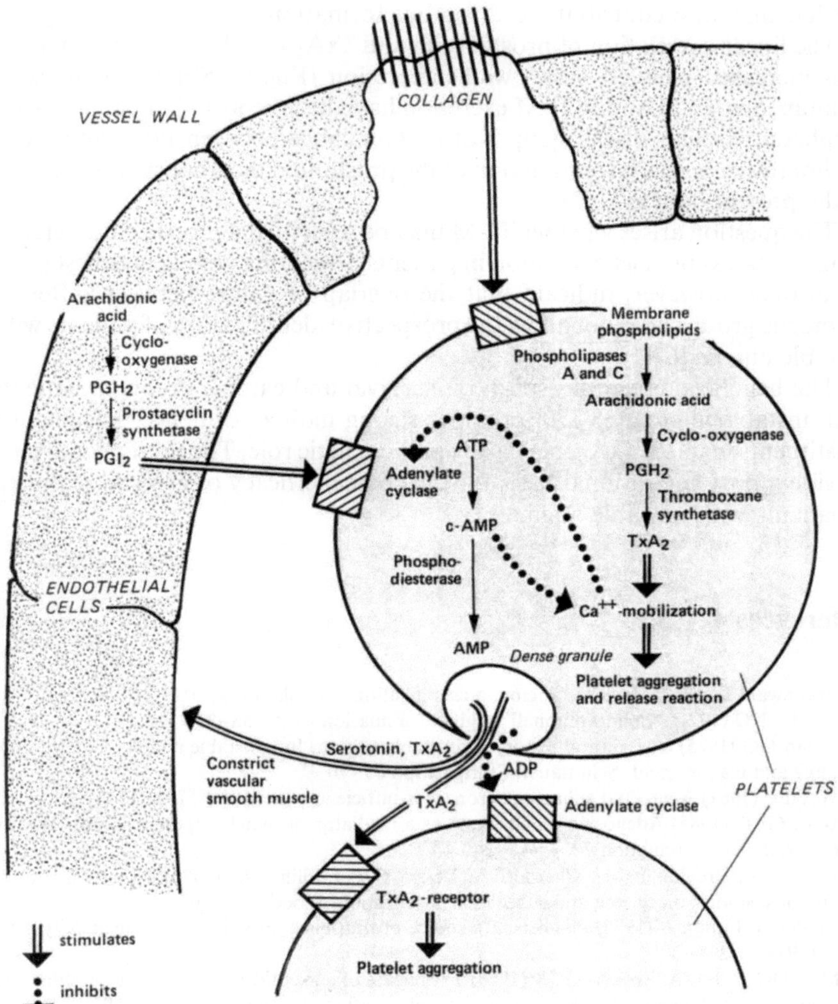

Fig. 5. Platelet–vessel wall interaction

Conclusion and Perspectives

Increased excretion of thromboxane metabolites documented in two independent studies by reliable analytical methods confirmed periodic platelet activation in patients with unstable angina. Consistently elevated levels of Tx-M were found in patients with angina resistant to medical therapy, which is the most severe form of unstable angina [1] associated with a poor prognosis [64]. However, in the chain of events originating from plaque rupture and subsequent exposure of subintimal thrombogenic material [28, 31], thromboxane may represent only one amplification factor inducing and sustaining platelet activation and aggregation. Substances such as adenosine diphosphate, platelet-activating factor, serotonin, and others released from activated platelets may also contribute to thrombus formation and vasoreaction [65].

The linear correlation of prostacyclin and TxA_2 metabolite excretion indicates increased platelet–vessel wall interaction (Fig. 5). Similar findings of simultaneous Tx-M and PGI-M excretion have been reported in patients with peripheral vascular disease [59]. Not an imbalance between PGI_2 and TxA_2 [66] but rather a general stimulation of the prostanoid metabolism is suggested by the present data [59, 63].

The question arises whether Tx-M may be a useful diagnostic parameter to routinely assess platelet activation in patients presenting with acute chest pain. Initial data, however, indicate that the overlap of values between different diagnostic groups does not allow the prospective identification of patients with unstable angina [67].

The beneficial effect of aspirin on survival and cardiac events in patients with unstable angina [68–70] provides strong indirect evidence that platelet constituents, namely TxA_2, play a key pathogenetic role. The present data may provide a post hoc rational basis for the clinical efficacy of aspirin treatment in patients with unstable angina.

References

1. Braunwald E (1989) Unstable angina, a classification. Circulation 80:410–414
2. Fowler NO (1971) "Preinfarctional" angina. Circulation 44, 5:755–758
3. Julian DG (1985) The natural history of unstable angina. In: Unstable angina. Current concepts and management. Schattauer, Stuttgart, pp 65–70
4. Wood P (1961) Acute and subacute coronary insufficiency. Br Med J 1779–1782
5. Born GVR (1985) Adenosine diphosphate as a mediator of platelet aggregation in vivo: an editorial view. Circulation 72, 4:741–746
6. Kaplan K, Broekman MJ, Chernoff A, Leszni GR, Drillings M (1979) Platelet a-granule proteins: studies on release and subcellular localization. Blood 53, 4:604–618
7. Kohler N, Lipton A (1974) Platelets as a source of fibroblast growth-promoting activity. Exp Cell Res 87:297–301
8. Mills DC, Robb JA, Roberts GCK (1968) The release of nucleotides, 5-hydroxytryptomine and enzymes from human blood platelets during aggregation. J Physiol 195:715–729

9. Needleman P, Moncada S, Bunting S, Vane JR, Hamberg M, Samuelsson B (1976) Identification of an enzyme in platelet microsomes which generates thromboxane A_2 from prostaglandin endoperoxides. Nature 261:558
10. Libby P, Warner St, Salomon R, Birinyi L (1988) Production of platelet-derived growth factor-like mitogen by smooth-muscle cells from human atheroma. N Engl J Med 318, 23:1493–1498
11. Ross R, Glomset J, Kariya B, Harker L (1974) A platelet-dependent serum factor that stimulates the proliferation of arterial smooth muscle cells in vitro. Proc Natl Acad Sci USA 71, 4:1207–1210
12. Cazenave JP, Benveniste J, Mustard JF (1979) Aggregation of rabbit platelets by platelet-activating factor is independent of the release reaction and the arachidonate pathway and inhibited by membrane-active drugs. Lab Invest 41, 3:275–285
13. Kaplan KL, Owen J (1981) Plasma levels of β-thromboglobulin and platelet factor 4 as indices of platelet activation in vivo. Blood 57, 2:199–202
14. Moncada S, Gryglewski R, Bunting S, Vane JR (1976) An enzyme isolated from arteries transforms prostaglandin endo-peroxides to an unstable substance that inhibits platelet aggregation. Nature 263:663
15. Kinlough-Rathbone RL, Mustard JF, Perry DW, Dejana E, Cazenave JP, Packham MA, Harfenist EJ (1983) Factors influencing the deaggregation of human and rabbit platelets. Thromb Haemostas 49, 3:162–167
16. Shattil SJ, Bennett JS (1980) Platelet and their membranes in hemostasis: physiology and pathophysiology. Ann Int Med 94:108–118
17. Adams PH, Fuster V, Badimon L, Badimon JJ, Chesebro J (1987) Platelet/vessel wall interactions, rheologic factors and thrombogenic substrate in acute coronary syndromes: preventive strategies. Am J Cardiol 60:9G–16G
18. Kramer C, Gerhardt HJ, Bleifeld W (1974) A model for closure of arterial vessels with special regard to the coronary arteries. Bas Res Cardiol 69:585–596
19. Wurzinger L, Blasberg P, Schmid-Schönbein H (1984) Rheologische Betrachtung der Abscheidungsthrombose. VASA 13:305–310
20. Folts JD, Crowell EB, Rowe GG (1976) Platelet aggregation in partially obstructed vessels and its elimination with aspirin. Circulation 54:365–370
21. Falk E (1985) Unstable angina with fatal outcome: dynamic coronary thrombosis leading to infarction and/or sudden death. Circulation 71:699–708
22. Davies MJ, Thomas AC (1985) Plaque fissuring – the cause of acute myocardial infarction, sudden ischaemic death, and crescendo angina. Br Heart J 534:363–373
23. The TIMI Study Group (1985) The thrombolysis in myocardial infarction (TIMI) trial. Phase I findings. N Engl J Med 312:932–936
24. Alison HW, Russell RO, Mantle JA, Kouchoukos N, Moraski RE, Rackley GH (1978) Coronary anatomy and arteriography in patients with unstable angina pectoris. Am J Cardiol 41:204–209
25. Neill WA, Ritzmann LW, Selden R (1977) The pathophysiologic basis of acute coronary insufficiency. Observations favoring the hypothesis of intermittent reversible coronary obstruction. Am Heart J 94:439–444
26. Ambrose JA, Hjemdahl-Monsen CE, Borrico S, Gorlin R, Fuster V (1988) Angiographic demonstration of a common link between unstable angina pectoris and non-Q-wave acute myocardial infarction. Am J Cardiol 61:244–247
27. Nellessen U, Hecker H, Danciu V, Specht S, Lichtlen PR, Borst HG (1986) Instabile Angina pectoris: Krankheitsbild und Verlauf neu überprüft. Z Kardiol 75:707–718
28. Fuster V, Badimon L, Cohen M, Ambrose J, Badimon JJ, Chesebro J (1988) Insights into the pathogenesis of acute ischemic syndromes. Circulation 77:1213–1220
29. Vermylen J, Verstraete M, Fuster V (1986) Role of platelet activation and fibrin formation in thrombogenesis. J Am Coll Cardiol 8:2B–9B
30. Terres W, Hamm CW, Kupper W, Bleifeld W (1988) Thrombozytenfunktion bei instabiler Angina pectoris. Dtsch Med Wschr 113:1182–1186
31. Chesebro JH, Fuster V (1987) The therapeutic challenge of plaque rupture: value of biochemical markers. J Am Coll Cardiol 10:1005–1006

32. Hamm CW, Bleifeld W (1988) Unstable angina; current concepts of medical management. Cardiovasc Drugs Therapy 2:333–339
33. Granström E, Diczfalusy U, Hamberg M, Hansson G, Malmsten C, Samuelsson B (1982) Thromboxane A_2: biosynthesis and effects on platelets. Prostaglandins and the Cardiovascular System 15–59
34. Patrono C, Ciabattoni G, Pugliese F, Perucci A, Blair IA, FitzGerald GA (1986) Estimated rate of thromboxane secretion into the circulation of normal humans. J Clin Invest 77:1–6
35. Roberts JL, Brash AR, Oates JA (1982) Metabolic fate of thromboxane A_2 and prostacyclin. Prostaglandins and the Cardiovascular System 213–223
36. Oates JA, FitzGerald GA, Branch RA, Jackson EK, Knapp HR, Roberts LJ (1988) Clinical implications of prostaglandin and thromboxane A_2 formation. New Engl J Med 319:689–698
37. Roberts JL, Sweetman BJ, Oates JA (1981) Metabolism of thromboxane B_2 in man. Identification of twenty urinary metabolites. J Biol Chem 256:8384–8393
38. Nichols AB, Owen J, Grossman BA, Marcella JJ, Fleisher LN, Lee MML (1984) Effect of heparin bonding on catheter induced fibrin formation and platelet activation. Circulation 70:843–850
39. Sobel M, Salzman EW, Davies GC, Handin RI, Sweeney RN, Ploetz J, Kurland G (1981) Circulating platelet products in unstable angina pectoris. Circulation 63:300–306
40. De Boer AC, Turpie AG, Butt RW, Johnston RV, Genton E (1982) Platelet release and thromboxane synthesis in symptomatic coronary artery disease. Circulation 66:327–333
41. Hirsch PD, Hillis D, Campbell WB, Firth BG, Willerson JT (1981) Release of prostaglandins and thromboxane into the coronary circulation in patients with ischemic heart disease. N Engl J Med 304:685–691
42. Mehta J, Mehta P, Feldman R, Horalek C (1984) Thromboxane release in coronary artery disease: spontaneous versus pacing-induced angina. Am Heart J 107:286–292
43. Neri Serneri GG, Gensini GF, Abbate R, Prisco D, Rogasi PG, Laureano R, Casolo GC, Fantini F, Donato MD, Dabizzi RP (1985) Abnormal cardiocoronary thromboxane A_2 production in patients with unstable angina. Am Heart J 109:732–738
44. Lawson JA, Patrono C, Ciabattoni G, FitzGerald GA (1986) Long-lived enzymatic metabolites of thromboxane B_2 in the human circulation. Analyt Biochem 155:198–205
45. Westlund P, Kumlin M, Nordenström A, Granström E (1986) Circulating and urinary thromboxane B_2 metabolites in the rabbit: 11-dehydro-thromboxane B_2 as parameter of thromboxane production. Prostaglandins 31:413–444
46. Patrono C, Ciabattoni G, Patrignani P, Filabozzi P, Pinca E, Satta MA, Van Dorne D, Cinotti GA, Pugliese F, Pierucci A, Simonetti BM (1983) Evidence for a renal origin of urinary thromboxane B_2 in health and disease. Adv Prostaglandin, Thromboxane, Leukotriene Res 11:493–498
47. FitzGerald GA, Pedersen AK, Patrono C (1983) Analysis of prostacyclin and thromboxane biosynthesis in cardiovascular disease. Circulation 67:1174–1177
48. Siess W, Lorenz R, Roth P, Weber PC (1982) Plasma catecholamines, platelet aggregation and associated thromboxane formation after physical exercise, smoking or norepinephrine infusion. Circulation 66:44–48
49. Gallino A, Haeberli A, Baur HR, Straub PW (1985) Fibrin formation and platelet aggregation in patients with severe coronary artery disease: relationship with the degree of myocardial ischemia. Circulation 72:27–30
50. Théroux P, Latour JG, Léger-Gauthier C, De Lara J (1987) Fibrinopeptide A and platelet factor levels in unstable angina pectoris. Circulation 5:156–162
51. Smitherman T, Milam M, Woo J, Willerson JT, Frenkel EP (1981) Elevated beta thromboglobulin in peripheral venous blood of patients with acute mocardial ischemia: Direct evidence for enhanced platelet reactivity in vivo. Am J Cardiol 48:395–402
52. Bugiardini R, Chierchia S, Crea F, Gallino A, Wild ST, Roskove A, Lenzi S, Maseri A (1984) Evaluation of the effects of catheter sampling for the study of platelet behavior in the pulmonary and coronary circulation. Am Heart J 108:255–260
53. Dusting GJ, Moncada S, Vane JR (1979) Prostaglandins, their intermediates and precursors: cardiovascular actions and regulatory roles in normal and abnormal circulatory systems. Prog Cardiovasc Dis 21:405–430

54. Weksler B (1984) Prostaglandins and vascular function. Circulation 70 (Suppl III):63–71
55. Needelmann P, Kaley G (1978) Cardiac and coronary prostaglandin synthesis and function. N Engl J Med 298:1122–1128
56. Roy L, Knapp HR, Robertson RM, FitzGerald GA (1985) Endogenous biosynthesis of prostacyclin during cardiac catheterization and angiography in man. Circulation 71:434–440
57. Falardeau P, Oates A, Brash AR (1981) Quantitative analysis of two dinor urinary metabolites of prostaglandin I_2. Analyt Biochem 115:359–367
58. Fischer S, Scherer B, Weber PC (1983) Prostacyclin metabolism in adults and neonates. Urinary profiles of 6-ketoprostaglandin $F_{1\alpha}$ and 2,3-dinor-6-ketoprostaglandin $F_{1\alpha}$ studied by gas chromatography – mass spectrometry. Biochim Biophys Acta 750:127–133
59. FitzGerald GA, Smith B, Pedersen AK, Brash A (1984) Increased prostacyclin biosynthesis in patients with severe atherosclerosis and platelet activation. New Engl J Med 310:1065–1068
60. FitzGerald GA, Reilly IA, Pedersen AK (1985) The biochemical pharmacology of thromboxane synthetase inhibition in man. Circulation 72:1194–1201
61. Patrono C, Ciabattoni G, Patrignani P, Pugliese F, Filabozzi P, Catella F, Davi G, Forni L (1985) Clinical pharmacology of platelet cyclooxygenase inhibition. Circulation 72:1177–1184
62. Fitzgerald DJ, Roy L, Catella F, FitzGerald GA (1986) Platelet activation in unstable coronary disease. New Engl J Med 315:983–989
63. Hamm CW, Lorenz R, Bleifeld W, Kupper W, Wober W, Weber PC (1987) Biochemical evidence of platelet activation in patients with persistent unstable angina. J Am Coll Cardiol 10:998–1004
64. Gazes PC, Mobley EM, Faris HM, Duncan RC, Humphries GB (1973) Preinfarction (unstable) angina – a prospective study – ten year follow-up. Circulation 48:331–337
65. Hook BG, Schumacher WA, Lee DL, Jolly StR, Lucchesi BR (1985) Experimental coronary artery thrombosis in the absence of thromboxane A_2 synthesis: evidence for alternate pathways for coronary thrombosis. J Cardiovasc Pharmacol 7:174–181
66. Bunting S, Monada S, Vane JR (1983) The prostacyclin-thromboxane A_2 balance: pathophysiological and therapeutic implications. British Med Bull 39:271–276
67. Lorenz R, Hamm CW, Riesner H, Bleifeld W, Weber PC (1990) Urinary thromboxane excretion in patients presenting with acute severe chest pain. J Int Med
68. Cairns JA, Gent M, Singer J, Finnie KJ, Froggatt GM, Holder DA, Hablonsky G, Kostuk WJ, Melendez LJ, Myers MG, Sackett DL, Sealey JB, Tanser PH (1985) Aspirin, sulfinpyrazone, or both in unstable angina. N Engl J Med 313:1369–1375
69. Lewis HD, Davies JW, Archibald DG, Steinke WE, Smithermann TC, Doherty JE, Schnaper HW, Le Winter MM, Linares E, Pouget JM, Sabharwal SC, Chesler E, DeMots H (1983) Protective effects of aspirin against acute myocardial infarction and death in men with unstable angina. N Engl J Med 309:396–403
70. Théroux P, Ouimet H, McCans J, Latour JG, Joly P, Lévy G, Pelletier E, Juneau M, Stasiak J, DeGuise P, Pelletier GB, Rinzler D, Waters DD (1988) Aspirin, heparin, or both to treat acute unstable angina. New Engl J Med 319:1105–1111

Detection of Myocardial Cell Damage in Patients with Unstable Angina by Serodiagnostic Tools

H.A. KATUS and W. KÜBLER [1]

Introduction

Patients with unstable angina represent a heterogeneous group. While in some patients no coronary artery disease is present, in others one finds severe coronary artery narrowing that leads to rather severe myocardial ischemia. In the latter subgroup of patients a release of myocardial cell constituents can be expected due to ischemic cell damage. Diagnostic tools of high sensitivity and specificity must be employed for its detection. This chapter therefore begins with a discussion of the determinants of diagnostic efficacy in serological tests.

Sensitive Detection of Myocardial Cell Damage by Serological Techniques

Table 1 presents schematically the characteristics of marker proteins in myocardium and circulation. A suitable marker protein should be present in the myocardium in high concentrations to allow the detection of even small areas of damage. Following the loss of membrane integrity most of the protein should arrive unaltered in the serum, i.e., the serum entry ratio should be high. To achieve a high sensitivity no marker protein should be detected in the serum compartment under normal conditions. If marker protein levels are present under normal conditions, a serum value must be defined that discriminates between the normal and the pathologically elevated. Due to individual variability in normal serum levels, this discriminating value must always be a compromise between sensitivity and specificity. As a consequence, minor elevations of marker protein in serum may not signify myocardial necrosis since they can be expected to be in the normal range of variance.

However, it is not only the intracellular concentration of a marker protein and its serum entry ratio but much more its intracellular compartmentation and its release kinetics that greatly contribute to the diagnostic sensitivity of a serological test. Ongoing release of a marker protein from infarcting

[1] Abteilung Innere Medizin III, Klinikum der Universität, Bergheimer Strasse 58, 6900 Heidelberg 1, West Germany

W. Bleifeld et al. (Eds.)
Unstable Angina

Table 1. Determinants of diagnostic efficacy in serological tests

Myocardium	
	Concentrations and serum entry ratio
	Compartmentation and release kinetics
	Tissue specificity
Circulation	
	Normal serum concentrations
	Elimination rate
In vitro assay	
	Sensitivity
	Specificity
	Accuracy

myocardium for a longer period of time results in an extended period of elevated marker protein levels in serum. Moreover, a low elimination rate of the marker protein from serum further increases the likelihood of a positive test result after an ischemic attack. Mainly for the detection of minor myocardial cell necrosis antigens unique to myocardium, i.e., cardiospecific marker proteins, must to measured. The sensitivity of the test system can be further improved if the protein concentration itself is measured, rather than its biological activity.

Immunological techniques such as radioimmunoassays and enzyme immunoassays are particularly useful for the detection of trace amounts of antigens. In these test systems high specificity can be achieved by the application of preselected monoclonal antibodies. The test system itself must be manufactured so as to yield an accurate, reproducible test result with essentially no unspecific interaction by any other serum proteins.

If the cardiac enzymes creatine kinase (CK) and lactate dehydrogenase are tested according to these criteria, it is quite obvious that these molecules are by no means ideal markers for the detection of myocardial cell necrosis especially if small areas are affected. Even the measurement of MBCK, which greatly improved diagnostic efficacy of enzyme measurements over that of total CK [8], suffers serious limitations: MBCK is not absolutely cardiospecific [13], following an ischemic episode elevated serum levels are only found for a brief period [7], and most importantly the normal serum levels are quite variable.

In spite of all limitations several groups of investigators were able to identify a subgroup of patients with unstable angina by means of increased serum levels of CK or MBCK. These patients with unstable angina and elevated cardiac enzymes had a worse prognosis [1, 3, 25]. Similar findings were reported in patients with suspected myocardial infarction. Those patients showing normal electrocardiogram and total CK activity but significantly elevated MBCK levels had a risk comparable to most patients with acute Q-wave infarction [12, 29]. These data suggest release of myocardial cell constituents in some patients with unstable angina or suspected myocardial infarction.

To allow more efficient serodiagnosis even of minor myocardial cell damage, marker proteins with higher sensitivity and specificity than that of cardiac enzymes should be applied. The specific contractile behavior of cardiac muscle is caused partly by multiple isoform expression of the contractile proteins myosin and actin and the regulative proteins tropomyosin and troponin complex [11, 22, 30]. The skeletal and cardiospecific isoforms of these proteins can be differentiated by immunological techniques. This is illustrated in Fig. 1, where a cryostat section of a mixed skeletal muscle is incubated with a monoclonal antibody specific for the slow isoform of myosin. In the immunohistochemical reaction only myocytes containing slow myosin are stained.

Among the proteins of the contractile apparatus, troponin T, troponin I, and myosin light chains appear to be distinct cardiac antigens [4, 15, 18]. The isoforms of these proteins can be differentiated by monoclonal antibodies, which therefore can be used to develop cardiospecific tests. So far, specific enzyme immunoassays have been developed for troponin I and T with essentially no cross-reactivity with their skeletal isoforms.

Not only high cardiospecificity but also increased sensitivity must be expected from measurements of circulating contractile proteins. These are major constituents of cardiac tissue, and for myosin light chains and cardiac troponin T it could be shown, that they are not detectable in the serum of normal humans [16, 18]. Following loss of membrane integrity, the first event is the release of cytosolic constituents such as CK, together with the minor pool of unbound proteins of the contractile apparatus. Most of the contractile proteins, which are located in the myofilaments, are released only after severe acidosis or after activation of proteolytic lysosomal enzymes [2, 28]. This degradation process of myofilaments leading to the release of contractile proteins persists during evolution of the infarct. As a consequence, characteristic serum concentrations of contractile marker proteins are found in acute myocardial infarction [16, 19]. This is shown in Fig. 2, which presents the median serum concentrations of myosin light chains and troponin T and median CK activity in patients with Q-wave infarction. Myosin light chains are released continuously from insoluble myosin during the infarcting process, leading to persistently elevated serum levels. The kinetics of troponin T release is intermediate between that of myosin light chains and that of CK activity. Troponin T serum levels show not only the initial release characteristic for cytosolic proteins but also the ongoing release of compartmented proteins. This prolonged period of release of the contractile proteins troponin T and myosin light chains and the absence of these marker proteins in normal serum allow the detection even of minor myocardial cell necrosis.

According to the data of our group myosin light chains were found elevated in more than half of the patients with unstable angina [17]. Similar data were obtained for troponin T, which was detectable at least twice in 32% and at least once in 49% of patients with unstable angina. In fewer than 50% of these patients, however, total CK activity and/or myoglobin was found to be

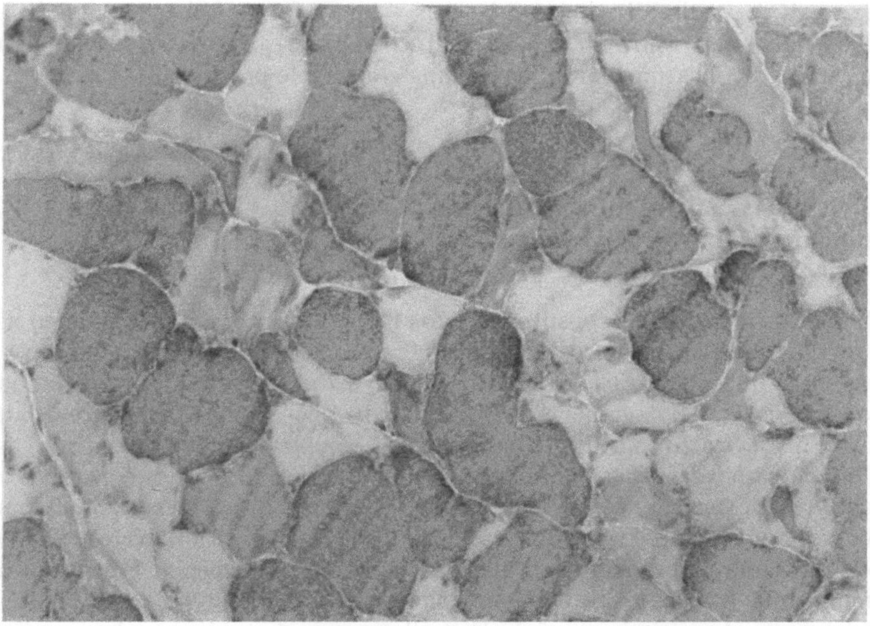

Fig. 1. Immunohistochemical staining of slow fibers of a mixed skeletal muscle. The tissue section was incubated with a monoclonal antibody specific for the slow myosin heavy chain isoform

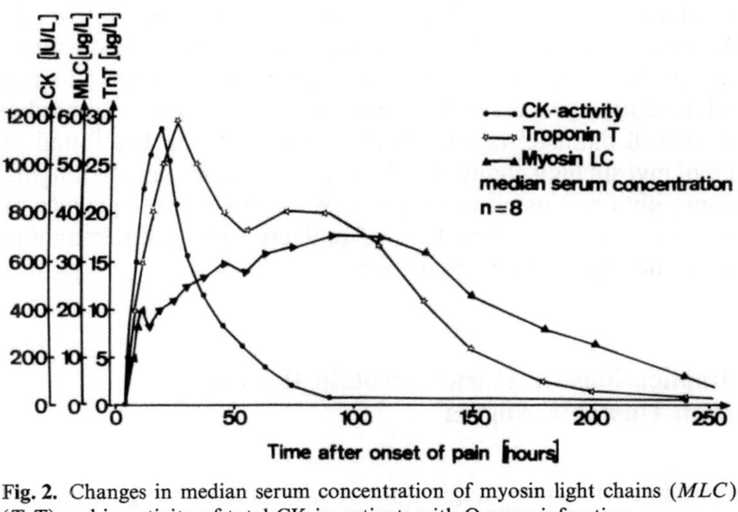

Fig. 2. Changes in median serum concentration of myosin light chains (*MLC*) and troponin T (*TnT*) and in activity of total CK in patients with Q-wave infarction

elevated above the discriminating serum value of 750 IU/l or 80 μg/l [10]. These data clearly show that myocardial cell damage can be detected with high sensitivity by measurement of circulating contractile proteins.

Does Marker Protein Release in Patients with Unstable Angina Indicate Cell Necrosis?

Release of intracellular constituents from myocytes is commonly regarded as a sign of irreversible myocardial cell damage, i.e., necrosis. This view, however, has been questioned. Using isolated myocytes in tissue culture Piper and coworkers [23, 24] documented release of cytosolic proteins from anoxic but viable myocytes. In contrast, for subcellularly compartmented proteins such as glutamate dehydrogenase no release could be found. More indirect evidence for cytosolic enzyme release from reversibly damaged myocytes comes from the work of Heyndricks and coworkers [9]. They observed a complete recovery of local contractile function in dogs after 30 min of ischemia in spite of a significant CK release. Histological examination of the hearts of these animals did not reveal any evidence of cardiac cell necrosis. According to these experimental findings, circulating cytosolic CK activity in patients with unstable angina must be assumed to originate at least partially from reversibly damaged myocytes. In these patients, therefore, increased serum levels of CK activity do not necessarily indicate myocardial cell necrosis.

Continuous elevation of contractile proteins in serum must result from the ongoing breakdown of myofilaments and cannot be attributed to a slow serum elimination rate, as their serum half-life ranges only between 75 and 120 min. This ongoing degradation process of the contractile apparatus can be used as a clinical sign for cell damage, i.e., necrosis. Our own group has found an ongoing release of myosin light chains in 27% of patients with unstable angina. Similar data were obtained using troponin T. With this marker protein biphasic release kinetics was found in 17% of patients with unstable angina, either of the crescendo type or angina at rest.

Prognostic Implications of Marker Protein Release in Patients with Unstable Angina

Compared to patients with stable angina, those with unstable angina have an increased risk of myocardial infarction and death [6, 20]. Therefore among these patients a high-risk subgroup may be identified. Several parameters, such as persisting anginal pain [21, 27], ST-segment and T-wave changes on the electrocardiogram [14, 26], elevations of cardiac enzymes [1, 3, 25], and positive scintiscans [5] have been used for identification of this high-risk subgroup.

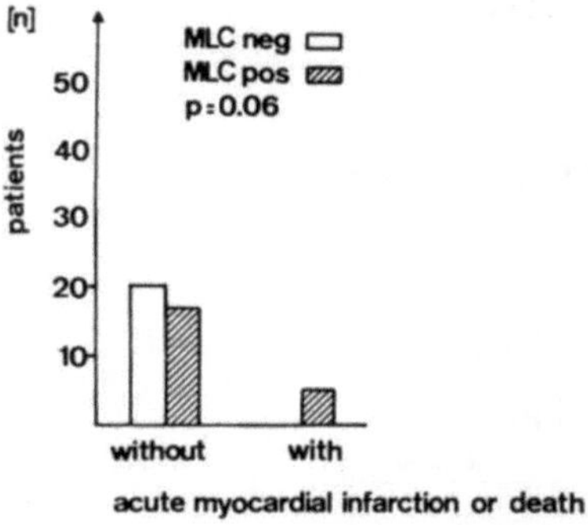

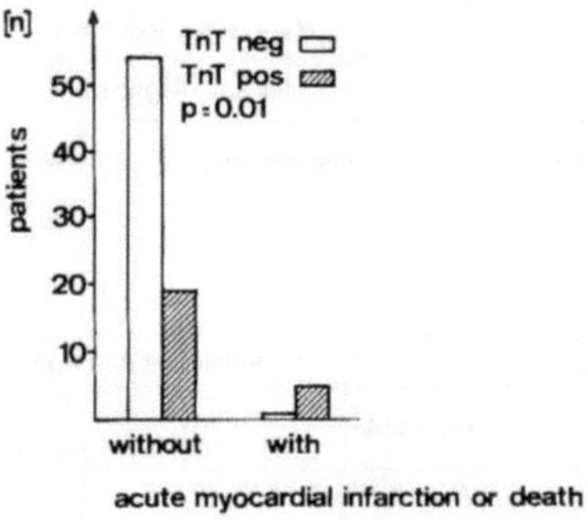

Fig. 3. Contractile protein release and in hospital complications in patients with unstable angina, at 1-month follow-up. *Left*, myosin light chain (*MLC*) release; *right*, troponin T (*TnT*)

Release of myosin light chains and troponin T could be observed only in patients with severe coronary artery narrowing, i.e., stenosis of over 75% in at least one major branch. It is, however, ischemia and not the presence of coronary artery disease which causes marker protein release. As might be expected in patients with unstable angina, marker protein release correlated with electrocardiographic signs of myocardial ischemia. As seen in Fig. 3, a positive test for troponin T or myosin light chains identifies a subgroup of patients with unstable angina and increased risk of acute myocardial infarction or death. Although the predictive value of such a positive test is low, complications occurred almost exclusively in this subgroup of patients. According to these results, elevated serum levels of contractile proteins in patients with unstable angina indicate a more serious prognosis and therefore demand a more careful observation of the patient and possibly a more extended indication for coronary angiography.

Conclusions

In unstable angina, cardiac enzymes should not be significantly elevated above the upper limit of normal, and no QRS changes indicative of acute myocardial infarction should be present on the electrocardiogram. However, neither the electrocardiogram nor the measurement of cardiac enzymes in serum are sufficiently sensitive to diagnose small areas of myocardial cell necrosis. Using more refined serodiagnostic procedures in patients with unstable angina, small amounts of myocardial necrosis may be detected. It therefore seems appropriate to consider unstable ischemic syndrome as a continuous spectrum extending between stable angina at the end to Q-wave infarction at the other (Fig. 4). In this spectrum ischemic cell damage may increase with release of cytosolic enzymes only at the beginning, being followed by a release of structurally bound marker proteins. This marker protein release results at the beginning

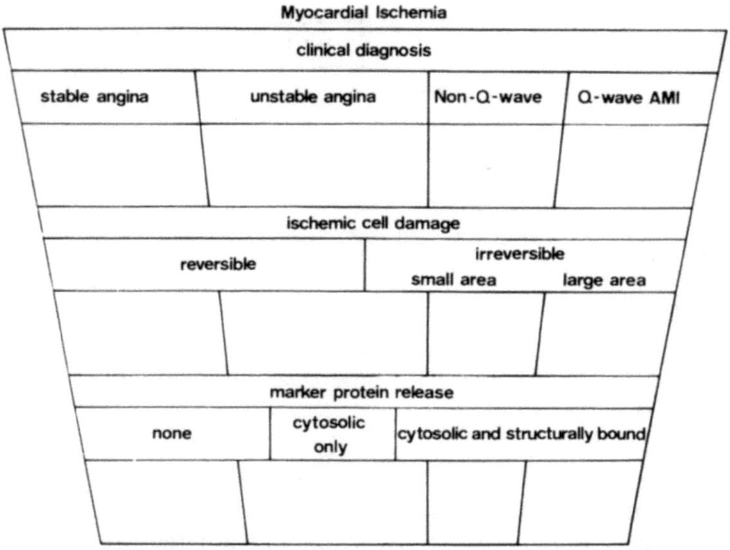

Fig. 4. Unstable angina: a continuous spectrum from no cell damage to non-Q-wave infarction

from reversible cell damage only in less severe ischemic episodes. More severe ischemia may induce irreversible cell damage leading to release of structurally bound marker proteins. If the area of myocardial necrosis is large enough to be detected by electrocardiographic changes or by the use of conventional cardiac enzyme criteria, then myocardial infarction is diagnosed.

The concept of unstable angina as lying on a spectrum between stable angina and myocardial infarction may explain many of the discrepancies and difficulties in defining unstable angina precisely in any individual patient.

The increased diagnostic efficacy of contractile protein measurements allows identification of patients with unstable angina and minor myocardial cell necrosis. These data demonstrate not only that minor degree of cell necrosis occur within the spectrum of unstable angina, but also that these microinfarcts are indicators of a more serious prognosis.

References

1. Armstrong PW, Chiong MA, Parker JO (1982) The spectrum of unstable angina: prognostic role of serum creatine kinase determination. Am J Cardiol 49:1849–1852
2. Bird JWC, Carter JH, Triemer RE et al. (1980) Proteinases in cardiac and skeletal muscle. Fed Proc 39:20–25
3. Boden WE, Bough EW, Benham I et al. (1983) Unstable angina with episodic ST segment elevation and minimal creatine kinase release culminating in extensive myocardial infarction. J Am Coll Cardiol 2:11–20

4. Cummins P, Young A, Auckland ML et al. (1987) Comparison of serum cardiac specific troponin-I with creatine kinase, creatine kinase-MB isoenzyme, tropomyosin, myoglobin and C-reactive protein release in marathon runners: cardiac or skeletal muscle trauma? Eur J Clin Invest 17:317–324
5. Freeman MR, Williams AE, Chisholm RJ et al. (1989) Role of resting thallium 201 perfusion in predicting coronary anatomy, left ventricular wall motion, and hospital outcome in unstable angina pectoris. Am Heart J 117:306–314
6. Gazes PC, Mobley EM, Faris HM et al. (1973) Preinfarction angina: a prospective study: ten years follow up. Prognostic significance of electrocardiographic changes. Circulation 48:331–337
7. Gerhardt W, Waldenström J, Hörder M et al. (1982) Creatine kinase and creatine kinase B-subunit activity in serum in cases of suspected myocardial infarction. Clin Chem 28:277–283
8. Grande P, Christiansen C, Pederson A et al. (1980) Optimal diagnosis in acute myocardial infarction. A cost-effectiveness study. Circulation 61:723–728
9. Hendrickx GR, Amano J, Kenna T et al. (1985) Creatine kinase release not associated with myocardial necrosis after short periods of coronary artery occclusion in conscious baboons. J Am Coll Cardiol 6:1299–1303
10. Hoberg E, Katus HA, Diederich KW et al. (1987) Myoglobin, creatine kinase-B isoenzyme, and myosin light chain release in patients with unstable angina pectoris. Eur Heart J 8:989–994
11. Hoh JFY, McGrath PA, Hale PT (1987) Electrophoretic analysis of multiple forms of rat cardiac myosin: effects of hypophysectomy and thyroxine replacement. J Mol Cell Cardiol 10:1076–1082
12. Hong RA, Licht JD, Wei JY et al. (1986) Elevated CKMB with normal total creatine kinase in suspected myocardial infarction: associated clinical findings and early prognosis. Am Heart J 111:1041–1147
13. Jockers-Wretou E, Pfleiderer G (1975) Quantitation of creatine kinase in human tissues and sera by an immunological method. Clin Chim Acta 58:223–229
14. Johnson SM, Mauritson DR, Winniford MD et al. (1982) Continuous electrocardiographic monitoring in patients with unstable angina pectoris: identification of a high risk subgroup with severe coronary artery disease, variant angina, and/or impaired early prognosis. Am Heart J 103:4–12
15. Katus HA, Hurrell J, Matsueda G et al. (1982) Increased specificity in human cardiac myosin radioimmunoassays utilizing two monoclonal antibodies in a double sandwich assay. J Mol Immun 19:451–455
16. Katus HA, Diederich KW, Schwarz F et al. (1987) Influence of reperfusion on serum concentrations of cytosolic creatine kinase and structural myosin light chains in acute myocardial infarction. Am J Cardiol 60:440–445
17. Katus HA, Diederich KW, Hoberg E et al. (1988) Circulating cardiac myosin light chains in patients with angina at rest: identification of a high risk subgroup. J Am Coll Cardiol 3:487–493
18. Katus HA, Remppis A, Looser S et al. (1989) Enzyme linked immuno assay of cardiac troponin T for the detection of acute myocardial infarction in patients. J Mol Cardiol 21:1349–1353
19. Khaw BA, Gold HK, Fallon JT et al. (1979) Detection of serum cardiac myosin light chains in acute experimental myocardial infarction. Circulation 58:1130–1136
20. Krauss KR, Hutter AM, DeSanctis RW (1972) Acute coronary insufficiency: course and follow up. Arch Intern Med 129:808–814
21. Nordlander R, Nyquist O (1979) Patients treated in a coronary care unit without acute myocardial infarction. Identification of high risk subgroup for subsequent myocardial infarction and/or cardiovascular death. Br Heart J 41:647–653
22. Pearlstone JR, Carpenter MR, Smilie LB (1986) Amino acid sequence of rabbit cardiac troponin T. J Biol Chem 261:16795–16810
23. Piper HM, Schwartz P, Spahr R et al. (1984) Early enzyme release from myocardial cells is not due to irreversible cell damage. J Mol Cell Cardiol 16:385–388
24. Piper HM, Schwartz P, Hütter JF et al. (1984) Energy metabolism and enzyme release of cultured adult rat heart muscle cells during anoxia. J Mol Cell Cardiol 16:995–1007

25. Quale J, Kimmelstiel C, Lipschik G et al. (1988) Use of sequential cardiac enzyme analysis in stratification of risk for myocardial infarction in patients with unstable angina. Arch Intern Med 148:1277–1279
26. Scarlovsky S, Rechavia E, Strasberg B et al. (1988) Unstable angina: ST segment depression with positive versus negative T wave deflections – clinical course, ECG evolution, and angiographic correlation. Am Heart J 116:933–941
27. Schroeder JS, Lamb IH, Harrison DC (1977) Patients admitted to the coronary care unit for chest pain: high risk subgroup for subsequent cardiac death. Am J Cardiol 39:829–832
28. Smitherman TC, Dycus DW, Richards EG (1980) Dissociation of myosin light chains and decreased myosin ATPase activity with acidification of synthetic myosin filaments: possible clues to the fate of myosin in myocardial ischemia and infarction. J Mol Cell Cardiol 12:149–164
29. White RD, Grande P, Califf L et al. (1985) Diagnostic and prognostic significance of minimally elevated creatine kinase MB in suspected acute myocardial infarction. Am J Cardiol 55:1478–1484
30. Wilkinson JM, Grand RJA (1978) Comparison of amino acid sequence of troponin I from different striated muscles. Nature 271:31–35

II. Clinical Findings in Unstable Angina

Unstable Angina: A Classification *

E. BRAUNWALD [1]

Introduction

The establishment of a prognosis and the approach to the treatment of many diseases is aided greatly by a logical classification. For example, classification of a wide variety of neoplasms by anatomic extent, microscopic appearance, and the presence of special markers now forms the basis for selecting appropriate therapy. In cardiology, the classification of patients with acute myocardial infarction and congestive heart failure has been of enormous value in following the progress and in selecting therapy of individual patients and in comparing the outcome of similar patients treated at different locations and at different times. The purpose of this article is to provide a classification of unstable angina. This classification is designed to facilitate communication about these patients, to aid in the decision regarding diagnostic measures and therapy of individual patients, and to provide a more precise basis for including patients in and for evaluating the outcome of clinical trials.

Unstable angina is a complex condition. Early in this century, the clinical-pathologic features of two of the principal manifestations of ischemic heart disease – acute myocardial infarction and chronic stable angina – had already been well described. It has taken much longer to define a syndrome that is intermediate in severity between these two conditions. In 1923, Wearn [1] described, in a group of 19 patients with acute myocardial infarction confirmed at necropsy, attacks of angina pectoris that may precede myocardial infarction and serve as warnings of the presence of coronary artery disease. In 1937, Sampson and Eliaser [2] and Feil [3] separately described a syndrome consisting of severe, prolonged anginal pain that often led to acute myocardial infarction, and they termed it "impending acute myocardial infarction." Other terms that have been used for this condition include "preinfarction angina," "crescendo angina," "status anginosus," "accelerated angina," "acute coronary insufficiency," and "intermediate coronary syndrome" [4–7]; the term most frequently used now, "unstable angina," was used by Fowler [8] and Conti et al. [9] in 1971. This large number of designations, as well as the lack

* This paper was originally published in *Circulation* 80:410–414, 1989, and it is reproduced here by permission of the American Heart Association, Inc.

[1] Department of Medicine, Brigham and Women's Hospital, Harvard Medical School, 75 Francis Street, Boston, MA 02115, USA

W. Bleifeld et al. (Eds.)
Unstable Angina

of a clear, agreed-upon definition, reflects the ambiguity that has continued to be associated with this "catch-all" syndrome. Unstable angina probably consists of a number of conditions, all characterized by severe transient myocardial ischemia [10–13].

Unstable angina is very common and often quite serious; it is responsible for more than 750000 hospitalizations annually in the United States [14] and thus ranks among the most frequent causes of hospitalization in this country. More than 70000 of these hospitalized patients develop myocardial infarction [13], and some die suddenly [15]. An unknown, but probably large, number of patients with unstable angina are not hospitalized but are treated at home. Many patients with unstable angina do not develop serious complications, but after recovery from the acute episode, they are left with chronic stable angina of varying severity. A minority of patients recover without developing either complications or chronic angina. In addition, a substantial percentage of patients who develop acute myocardial infarction, ranging from 30% to 60% in most series [16], experience a prodrome of unstable angina before reaching the hospital. A significant percentage of patients with acute myocardial infarction develop unstable angina in the early postinfarction period.

There is currently intense interest in elucidating the pathogenesis of unstable angina [10, 17]. Maseri [18] has emphasized that both increased myocardial oxygen demand in the presence of severely restricted coronary reserve and dynamic stenosis caused by coronary vasoconstriction may be responsible. Coronary arteriographic examinations have revealed that rapid progression of coronary stenosis often precedes the development of unstable angina [19], and that this stenosis is frequently caused by eccentric, irregular lesions [20] often associated with filling defects thought to be caused by coronary thrombi [21–24]. Angioscopic studies at operation have revealed that many patients with unstable angina have disrupted, fissured plaques often associated with mural thrombi [25]; the latter finding has been confirmed by pathologic examination [26]. Also, evidence exists that abnormal coronary vasoconstriction [18] and activation of platelets [27] and of the clotting system [10] may occur during and be of pathogenetic importance in unstable angina. Coronary thrombi causing variable degrees of coronary obstruction may develop and regress rapidly, reflecting the opposing actions of the hemostatic and fibrinolytic systems. Platelet emboli may cause arrhythmias and sudden death in these patients [28]. Unstable angina occurring soon after acute myocardial infarction is particularly dangerous, often heralds infarct extension, and is associated with a high incidence of recurrent events [29–32]; the latter also occur more frequently in patients whose episodes of chest pain are accompanied by transient electrocardiographic changes of ischemia [33–38].

Considerable efforts are also underway to improve the treatment of unstable angina, and a variety of therapeutic approaches are being actively used and investigated. In addition to anti-ischemic pharmacologic agents (nitrates, β-adrenergic blockers, and calcium antagonists), therapeutic options include anticoagulants, antiplatelet aggregating agents, thromboxane synthesis inhibitors, thromboxane receptor blockers, thrombolytic agents, percutaneous transluminal angioplasty, and coronary artery bypass surgery [11, 39–48]. New methods of revascularization, such as coronary atherectomy, balloon angioplasty with stents, and laser angioplasty, are being actively investigated. These modes of therapy are being tested in various combinations and sequences, and a major challenge will be to select individual patients with unstable angina for various treatment options.

One impediment to obtaining a clearer understanding of the natural history of unstable angina and to evaluating therapeutic strategies is the heterogeneous nature of the syndrome and the lack of general agreement about its precise definition. Currently, a broad spectrum of patients with ischemic episodes varying widely in cause, severity, prognosis, and responsiveness to therapy are lumped together under the broad umbrella of unstable angina pectoris. These patients can be described by using information obtained not only from the clinical examination and routine electrocardiogram but also from a variety of specialized tests, including coronary arteriography, left ventriculography, continously recorded (Holter) electrocardiography, and perfusion scintigraphy. Characterization of patients by all of these methods can lead to the classification of unstable angina into an almost infinite number of subgroups. Such fine classification is almost as useless to the clinician as is the lumping of all patients into a single category.

To separate patients with unstable angina into a manageable number of meaningful and easily understood subgroups based on the severity, the presumed precipitating cause, and the presence of electrocardiographic changes, a clinical classification of this condition is proposed (Table 1). This classification focuses on three important aspects of unstable angina: (a) the severity of the clinical manifestations, (b) the clinical circumstances in which unstable angina occurs, and (c) whether or not the symptomatic ischemic episodes are accompanied by transient electrocardiographic changes. The classification can be made before obtaining the above-mentioned specialized laboratory tests, and once the tests are performed, the results may then be used to supplement the clinical information and the standard electrocardiogram. This classification of unstable angina is based on two premises: (a) the patient's symptoms are actually caused by myocardial ischemia, and (b) in patients with prolonged ischemia, the diagnosis of acute myocardial infarction is excluded by electrocardiography or serum enzyme determinations. Often, this exclusion must be retrospective.

Classification

Severity

Class I. New onset severe or accelerated angina. Patients with new onset (<2 months in duration) exertional angina pectoris that is severe or frequent (≥3 episodes/day) or patients with chronic stable angina who develop acceler-

Table 1. Classification of unstable angina

Severity	Clinical circumstances		
	A. Develops in presence of extracardiac condition that intensifies myocardial ischemia (secondary UA)	B. Develops in absence of extracardiac condition (primary UA)	C. Develops within 2 weeks after AMI (postinfarction UA)
I. New onset of severe angina or accelerated angina; no rest pain	IA	IB	IC
II. Angina at rest within past month but not within preceding 48 h (angina at rest, subacute)	IIA	IIB	IIC
III. Angina at rest within 48 h (angina at rest, acute)	IIIA	IIIB	IIIC

Patients with UA may also be divided into three groups depending on whether UA occurs (a) in the absence of treatment for chronic stable angina, (b) during treatment for chronic stable angina, or (c) despite maximal anti-ischemic drug therapy. These three groups may be designated by subscripts 1, 2, or 3, respectively. Patients with UA may be divided further into those with and without transient ST-T wave changes during pain. UA, unstable angina; AMI, acute myocardial infarction.

ated angina (that is, angina distinctly more frequent, severe, longer in duration, or precipitated by distinctly less exertion than previously), but who have not experienced pain at rest during the preceding 2 months.

Class II. Angina at rest, subacute. Patients with one or more episodes of angina at rest during the preceding month but not within the preceding 48 hours.

Class III. Angina at rest, acute. Patients with one or more episodes of angina at rest within the preceding 48 h.

In classes II and III, manifestations described in class I may also occur. Unstable angina is no longer considered to be present when a patient has been asymptomatic or suffers angina that has been stable for more than 2 months.

Clinical Circumstances in which Unstable Angina Occurs

Class A. Secondary unstable angina. Patients in whom unstable angina develops secondary to a clearly identified condition extrinsic to the coronary vascular bed that has intensified myocardial ischemia. Such conditions reduce myocardial oxygen supply or increase myocardial oxygen demand and include anemia, fever, infection, hypotension, uncontrolled hypertension, tachyarrhythmia, unusual emotional stress, thyrotoxicosis, and hypoxemia secondary to respiratory failure.

Class B. Primary unstable angina. Patients who develop unstable angina pectoris in the absence of an extracardiac condition that has intensified ischemia, as in class A.

Class C. Postinfarction unstable angina. Patients who develop unstable angina within the first 2 weeks after a documented acute myocardial infarction.

Electrocardiographic Changes

If an electrocardiogram has been recorded during an episode of chest pain, the presence or absence of transient ST-T abnormalities is noted. (The presence of such abnormalities is associated with more severe underlying disease [33–38]).

Intensity of Treatment

For research purposes, especially clinical trials, it may be helpful also to classify patients by the intensity of treatment as follows: (a) unstable angina occurring in the absence of or with minimal antianginal therapy; (b) unstable angina occurring in the presence of appropriate therapy for chronic stable angina (the administration of conventional oral doses of antianginal drugs, i.e., β-adrenergic blockers, long-acting nitrates, and calcium antagonists); and (c) unstable angina occurring in the presence of maximally tolerated doses of all three categories of anti-ischemic drugs, including intravenous nitroglycerin [49].

These three levels of treatment may be designated by the subscripts 1, 2, and 3.

Discussion

This classification of unstable angina, which should be tested prospectively, permits the grading of patients with unstable angina from the mildest to the most severe condition. An example of the mildest form would be a patient with chronic stable angina who develops marked intensification of exertion-induced angina pectoris after blood loss and who has no ST segment or T wave changes during angina. This patient would be in class I A without transient electrocardiographic changes (I, accelerated angina; A, secondary unstable angina). At the other end of the spectrum is the patient who experiences recurrent angina at rest with transient ST segment depressions several days after an acute myocardial infarction. This patient would be in class III C with transient electrocardiographic changes (class III, angina at rest, acute; C, postinfarction unstable angina).

Unstable angina is a dynamic condition, and patients may initially be in one class and move to another as the underlying disease changes or as response to treatment occurs. For example, a patient with the new onset of severe and frequent exertional angina without an apparent provocative extracardiac condition is in class I B. If that patient then developed an episode of angina at rest, he would be in class III B. If no pain recurred for 48 h, he would be in class II B.

The classification of the intensity of treatment may be used as follows. A patient with a history of primary unstable angina at rest during convalescence from a myocardial infarction who is receiving no anti-ischemia therapy is in class III C_1. If episodes of pain persist despite treatment with usual doses of antianginal agents, the patient would advance to III C_2; if during treatment with intravenous nitroglycerin the episodes disappeared for more than 48 h, the patient would be classified as II C_3.

Although the proposed classification of unstable angina is clinical, it can be related to the underlying disease. Angioscopic observations performed during operation suggest a good correlation between the presence of nonocclusive thrombi and the recent occurrence of angina at rest [25]. Such thrombi usually undergo rapid spontaneous lysis and therefore become less prevalent with the passage of time. Thrombolytic or anticoagulant therapy may therefore be of great value in patients in class III, of less value in class II, and of little value in class I. The precipitation of unstable angina by changes in conditions extrinsic to the coronary artery bed that have intensified ischemia (class A) is compatible with fixed, severe coronary obstruction, and the presence of a fissured plaque or thrombus need not be presumed (but cannot, of course, be excluded). Unstable angina secondary to an increase in myocardial oxygen needs or abnormal coronary vasoconstriction generally responds to bed rest, mild sedation, and vigorous treatment with multiple anti-ischemic drugs; failure to respond to such vigorous therapy suggests total or subtotal coronary occlusion, sometimes by a thrombus.

It is hoped that this classification will aid in the clear description of and communication about patients with unstable angina, in the elucidation of the natural history and prognosis of the various subgroups, in the precise definition of patients selected for clinical trials so that therapy can be evaluated in comparable patients, and ultimately in the development of treatment regimens that are appropriate for each subgroup.

Acknowledgements. The aid of a number of colleagues who reviewed this manuscript is gratefully acknowledged. Particularly valuable suggestions were made by Drs. C.R. Conti, S. Epstein, V. Fuster, L. Goldman, R. Gorlin, S. Gottlieb, R. Helfant, A. Maseri, R. Ross, and T. Ryan.

References

1. Wearn JT (1923) Thrombosis of the coronary arteries, with infarction of the heart. Am J Med Sci 165:250–276
2. Sampson JJ, Eliaser M Jr (1937) The diagnosis of impending acute coronary artery occlusion. Am Heart J 13:675–686
3. Feil H (1937) Preliminary pain in coronary thrombosis. Am J Med Sci 193:42–48
4. Scanlon PJ, Nemickas R, Moran JF, Talano JV, Amirparviz F, Pifarre R (1973) Accelerated angina pectoris: clinical hemodynamic, arteriographic, and therapeutic experience in 85 patients. Circulation 47:19–26
5. Wood P (1961) Acute and subacute coronary insufficiency. Br Med J I:1779–1782
6. Vakil RJ (1961) Intermediate coronary syndrome. Circulation 24:557–571
7. Vakil RJ (1964) Preinfarction syndrome: management and follow-up. Am J Cardiol 14:55–63
8. Fowler NO (1971) "Preinfarctional" angina: A need for an objective definition and for a controlled clinical trial of its management. Circulation 44:755–758
9. Conti CR, Greene B, Pitt B, Griffith L, Humphries O, Brawley R, Taylor D, Bender H, Gott V, Ross RS (1971) Coronary surgery in unstable angina pectoris (abstract). Circulation 44 (Suppl II):II-154
10. Patterson DLH (1988) Unstable angina. Postgrad Med J 64:196–200
11. Patterson DLH (1988) Management in unstable angina. Postgrad Med J 64:271–277
12. Bertolasi CA, Tronge JE, Mon GA, Turri D, Lugones MI (1979) Clinical spectrum of "unstable angina." Clin Cardiol 2:113–120
13. Julian DG (1985) The natural history of unstable angina, in Hugenholtz PG, Goldman BS (eds) Unstable angina: current concepts and management. Stuttgart, Schattauer, pp 65–70
14. National Center for Health Statistics (1987) Vital and health statistics: detailed diagnosis and procedures for patients discharged from short stay hospitals. US Department of Health and Human Services, Public Health Service, Series 13, No. 90, Hyattsville, Md.
15. Falk E (1985) Unstable angina with fatal outcome: dynamic coronary thrombosis leading to infarction and/or sudden death. Circulation 71:699–708
16. Harper RW, Kennedy G, DeSanctis RW, Hutter AM (1979) The incidence and pattern of angina prior to acute myocardial infarction: a study of 577 cases. Am Heart J 97:178–183
17. Fuster V, Badimon L, Cohen M, Ambrose JA, Badimon JJ, Chesebro J (1988) Insights into the pathogenesis of acute ischemic syndromes. Circulation 6:1213–1220
18. Maseri A (1986) Pathogenetic classifications of unstable angina as a guideline to individual patient management and prognosis. Am J Med 80 (Suppl 4C):48–55
19. Moise A, Theroux P, Taeymans Y, Descoings B, Lesperance J, Waters DD, Pelletier GB, Bourassa M (1983) Unstable angina and progression of coronary atherosclerosis. N Engl J Med 309:685–689
20. Ambrose JA, Winters SL, Arora RR, Eng A, Ricco A, Gorlin R, Fuster V (1986) Angiographic evolution of coronary artery morphology in unstable angina. J Am Coll Cardiol 7:472–478
21. Holmes DR Jr, Hartzler GO, Smith HC, Fuster V (1981) Coronary artery thrombosis in patients with unstable angina. Br Heart J 45:411–416
22. Vetrovec GW, Cowley MJ, Overton H, Richardson DW (1981) Intracoronary thrombus in syndromes of unstable myocardial ischemia. Am Heart J 102:1202–1208
23. Capone G, Wolf NM, Meyer B, Meister SG (1985) Frequency of intracoronary filling defects by angiography in angina pectoris at rest. Am J Cardiol 56:403–406
24. Gotoh K, Katoh K, Fukui S, Hamano Y, Minamino T (1985) Angiographic visualization of coronary thrombus during anginal attack in unstable angina (abstract). Circulation 72 (Suppl III):III-112
25. Sherman CT, Litvack F, Grundfest ME, Lee M, Hickey A, Chaux A, Kass R, Blanche C, Matloff J, Morgenstern L, Ganz W, Swan HJC, Forrester J (1986) Coronary angioscopy in patients with unstable angina pectoris. N Engl J Med 315:913–919
26. Falk E (1983) Plaque rupture with severe pre-existing stenosis precipitating coronary thrombosis: characteristics of coronary atherosclerotic plaques underlying fatal occlusive thrombi. Br Heart J 50:127–134

27. Fitzgerald DJ, Roy L, Catella F, Fitzgerald GA (1986) Platelet activation in unstable coronary disease. N Engl J Med 315:983–989
28. Haerem JW (1974) Mural platelet microthrombi and major acute lesions of main epicardial arteries in sudden coronary death. Atherosclerosis 19:529–541
29. Ross J Jr, Gilpin EA, Madsen EB, Henning H, Nicod P, Dittrich H, Engler R, Rittelmeyer J, Smith SC, Viquerat C (1989) A decision scheme for coronary angiography after acute myocardial infarction. Circulation 79:292–303
30. Ross J Jr, Bradenburg RO, Dinsmore RE, Friesinger GC II, Hultgren HH, Pepine CJ, Rapaport E, Ryan TJ, Weinberg SL, Williams JF (1987) Guidelines for coronary angiography: Report of the Joint American College of Cardiology/American Heart Association Task Force on Assessment of Cardiovascular Procedures. J Am Coll Cardiol 10:935–950 and Circulation 76:963A–977A
31. Breyer RH, Engelman RM, Rousou JA, Lemeshow S (1985) Postinfarction angina: an expanding subset of patients undergoing coronary artery bypass. J Thorac Cardiovasc Surg 90:532–540
32. DeBusk RF, Blonqvist CG, Kochoukos NT, Luepker RV, Miller HS, Moss AJ, Pollock ML, Reeves TJ, Selvester RH, Stason WB, Wagner GS, Willman VL (1986) Identification and treatment of low-risk patients after acute myocardial infarction and coronary-artery bypass graft surgery. N Engl J Med 314:161–166
33. Gazes PC, Mobley EM Jr, Farris HM Jr, Duncan RC, Humphries GB (1973) Preinfarctional (unstable) angina – a prospective study: ten year follow-up. Circulation 48:331–337
34. Haines DE, Raabe DS, Gundel WD, Wackers FJ (1983) Anatomic and prognostic significance of new T-wave inversion in unstable angina. Am J Cardiol 52:14–18
35. Sclarovsky S, Davidson E, Lewin RF, Strasberg B, Arditti A, Agmon J (1986) Unstable angina pectoris evolving to acute myocardial infarction: significance of ECG changes during chest pain. Am Heart J 112:459–462
36. Sclarovsky S, Davidson E, Strasberg B, Lewin RF, Arditti A, Wurtzel M, Agmon J (1986) Unstable angina: the significance of ST segment elevation or depression in patients without evidence of increased myocardial oxygen demand. Am Heart J 112:463–467
37. Plotnick GD, Greene HL, Carliner NH, Becker LC, Fisher ML (1979) Clinical indicators of left main coronary artery disease in unstable angina. Ann Intern Med 91:149–153
38. Papapietro SE, Niess GS, Paine TD, Mantle JA, Rackley CE, Russell RO, Rogers WJ (1980) Transient electrocardiographic changes in patients with unstable angina: relation to coronary arterial anatomy. Am J Cardiol 46:28–33
39. Lewis HD, Davis JW, Archibald DG, Steinke WE, Smitherman TC, Doherty JE III, Schnaper HW, LeWinter MM, Linares E, Pouget JM, Sabharwal SC, Chester E, DeMots H (1983) Protective effects of aspirin against acute myocardial infarction and death in men with unstable angina. N Engl J Med 309:396–403
40. Theroux P, Ouimet H, McCans J, Latour JG, Joly P, Levy G, Pelletier E, Juneau M, Stasiak J, DeGruise P, Pellitier GB, Rinzler D, Waters DD (1988) Aspirin, heparin, or both to treat acute unstable angina. N Engl J Med 319:1105–1111
41. Gold HK, Johns JA, Leinbach RC, Yasuda T, Grossbard E, Zusman R, Collen D (1987) A randomized, blinded, placebo-controlled trial of recombinant human tissue-type plasminogen activator in patients with unstable angina pectoris. Circulation 75:1192–1199
42. Topol EJ, Nicklas JM, Kander NH, Walton JA, Ellis SG, Gorman L, Pitt B (1988) Coronary revascularization after intravenous tissue plasminogen activator for unstable angina pectoris: results of a randomized double-blind, placebo-controlled trial. Am J Cardiol 62:368–371
43. de Zwaan C, Bar FW, Janssen JHA, de Swart HB, Vermeer F, Wellens HJJ (1988) Effects of thrombolytic therapy on unstable angina: clinical and angiographic results. J Am Coll Cardiol 12:301–309
44. Williams DO, Riley RS, Singh AK, Gerwitz H, Most AS (1981) Evaluation of the role of coronary angioplasty in patients with unstable angina pectoris. Am Heart J 102:1–90
45. De Feyter PJ, Suryapranata H, Serruys PW, Beatt K, van Domburg R, van den Brand M, Tijssen JJ, Azar AJ, Hugenholtz PG (1988) Coronary angioplasty for unstable angina: immediate and late results in 200 consecutive patients with identification of risk factors for unfavorable early and late outcome. J Am Coll Cardiol 12:324–333

46. Favaloro RG, Effler DB, Cheanvechai C, Quint RA, Sones FM Jr (1971) Acute coronary insufficiency (impending myocardial infarction and myocardial infarction). Am J Cardiol 28:598–607
47. Unstable Angina Pectoris Study Group: Unstable angina pectoris (1978) National cooperative study group to compare surgical and medical therapy. II. In-hospital experience and initial follow-up results in patients with one, two and three vessel disease. Am J Cardiol 42:839–848
48. Luchi RJ, Scott SM, Deupree RH, and the Principal Investigators and Their Associates of Veterans Administration Cooperative Study No. 28 (1987) Comparison of medical and surgical treatment for unstable angina pectoris. N Engl J Med 316:977–984
49. Curfman GD, Heinsimer JA, Lozner EC, Ho-Leung F (1983) Intravenous nitroglycerin in the treatment of spontaneous angina pectoris: a prospective, randomized trial. Circulation 67:276–282

Coronary Angiographic Findings in the Acute Coronary Syndromes

J. A. AMBROSE [1]

Introduction

Over the past few years research in several related cardiac disciplines has shed new light concerning the pathogenesis of the acute coronary syndromes of unstable angina, myocardial infarction, and sudden cardiac death. Data obtained by careful pathologic analysis of the coronary arteries at postmortem examination along with analysis of coronary morphology at angiography, serial angiographic evaluations in patients before and after the development of an acute syndrome, coronary angioscopy, and biochemical studies of platelet activation and fibrin formation from peripheral and coronary sinus blood have provided new and interesting information concerning these syndromes. A unifying theory can now be proposed in which plaque disruption with thrombus formation is the common substrate in the majority of patients presenting with either unstable angina, non-Q-wave infarction, Q-wave infarction, or sudden cardiac death [1, 2]. In this paper we review the coronary angiographic findings in these conditions and speculate as to the pathogenetic differences between syndromes. In particular, we try to answer the question of why a patient develops a particular syndrome following disruption of a plaque.

Unstable Angina

Unstable angina is a clinical syndrome that is usually defined as either the new onset of angina occurring at low workloads or at rest or the presence of crescendo angina. In the majority of cases there has been an abrupt onset or change in symptoms culminating in angina at rest. The clinical presentation is often quite similar to that of myocardial infarction except that the duration of ischemia is less, and there has no been no release of cardiac enzymes indicating myocardial necrosis. However, in fact, very sensitive biochemical assays often indicate some myocardial necrosis in patients with unstable angina and rest pain [3].

[1] Division of Cardiology, Mount Sinai Hospital, One Gustave L. Levy Place, New York, NY 10029, USA

W. Bleifeld et al. (Eds.)
Unstable Angina

Coronary Angiographic Findings

Coronary arteriographic studies in the 1970s indicated no difference in angiographic findings between stable and unstable angina in the number of vessels with significant disease or in the percentage stenosis in the affected vessels [4, 5]. A higher incidence of left main stenosis in unstable angina has been shown in some studies. In patients with crescendo angina and both rest and exertional chest pain, Plotnick et al. found significant left main stenosis in 25% of patients [6]. While most patients with unstable angina have multivessel disease, single-vessel disease has been common in some studies. Victor et al. found a 52% incidence of single-vessel disease in patients with new-onset angina who underwent angiography within 90 days of onset of symptomatology [7]. Of these patients 77% had involvement of the left anterior descending artery. In other studies the incidence of single-vessel disease has varied between 12% and 33% [8, 9]. In most angiographic studies of unstable angina approximately 10%–15% of patients have had normal or nonobstructive coronary arteries. In these patients either the clinical diagnosis was incorrect, or ischemia unrelated to fixed obstruction of the epicardial coronary arteries was present.

Progression of Coronary Disease

In 1983, Moise et al. reported progression of coronary artery disease in 76% of patients with unstable angina in whom a prior angiogram was available for comparison before the onset of instability [10]. This incidence of progression was significantly higher than in patients with stable angina. These findings were corroborated by Ambrose et al. 3 years later [11]. Of interest, in 38% of patients with progression Moise et al. found that this progression occurred in coronary segments that were previously "healthy." In our study 72% of lesions with progression occurred from vessels which initially were less than 50% occlusive (diameter reduction) [11]. While about 75% of patients with unstable angina demonstrate progression of coronary disease on angiography, one-quarter do not show a significant difference between studies. In these latter patients, either transient increases in myocardial oxygen demand, transient thrombus formation which has spontaneously dissipated by the time of angiography, or lesser degrees of progression which were by definition insignificant although still hemodynamically important might be responsible for the increase in symptomatology. It should be remembered that once an artery contains a critical lesion, only a small transient decrease in diameter is all that is required to cause a profound drop in pressure across the lesion (pressure gradient across a stenosis $\sim$ flow^2/diam^4) and be responsible for ischemia [12].

Over the past few years there have been a number of new angiographic observations in patients presenting with unstable angina. It has been shown that the coronary morphology of lesions in unstable angina is distinct from that of patients with stable angina. Coronary morphology qualitatively analyzes the shape of coronary lesions at angiography with special emphasis on lesion symmetry and border regularity. To appreciate differences in morphology between different coronary syndromes, one must first consider the concept of the angina or ischemia-related vessel [13]. In patients with single-vessel disease and in about one-half of patients with multivessel disease, the vessel responsible for unstable angina can be identified. Identification of this vessel is based on a number of factors including analysis of EKG changes during pain, in addition to the coronary anatomical findings. This concept of an ischemia-related vessel is corroborated by angiographic studies of progression of coronary disease in unstable angina. Often, there is only one "new" lesion or only one lesion exhibiting progression while other lesions have remained stable.

Coronary Morphology in Unstable Angina

Asymmetric or eccentric stenoses with irregular borders and/or overhanging edges have been found in about two-thirds to three-fourths of angina or ischemia-producing vessels in unstable angina (Fig. 1). These eccentric stenoses which have been called type II eccentric lesions occur in only 10%–20% of the patients with stable angina [13]. These angiographic observations have been confirmed by other authors although some have referred to a similarly appearing lesion as one with a complex morphology [14], a T lesion [15],

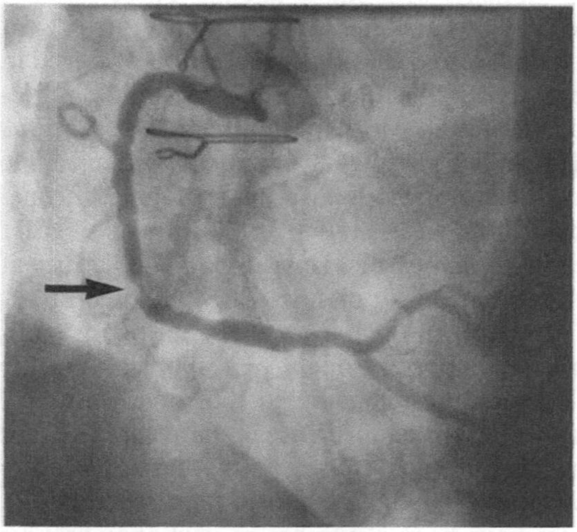

Fig. 1. Right coronary artery in LAO projection showing the typical angiography features (*arrow*) of a complex lesion (type II eccentric). The patient had recent onset of unstable angina and was admitted to the hospital with rest pain

or an intracoronary thrombus [16]. Type II eccentric lesions are similar in appearance to complicated plaques found on postmortem angiography by Levin and Fallon [17]. On pathologic analysis these complicated plaques demonstrate the typical acute coronary syndrome substrate of plaque disruption with thrombus formation. In patients with unstable angina in whom type II eccentric lesions are not found, either smooth concentric or eccentric lesions are usually noted. Concentric or eccentric lesions with ulcerations are occasionally found in unstable angina. While insensitive, they are specific as "culprit lesions" in the acute coronary syndromes [18]. Therefore, since angina-producing lesions in unstable angina are not necessarily eccentric, we now prefer the more general terminology of complex lesions rather than type II eccentric lesions.

Analysis of coronary morphology was not used as a criterion to identify the ischemia-producing vessel in our original study of unstable angina. We now believe that the presence of a complex lesion and/or a filling defect proximal or distal to a significant lesion (indicative of thrombus) can identify the ischemia-related vessel with reasonable certainty.

Angiographic Evidence of Thrombus Formation in Unstable Angina

The incidence of intracoronary thrombus on angiography in unstable angina varies widely according to the study quoted. This incidence has ranged between 1% and 52% [19]. Two more recent publications have noted an incidence of 45% [20] and 41% [21]. The incidence of intracoronary thrombus appeared increased when patients were studied soon after an episode of rest pain, and in some studies when angiography was performed within 24 h of admission to the hospital. Unfortunately, some of these differences in the incidence of intracoronary thrombi in unstable angina between studies may be spurious. There is no standardized definition for intracoronary thrombus especially when the ischemia-related vessel is less than 100% occluded. What one angiographer calls a type II eccentric or complex lesion another may classify as an intracoronary thrombus [22]. Only when a filling defect is located proximal or distal to a significant stenosis, or a lesion irregularity disappears following thrombolytic therapy, can one be sure that there is an intracoronary thrombus (Fig. 2). As complex lesions also contain thrombus, this distinction may be nothing more than semantics. However, it has been our anecdotal experience and that of others that these proximal or distal filling defects are risk factors for acute closure during angioplasty. The presence of a complex lesion in unstable angina by itself is not usually a risk factor for closure.

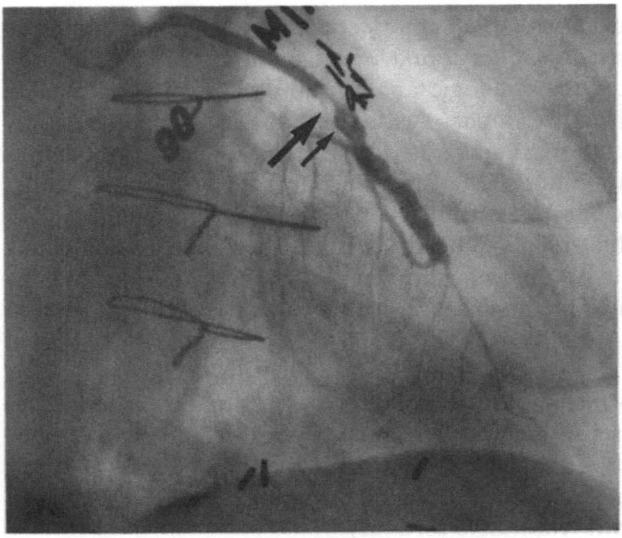

Fig. 2. Saphenous vein graft to the left anterior descending artery showing a complex lesion (*large arrow*) with filling defects distal to the lesion (*small arrow*). The patient received an intracoronary infusion of t-PA with partial resolution of filling defect on a later film

Percentage Stenosis of Coronary Lesions in Unstable Angina

Coronary artery perfusion in unstable angina is very dynamic. During episodes of rest pain in many patients a primary decrease in coronary blood flow is the most common mechanism for ischemia [23]. This is related to either intermittent thrombus formation with spontaneous lysis/embolization and/or a transient increase in vasomotor tone [24]. When patients are pain free, angiography usually shows a patent ischemia-related vessel which contains a significant lesion with at least a 70% but less than 100% diameter reduction. This degree of stenosis is similar to that found in patients with stable angina. Total occlusion of the ischemia-related vessel is found in about 8%–13% [20, 25] of unstable patients at angiography following chest pain. In these patients with total occlusion, distal collaterals are usually present preventing myocardial necrosis following permanent occlusion.

Prognostic Importance of Coronary Morphology in Unstable Angina

There have been, until recently, few prospective data on the importance of different morphologies in unstable angina. Sansa et al. found that patients with complex morphology or thrombus were more likely to have unstable angina refractory to medical therapy [26]. Freeman et al. have recently shown that the angiographic detection of intracoronary thrombus in unstable angina is strongly predictive of cardiac events (urgent revascularization, myocardial infarction, death). From analysis of patients in the CASS Registry who subsequently developed myocardial infarction over a 3-year period, Ellis et al. found that lesion roughness (irregularity) ranked second in importance to quantitative measurements of percentage stenosis as predictors of subsequent infarction in the distribution of the original lesion [27]. While in this study patients who subsequently developed infarction did not necessarily have unstable angina at the time of angiography, these data suggest the possibility that irregularity rather than eccentricity may be the more important variable in analyzing cardiac events in relationship to coronary morphology. Analysis of morphology may therefore have some predictive importance as to the clinical outcome of the patient.

Non-Q-Wave Infarction

By definition, non-Q-wave infarction includes patients with resting ischemia and either new and persistent ST- and T-wave changes, without new Q-waves, and/or transient increases in cardiac enzymes following episodes of ischemic rest pain. By convention, creatine kinase must be at least twice normal, with a concomitant increase in CPK-MB to be considered diagnostic for a non-Q-wave infarction. While non-Q-wave infarction has also been referred to as nontransmural infarction, the two are not synonymous [28]. Nontransmural infarction is a pathologic term, and it does not necessarily correspond to the ECG of non-Q-wave infarction. Non-Q-wave infarction may demonstrate transmural infarction at autopsy while Q-wave infarction by ECG may be nontransmural. Clinically, the distinction between non-Q-wave infarction and unstable angina is not always absolute. While this can be at times confusing, these similarities between syndromes are further evidence suggesting that the acute coronary syndromes form a continuous clinical spectrum of ischemia from unstable angina through Q-wave infarction and sudden coronary death.

Angiographic Findings in Non-Q-Wave Infarction

The incidence of one-, two-, and three-vessel disease is similar among patients with unstable angina, non-Q-wave infarction and Q-wave infarction [5, 29]. In addition, pathologic studies have shown similar degrees of coronary artery disease between nontransmural and transmural myocardial infarction [30]. Angiographically, total occlusion of the infarct-related vessel occurs more frequently in non-Q-wave infarction than in unstable angina. The incidence of total occlusion ranges from 20% to almost 50% when angiography is performed soon after infarction [25, 29, 31]. In patients with less than total occlusion, coronary morphology of infarct-related vessels in non-Q-wave infarction is similar to that of patients with unstable angina. Complex (type II eccentric) lesions are found in approximately two-thirds of these arteries [25].

In patients with recent non-Q-wave infarction in whom a prior angiographic study was available for analysis the angiographic findings are similar to those with unstable angina in that the majority of lesions developed de novo from vessels with less than significant stenoses [32]. However, we have also demonstrated that in some patients with non-Q-wave infarction severe lesions were present at a prior angiogram [33]. Perhaps, it is this same group of patients with a prior significant lesion in whom total occlusion of the infarct-related vessel is found on angiography after the clinical event. Total occlusion with partial collaterals limits the amount of myocardial infarction, preventing the development of more extensive infarction and therefore Q-waves.

Q-Wave Infarction

By definition, Q-wave infarction implies that myocardial necrosis is followed by the development of abnormal Q-waves on ECG. The relationship of Q-wave infarction to the pathologic diagnosis of transmural infarction has been considered in the previous section.

Angiographic Findings in Q-Wave Myocardial Infarction

When angiography is performed within 12 h after the onset of symptoms, total occlusion of the infarct-related vessel is found in approximately 75%–80% of patients although the incidence ranges between 67% and 95% in various studies. DeWood found total coronary occlusion in 87% of patients who underwent angiograms within 4 h of the new onset of symptoms [34]. This proportion decreased to 65% in patients studied 12–24 h after infarction, suggesting spontaneous reperfusion. In patients with an acute myocardial infarction but without total occlusion, stenoses of over 90% in the infarct-related vessel are usually found. Angiographic evidence of intracoronary thrombus on acute angiography usually accompanies coronary occlusion and is usually manifested by either dye staining of thrombus, convex borders to the occlusion, or one or multiple filling defects in the artery (Fig. 3). In patients with patent infarct-related vessels coronary morphology is similar to that found in the other acute syndrome with a predominance of complex lesions [35]. However, filling defects suggestive of thrombus are frequently found (Fig. 4).

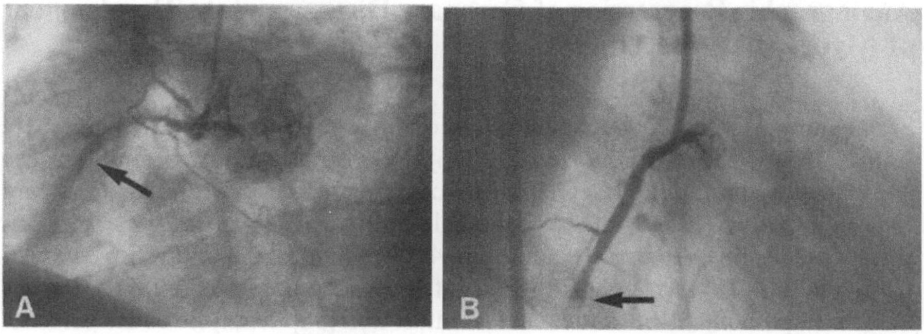

Fig. 3. **A** Dye staining (*arrow*) following significant lesion in middle right coronary artery in a patient with recent inferior wall infarction. **B** Right coronary artery in RAO projection of a different patient with total occlusion in the middle segment. The convex border to the occlusion (*arrow*) indicates acute thrombus formation

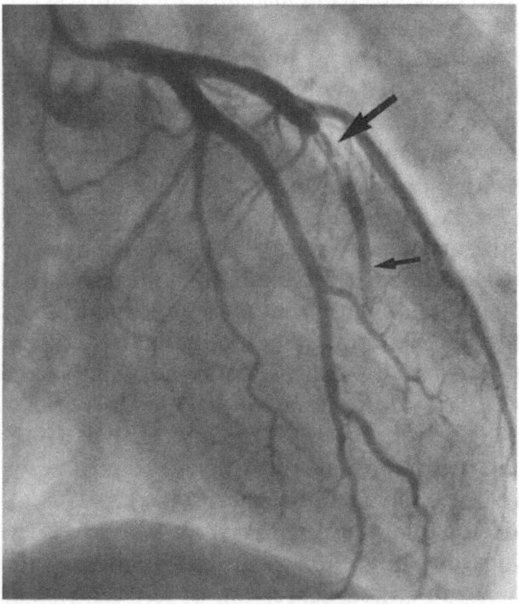

Fig. 4. Multiple filling defects in middle segment of left anterior descending artery indicating thrombus (*large arrow*) with slow antegrade filling of the distal left anterior descending artery (*small arrow*). The patient had a recent anterior wall infarction with recurrent rest pain

Angiographic Progression of Coronary Disease and the Development of Myocardial Infarction

Serial angiography in patients who subsequently developed myocardial infarction has been recently reported [33, 36]. While patients undergoing repeat angiography represent a selected group of patients, these studies also indicate that myocardial infarction, like unstable angina, often progresses from insignificant lesions. Ambrose et al. found 48% of myocardial infarction evolved from less than 50% lesions [33] while Little et al. found less than 50% lesions in 66% of patients prior to myocardial infarction [36]. Analysis of the percentage coronary stenosis following thrombolysis has revealed less than 50% lesions in up to 20% of patients with acute myocardial infarction. However, Hackett et al. found that nearly 60% had lesions between 50% and 70% occlusive, utilizing quantitative techniques immediately after thrombolysis [37]. As it may be difficult pathologically to quantitate the degree of underlying stenosis following plaque disruption even with thrombolysis [38], this later sort of angiographic analysis may overestimate the severity of the underlying plaque prior to infarction.

That myocardial infarction often develops from insignificant lesions is not supported by all the data. Moise et al. found new coronary occlusion in 31% of 313 patients restudied following medical therapy in coronary artery disease [39]. A new occlusion was strongly associated with an interim infarction and could be predicted by the presence of at least an 80% narrowing on initial study supplying a non-akinetic left ventricular segment. However, in 54% of arteries the site of occlusion was either distal to, or in a different segment of the same artery remote from, the 80% narrowing. Therefore, occlusion may not have occurred at the site of the original significant stenosis. Analysis of patients in the CASS Registry with left anterior descending lesions found that the quantitative severity of coronary lesions was the most important factor directly related to subsequent anterior infarction [40]. Unfortunately, repeat angiographic evaluation was not performed following infarction and so the "culprit lesion" was not determined. In addition, nearly half of the patients with a subsequent event had non-Q-wave infarction. Finally, Neill et al. repeated angiography in 34 patients with coronary insufficiency and known coronary artery disease. Nine of 30 severely stenotic arteries (80%–95% diameter narrowing) became occluded on follow-up angiography 4 months later. Five patients had an interim myocardial infarction in the distribution of the new occlusion, and three of these had marked depression of left ventricular function as a result. Therefore, three of nine patients with progression from a severe narrowing to total occlusion had a large myocardial infarction. However, in five of the other six patients, recurrent pain occurred without infarction or with only limited infarction [41]. Again, this suggests that collaterals likely prevent or limit infarction in patients with prior severe narrowings.

Ischemic Sudden Death

The reported incidence of plaque fissuring and thrombus formation on pathologic analysis of the coronary arteries in ischemic sudden death is quite variable. While older studies found these lesions to be infrequent [42, 43], more recent data utilizing careful serial sectioning of the coronary arteries suggest a much higher incidence [44, 45]. Davies and Thomas found that in 74% of cases there was recent thrombus present in the lumen while an additional 21% had plaque fissures with intraintimal thrombus formation [44]. However, patients studied at autopsy with sudden death from ischemic heart disease comprise two groups of patients. The first group includes patients with a new acute ischemic event, e.g., acute infarction, while in the second group the substrate is a scarred and/or hypertrophied left ventricle leading to a terminal ventricular arrhythmia. In an attempt to pathologically classify patients with sudden death, Davies et al. analyzed the autopsy findings in an additional 168 cases of sudden death due to ischemic heart disease [46]; 73% had either an occlusive intraluminal thrombus or a mural intraluminal thrombus. Single-vessel disease, the presence of an acute myocardial infarction at autopsy, or prodromal symptoms suggestive of an ischemic event prior to death was positively associated with the presence of coronary thrombosis. On the other hand, the presence of old myocardial infarction at autopsy, a prior history of ischemic heart disease, and three-vessel disease were associated with a significantly lower incidence of acute thrombus formation.

Angiography in Survivors of Sudden Death

Pathologic and clinical studies in patients with sudden death obviously deal with different subgroups. Clinical studies analyze patients who survived. Survivors of out-of-hospital sudden death have an incidence of acute myocardial infarction, as judged by the presence of new Q-waves, in 19–44% [47, 48]. In 64 out-of-hospital survivors of ischemic sudden death, Weaver et al. performed coronary arteriography and left ventricular angiography [49]. Of these, 94% had one or more coronary arteries with at least a 70% diameter reduction, and 61% had multivessel disease. At least one total coronary occlusion was found in 67%, and 70% had some degree of left ventricular dysfunction.

Two recent studies have examined the incidence of complex or acute lesions on angiography in survivors of sudden death [50, 51]. Stevenson et al., using angiographic criteria similar to those of Ambrose et al., found complex lesions in 64% of survivors without inducible ventricular tachycardia compared to only 25% of patients with inducible ventricular tachycardia ($p = 0.10$). Likewise, Lo et al. found eccentric irregular or long irregular lesions in 11 of 22 (50%) survivors of sudden death without inducible ventricular tachycardia compared to 5 of 27 (19%) patients with inducible ventricular tachycardia

($p<0.05$). Those without inducible tachycardia would be less likely to have a chronic substrate for the induction of ventricular arrhythmias. In these patients it is more likely to assume that acute ischemia led to an episode of ischemic ventricular tachycardia/ventricular fibrillation. Therefore, these data indicate a higher incidence of complex lesions on angiography in survivors of sudden death. However, both studies excluded patients with acute infarction – a group with a high incidence of complex lesions on angiography and at autopsy. It is likely that the exclusion of these patients in addition to other obvious differences in patient selection are responsible for the lower incidence of complex lesions on angiography after sudden cardiac death when compared to more recent autopsy studies.

Differences Between Acute Coronary Syndromes

If plaque disruption with thrombus formation is common to all the syndromes, how are they different? There are several possible explanations for these clinical differences. More than one factor is likely responsible for a given clinical presentation. These several possibilities include the following:

1. The degree of narrowing in the artery prior to the onset of the acute syndrome
2. The degree of narrowing following the onset of the acute syndrome
3. The acuteness of the obstruction
4. The duration of decreased perfusion, which may be translated into the duration of total coronary occlusion
5. Embolization of thrombotic material or platelet aggregates to the distal circulation
6. The ability acutely to recruit collaterals following occlusion
7. Myocardial oxygen demands

Degree of Coronary Artery Narrowing Prior to the Onset of the Acute Syndrome

There are few angiographic data to support the possibility that differences in the degree of coronary artery narrowing prior to the onset of an acute syndrome are primarily responsible for the particular syndrome. Serial angiographic studies in selected patients before and after an episode of either unstable angina or myocardial infarction have shown less than 50% narrowing in the majority of patients. As mentioned previously, some patients following a bout of unstable angina or non-Q-wave infarction have total occlusion of the "culprit lesion" on angiography. It is likely that in most of these patients severe narrowing of the "culprit lesion" preceeded the onset of the syndrome. Collaterals forming distal to the occlusion limited or prevented myocardial necrosis.

Degree of Narrowing Following the Onset of the Syndrome

In support of this premise is the fact that most patients undergoing angiography early after Q-wave infarction have total occlusion of the infarct-related vessel while in unstable angina total occlusion of the ischemia-related vessel is unusual. The incidence of total occlusion in non-Q-wave infarction is greater than that found in unstable angina but less than that seen in Q-wave myocardial infarction. However, this alone seems unlikely to explain the differences between syndromes, as transient decreases in perfusion are common to all syndromes and represent the major mechanism of ischemia.

Acuteness of Coronary Artery Obstruction

Clinically, most patients presenting with any one of these syndromes have an acute onset of symptoms. An acute total obstruction of a coronary artery which previously had a less than critical lesion would be likely to cause transmural infarction if the obstruction was prolonged. In this situation there would be little time for the recruitment of collaterals to limit the amount of myocardial necrosis. On the other hand, in unstable angina while the clinical presentation is often acute there are some pathologic data suggesting a more subacute course. Layering of thrombus at the site of plaque disruption is commonly found in patients with a history of unstable angina who develop coronary thrombosis and ultimately die [52]. It is possible that in some patients with unstable angina there is at first a change in geometry of the lesion following plaque disruption with thrombus forming under the fibrous cap of the plaque. This may be followed, at a later timer, by further thrombus formation which is possibly intraluminal. When the mass of thrombus reaches a critical size or when the lumen is significantly narrowed, symptoms may occur. Additionally, altered flow patterns caused by a critically narrowed stenosis may predispose to thrombus formation distal to the lesion. This is obviously an oversimplification of a very complex process which also includes changes in vasomotor tone and possibly embolization of thrombotic debris distal to the original site of thrombus formation as causes of ischemia.

Based on the positive response of coronary lesions to thrombolysis in acute myocardial infarction (i.e., reperfusion in about 70% of patients with total coronary occlusion) and the usually negative or only mildly successful results of thrombolysis in unstable angina, especially when the "culprit lesion" is less than 100% occluded, the amount of fresh intraluminal thrombus may be an important determinant of how acutely the obstruction develops [53]. In unstable angina there is usually little fresh intraluminal thrombus while in acute myocardial infarction intraluminal thrombus is more abundant. Acute closure in this latter group causes extensive infarction. This difference in the amount of acute intraluminal thrombus formation may be related to factors mentioned previously such as the rate of thrombus formation following plaque disruption or the location of thrombus (i.e., in unstable angina under the fibrous cap while intraluminally in myocardial infarction). Finally, differences in the amount of thrombus could be related to the degree of plaque disruption. A superficial plaque fissure or ulcer may be responsible for some cases of unstable angina while a disruption into the media may cause myocardial infarction. In this situation in unstable angina there is only a small amount of intraluminal thrombus which is intermittent and responsible for episodes of ischemia [2].

Duration of Total Coronary Occlusion

There are inferential data that the duration of coronary occlusion is an important factor in determining the clinical syndrome. Duration of total occlusion is the expression of the pathophysiologic events of plaque disruption with thrombus formation and altered vasomotor tone. The higher incidence of patent infarct-related vessels early after non-Q-wave infarction when compared to Q-wave infarction is likely related to spontaneous reperfusion in the former group of patients. Furthermore, early peaking of creatine phosphokinase in non-Q-wave infarction, which is similar to that seen following successful thrombolysis in Q-wave infarction, also supports the theory of a shorter duration of coronary artery occlusion in most patients with non-Q-wave infarction when compared to Q-wave myocardial infarction [54]. Likewise, in unstable angina with rest pain an even shorter duration of decreased coronary perfusion is responsible for the absence of myocardial necrosis. Recurrent cycles of occlusion/reperfusion have been found in some patients with acute infarction and could represent an important determinant of the amount of ischemia or myocardial necrosis following plaque disruption [55].

Recruitable Collaterals

Visible collaterals at angiography require the presence of a severe (usually $>90\%$) diameter narrowing in a coronary artery creating a pressure gradient between the distal vascular bed and other vessels [56]. Collaterals are preformed, anastamotic channels which dilate and become functional as the need arises. Early angiography after myocardial infarction with total coronary occlusion reveals collaterals to the distal vasculature in a minority of cases [57]. This probably is related to the rate of coronary obstruction, which may be too rapid in most cases of Q-wave infarction with total occlusion to open these vessels acutely. In unstable angina and non-Q-wave infarction with total coronary occlusion, collaterals are usually present at early angiography. As previously mentioned, these patients likely had a severe, preexisting lesion in the vessel that subsequently occluded.

Distal Embolization

Pathologic studies in patients dying suddenly from ischemic heart disease have often shown evidence of embolization of thrombotic debris or platelet aggregrates to the distal vascular bed [58, 59]. These emboli occur only distal to a plaque disruption with intraluminal thrombus formation and are closely associated with the presence of microscopic myocardial necrosis distributed throughout the thickness of the ventricular wall. While a cause-and-effect mechanism between platelet embolization and sudden death is pure speculation, a terminal ventricular arrhythmia could be precipitated by this or any other cause of myocardial necrosis. In vivo data supporting this possibility are not available. As far as I know, there have been no angiographic studies relating distal embolization to the appearance of ventricular fibrillation during angioplasty. Distal embolization has also been suggested, as mentioned previously, as a possible cause of rest ischemia in some patients with unstable angina.

Myocardial Oxygen Demands

There are few recent data suggesting that increased myocardial oxygen demand is an important pathogenetic mechanism in unstable angina or myocardial infarction. However, increased oxygen demands may be responsible for bouts of rest ischemia in unstable angina. Slight but significant increases in pressure-rate product have been recently reported by Langer et al. in some patients before an episode of ischemia in unstable angina [60]. While an acute lesion may be responsible for causing the particular syndrome, it must be recalled that there is a delicate balance between coronary blood supply and myocardial oxygen demand. Increasing demand can precipitate ischemia when coronary perfusion is limited.

One final point concerning these possible differences between syndromes must be reemphasized. Just as the clinical presentations represent a continuous spectrum of ischemia from unstable angina through Q-wave infarction and sudden death, these proposed pathophysiologic mechanisms are not all-or-none phenomena. The interaction between a number of the above factors is likely responsible for the expression of a particular clinical syndrome.

Conclusions

In this article, I have reviewed the angiographic findings in the acute coronary syndromes. While they share in the majority of cases a common pathologic substrate, the clinical expression of plaque disruption with thrombus is variable. Angiographic evaluation of the coronary arteries in each syndrome is similar, with a majority of cases showing the typical appearance of acute or complex lesions. The incidence of total coronary occlusion increases as the degree or amount of ischemia/infarction increases. In many patients with either unstable angina or myocardial infarction, progression of coronary disease occurs from lesions that were less than significant on prior angiography. Variability in the acuteness of obstruction which may be related to the amount of fresh intracoronary thrombus formation and differences in the duration of total coronary occlusion may explain this clinical variation. The precise mechanisms as to how plaque disruption leads to sudden death in the absence of myocardial infarction remains unclear at present.

References

1. Gorlin R, Fuster V, Ambrose JA (1986) Anatomic physiologic links between acute coronary syndromes. Circulation 74:6–9
2. Fuster V, Badimon L, Cohen M, Ambrose JA, Badimon JJ (1988) Insights into the pathogenesis of acute ischemic syndromes. Circulation 77:1213–1220
3. Hoberg E, Katus HA, Diederich KW, Kubler W (1987) Myoglobin, creatine kinase-B isoenzyme, and myosin light chain release in patients with unstable angina pectoris. Eur Heart J 8:989–994
4. Alison HW, Russel RO Jr, Mantle JA, Kouchoukos NT, Moraski RE, Rackley CE (1978) Coronary anatomy and arteriography in patients with unstable angina pectoris. Am J Cardiol 41:204–209
5. Fuster V, Frye RL, Connolly DC, Danielson MA, Elveback LR, Kurland LT (1975) Arteriographic patterns early in the onset of the coronary syndromes. Br Heart J 37:1250–1255
6. Plotnick GD, Greene HL, Carliner NH, Becker LC, Fisher ML (1979) Clinical indicators of left main coronary artery disease in unstable angina. Ann Intern Med 91:149–153
7. Victor MF, Likoff MJ, Mintz GS, Likoff W (1981) Unstable angina pectoris of new onset: a prospective clinical and arteriographic study of 75 patients. Am J Cardiol 47:228–232
8. Conti CR, Brawley RK, Griffith LSC, Pitt B, Humphries JO, Gott VL, Ross RS (1973) Unstable angina pectoris: morbidity and mortality in 57 consecutive patients evaluated angiographically. Am J Cardiol 32:745–750
9. Bertolasi CA, Tronge JE, Mon GA, Turri D, Lugones MI (1979) Clinical spectrum of "unstable angina". Clin Cardiol 2:113–120
10. Moise A, Theroux P, Taeymans Y, Descoings B, Lesperance J, Waters DD, Pelletier GB, Bourassa MG (1983) Unstable angina and progression of coronary atherosclerosis. N Engl J Med 309:685–689
11. Ambrose JA, Winters SL, Arora RR, Eng A, Riccio A, Gorlin R, Fuster V (1986) Angiographic evolution of coronary artery morphology in unstable angina. J Am Coll Cardiol 7:472–478
12. Gould KL (1980) Dynamic coronary stenosis. Am J Cardiol 45:286–292
13. Ambrose JA, Winters SL, Stern A, Eng A, Teichholz LE, Gorlin R, Fuster V (1985) Angiographic morphology and the pathogenesis of unstable angina pectoris. J Am Coll Cardiol 5:609–616
14. Williams AE, Freeman MR, Chisholm RJ, Patt NL, Armstrong PW (1988) Angiographic morphology in unstable angina pectoris. Am J Cardiol 62:1024–1027
15. Haft JI, Goldstein JE, Niemiera ML (1987) Coronary arteriographic lesion of unstable angina. Chest 92:609–612
16. DeZwaan C, Bar FW, Janssen JHA, DeSwart HB, Vermeer F, Wellens HJJ (1988) Effects of thrombolytic therapy in unstable angina: clinical and angiographic results. J Am Coll Cardiol 12:301–309
17. Levin DC, Fallon JT (1982) Significance of the angiographic morphology of localized coronary stenosis. Histopathologic correlations. Circulation 66:316–320
18. Wilson RF, Holida MD, White CW (1986) Quantitative angiographic morphology of coronary stenosis leading to myocardial infarction or unstable angina. Circulation 73:286–293

19. Suryapranata H, deFeyter PJ, Serruys PW (1988) Coronary angioplasty in patients with unstable angina pectoris: is there a role for thrombolysis? J Am Coll Cardiol 12 [Suppl A]:69A–77A
20. Cowley MJ, DiSciascio G, Rehr RB, Vetrovec GW (1989) Angiographic observations and clinical relevance of coronary thrombus in unstable angina pectoris. Am J Cardiol 63:108E–113E
21. Freeman MR, Williams AE, Chisholm RJ, Armstrong PW (1989) Intracoronary thrombus and complex morphology in unstable angina. Relation to timing of angiography and in-hospital cardiac events. Circulation 80:17–23
22. Ambrose JA (1989) Coronary arteriographic analysis and angiographic morphology. J Am Coll Cardiol 13:1492–1494
23. Rutherford JD, Braunwald E, Cohn PF (1988) Chronic ischemic heart disease. In: Braunwald E (ed) Heart disease: a textbook of cardiovascular medicine, 3rd edn. Saunders, Philadelphia, p 1355
24. Ambrose JA, Hjemdahl-Monsen CE (1987) Arteriographic anatomy and mechanisms of myocardial ischemia in unstable angina. J Am Coll Cardiol 9:1397–1402
25. Ambrose JA, Hjemdahl-Monsen CE, Borrico S, Gorlin R, Fuster V (1988) Angiographic demonstration of a common link between unstable angina pectoris and non-Q wave acute myocardial infarction. Am J Cardiol 61:244–247
26. Sansa M, Cernigliaro C, Bolognese L, Bongo SA, Rossi L, Rossi P (1988) Angiographic morphology and response to therapy in unstable angina. Clin Cardiol 11:121–126
27. Ellis S, Alderman EL, Cain K, Wright A, Bourassa M, Fisher L (1989) Morphology of left anterior descending coronary territory lesions as a predictor of anterior myocardial infarction: a CASS Registry study. J Am Coll Cardiol 13:1481–1491
28. Ogawa H, Hiramori K, Haze K, Saito M, Sumiyoshi T, Fukami K, Goto Y, Ikeda M (1985) Classification of non-Q-wave myocardial infarction according to electrocardiographic changes. Br Heart J 54:473–478
29. Huey BL, Gheorghiade M, Crampton RS, Beller GA, Kaiser DL, Watson DD, Nygaard TW, Craddock GB, Sayre SL, Gibson RS (1987) Acute non-Q wave myocardial infarction associated with early ST segment elevation: evidence for spontaneous coronary reperfusion and implications for thrombolytic trials. J Am Coll Cardiol 9:18–25
30. Freifeld AG, Schuster EH, Bulkley BH (1983) Nontransmural versus transmural myocardial infarction. A morphologic study. Am J Med 75:423–432
31. DeWood MA, Stifter WF, Simpson CS, Spores J, Eugster GS, Judge TP, Hinnen ML (1986) Coronary arteriographic findings soon after non-Q wave myocardial infarction. N Engl J Med 315:417–423
32. Little WC, Workman R, Burrows M, Kahl FR, Kutcher MA, Santamore WP, Applegate R (1989) Coronary anatomy preceding non-Q wave myocardial infarction (abstr). J Am Coll Cardiol 13:6A
33. Ambrose JA, Tannenbaum MA, Alexopoulos D, Hjemdahl-Monsen CE, Leavy J, Weiss M, Borrico S, Gorlin R, Fuster V (1988) Angiographic progression of coronary artery disease and the development of myocardial infarction. J Am Coll Cardiol 12:56–62
34. DeWood MA, Spores J, Notske R, Mouser LT, Burroughs R, Golden MS, Lang HT (1980) Prevalence of total coronary occlusion during the early hours of transmural myocardial infarction. N Engl J Med 303:897–902
35. Ambrose JA, Winters SL, Arora RR, Haft JI, Goldstein J, Rentrop KP, Gorlin R, Fuster V (1985) Coronary angiographic morphology in myocardial infarction: a link between the pathogenesis of unstable angina and myocardial infarction. J Am Coll Cardiol 6:1233–1238
36. Little WC, Constantinescu M, Applegate RJ, Kutcher MA, Burrows MT, Kahl FR, Santamore WP (1988) Can coronary angiography predict the site of a subsequent myocardial infarction in patients with mild-to-moderate coronary artery disease? Circulation 78:1157–1166
37. Hackett D, Davies G, Maseri A (1988) Pre-existing coronary stenoses in patients with first myocardial infarction are not necessarily severe. Eur Heart J 9:1317–1323
38. Davies MJ, Thomas AC (1985) Plaque fissuring – the cause of acute myocardial infarction, sudden ischaemic death, and crescendo angina. Br Heart J 53:363–373
39. Moise A, Lesperance J, Theroux P, Taeymans Y, Goulet C, Bourassa MG (1984) Clinical and

angiographic predictors of a new total coronary occlusion in coronary artery disease: analysis of 313 non-operated patients. Am J Cardiol 54:1176–1181
40. Ellis S, Alderman E, Cain K, Fisher L, Sanders W, Bourassa M, CASS Investigators (1988) Prediction of risk of anterior myocardial infarction by lesion severity and measurement method of stenoses in the left anterior descending coronary distribution: a CASS Registry study. J Am Coll Cardiol 11:908–916
41. Neill WA, Wharton TP, Fluri-Lundeen J, Cohen IS (1980) Acute coronary insufficiency – coronary occlusion after intermittent ischemic attacks. N Engl J Med 302:1157–1162
42. Roberts WC, Buja LM (1972) The frequency and significance of coronary arterial thrombi and other observations in fatal acute myocardial infarction. Am J Med 52:425–443
43. Warnes CA, Roberts WC (1984) Sudden coronary death: relation of amount and distribution of coronary narrowing at necropsy to previous symptoms of myocardial ischemia, left ventricular scarring and heart weight. Am J Cardiol 54:65–73
44. Davies MJ, Thomas AC (1984) Thrombosis and acute coronary artery lesions in sudden cardiac ischaemic death. N Engl J Med 310:1137–1140
45. Falk E (1989) Morphologic features of unstable atherothrombotic plaques underlying acute coronary syndromes. Am J Cardiol 63:114E–120E
46. Davies MJ, Bland JM, Hangartner JRW, Angelini A, Thomas AC (1989) Factors influencing the presence or absence of acute coronary artery thrombi in sudden ischaemic death. Eur Heart J 10:203–208
47. Cobb LA, Werner JA, Trobaugh GB (1980) Sudden cardiac death. I. A decade's experience with out-of-hospital resuscitation. II. Outcome of resuscitation, management, and future directions. Mod Concepts Cardiovasc Dis 49:31–42
48. Goldstein S, Landis JR, Leighton R, Ritter G, Vasu M, Lantis A, Serokman R (1981) Characteristics of the resuscitated out-of-hospital cardiac arrest victim with coronary heart disease. Circulation 64:977–984
49. Weaver WD, Lorch GS, Alvarez HA, Cobb LA (1976) Angiographic findings and prognostic indicators in patients resuscitated from sudden cardiac death. Circulation 54:895–900
50. Stevenson WG, Wiener I, Yeatman L, Wohlgelernter D, Weiss JN (1988) Complicated atherosclerotic lesions: a potential cause of ischemic ventricular arrhythmias in cardiac arrest survivors who do not have inducible ventricular tachycardia? Am Heart J 116:1–6
51. Lo Y-SA, Cutler JE, Blake K, Wright AM, Kron J, Swerdlow CD (1988) Angiographic coronary morphology in survivors of cardiac arrest. Am Heart J 115:781–785
52. Falk E (1985) Unstable angina with fatal outcome: dynamic coronary thrombosis leading to infarction and/or sudden death. Circulation 71:699–708
53. Ambrose JA, Alexopoulos D (1989) Thrombolysis in unstable angina: will the beneficial effects of thrombolytic therapy in myocardial infarction apply to patients with unstable angina? J Am Coll Cardiol 13:1666–1671
54. Gibson RS (1987) Clinical, functional and angiographic distinctions between Q wave and non-Q wave myocardial infarction: evidence of spontaneous reperfusion and implications for intervention trials. Circulation 75 [Suppl V]: V–128–V–138
55. Hackett D, Davies G, Chierchia S, Maseri A (1987) Intermittent occlusion in acute myocardial infarction. Value of combined thrombolytic and vasodilator therapy. N Engl J Med 317:1055–1059
56. Levin DC (1974) Pathways and functional significance of the coronary collateral circulation. Circulation 50:831–837
57. Cohen M, Sherman W, Rentrop KP, Gorlin R (1989) Determinants of collateral filling observed during sudden controlled coronary artery occlusion in human subjects. J Am Coll Cardiol 13:297–303
58. Davies MJ, Thomas AC, Knapman PA, Hangartner JR (1986) Intramyocardial platelet aggregation in patients with unstable angina suffering sudden ischemic cardiac death. Circulation 73:418–427
59. Haerem JW (1972) Platelet aggregates in intramyocardial vessels of patients dying suddenly and unexpectedly of coronary artery disease. Atherosclerosis 15:199–213
60. Langer A, Freeman MR, Armstrong PW (1989) ST segment shift in unstable angina: pathophysiology and association with coronary anatomy and hospital outcome. J Am Coll Cardiol 13:1495–1502

The Value of Coronary Endoscopy in Patients with Stable and Unstable Angina Pectoris

V. Hombach, M. Höher, M. Kochs, T. Eggeling, A. Schmidt, W. Haerer, and S. Wieshammer [1]

Introduction

Coronary angiography is the method of choice for documenting the extent and degree of coronary atherosclerotic lesions. Estimating lesion length and degree of stenosis (diameter and cross-section) provides qualitative and quantitative data for estimating the impairment of coronary flow distal to the stenotic coronary artery [2]. However, coronary angiography provides little information about the nature and surface of atherosclerotic plaques, and particularly about additional pathoanatomical processes at the site of the atheroma [1, 25, 27]. Some pathoanatomical postmortem studies have shown that in about 60%–70% of patients with myocardial infarctions thrombotic processes, fissures, and dissections of the atherosclerotic plaques may be present and may account for occlusion of a coronary vessel [3, 4, 6, 7]. Thus, it seems valuable from a clinical point of view to use endoscopic methods to visualize directly the atherosclerotic lesion for documenting such complications.

Cardiac endoscopy is not a recently developed investigational tool (Table 1) [9, 11, 15, 26, 33, 38]. The direct endoscopic imaging of endovascular atherosclerotic processes was first presented by Greenstone et al. 1966 [9] in an animal

Table 1. History of angioscopy

1913	Rhea and Walker	Metal tube with lens
1936	Sakakibara	Saline flushing
1951	Butterworth	Rigid fiberscope
1966	Greenstone et al.	Flexible fiberscope
1969	Vollmar	Intraoperative angioscopy
1982	Lee	Angioscopically controlled laser angioplasty in dogs
1983	Spears et al.	Percutaneous angioscopy of occluded coronary vessels
1985	Höher et al.	Percutaneous angioscopy of peripheral arteries in the catheterization laboratory
1986	Hombach et al.	Percutaneous coronary angioscopy in the catheterization laboratory
1987	Forrester et al.	Percutaneous coronary angioscopy in the catheterization laboratory
1986	Sherman et al.	Angioscopy in patients with unstable angina

[1] Abteilung Innere Medizin IV, Medizinische Universitätsklinik und Poliklinik, Robert-Koch-Strasse 8, 7900 Ulm, West Germany

W. Bleifeld et al. (Eds.)
Unstable Angina

model. Since that time several groups have used this technique during vascular surgical procedures [38, 39]. In recent years new fiberoptic technologies have enabled the production of ultrathin and flexible fiberscopes with diameters of under 1 mm. Applications of endovascular fiberoptic studies in the catheter laboratory have been reported by Höher and coworkers [11] for peripheral vessels and most recently by Hombach et al. [15] and Forrester et al. [5] for coronary arteries. Due to improvements in endoscopic technology it is now feasible to perform endovascular endoscopy in coronary arteries and peripheral arteries both in the operating room and in the catheterization laboratory [5, 10–12, 13, 15, 18, 20, 30, 39].

Clinical Applications of Coronary Endoscopy

There are many questions that can be answered by direct endoscopic visualization and many clinical situations, in which coronary endoscopy may help to improve and confirm special therapeutic interventions. It may also help to preselect certain methods of angioplasty for specific treatment of different types of coronary artery stenoses. These special indications of coronary endoscopy (Table 2) are discussed briefly below.

Characterization of Coronary Atherosclerotic Lesions

For several decades early in this century researchers questioned the role of occluding coronary thrombus in the development of acute myocardial infarction. From the extensive pathoanatomical postmortem studies of Davies et al.

Table 2. Clinical applications of coronary angioscopy

Characterization of the atherosclerotic lesion
– Criteria in addition to angiography
– Pathophysiology of the different anginal syndromes
Control of coronary angioplasty
– Selection of different angioplasty techniques, depending on gross anatomy of the plaque
– Direct visual control of the effect of the angioplasty technique (balloon, radiofrequency, laser)
Control during coronary artery bypass surgery
– Native coronary artery to be by-passed
– Proximal and distal bypass anastomosis
Visual guidance of new angioplasty techniques
– Radiofrequency angioplasty
– Laser angioplasty
– Atherectomy

[3], Fulton [7], and Friedman [6] it became apparent that complications such as fissures, dissections, and bleeding into the disrupted atheroma are associated in a high percentage of cases with partially or totally occluding coronary thrombi. Therefore, these authors maintained that an acute myocardial infarction may be induced by an active and progressive process at the site and within the atheroma itself, which may induce thrombus formation with the potential of obstructing the vessel. These studies have been confirmed by results of coronary endoscopy in living humans, both by Forrester and coworkers [5] and by our own group [15, 17, 18]. In the first series of coronary endoscopic studies Sherman and coworkers [33] investigated a total of 27 coronary arteries, 17 in patients with stable and 10 in patients with unstable angina. In none of the 17 coronary segments of patients with stable angina was a complicated plaque found. On the other hand, in the ten coronary segments of patients with unstable angina three were found to have fissures or dissections, and another seven revealed thrombus formation on the plaque.

Based on these results, Forrester and coworkers described the so-called ulceration-thrombosis cycle [5, 20]. They noted that results from pathoanatomical studies and from coronary endoscopy show patients with stable angina to have a stable smooth atheroma. When an ulceration of the atheroma occurs, the patient may reveal an accelerated angina, and with further platelet aggregation he may develop sudden cardiac death or ischemic cardiomyopathy. These lesions may heal, and the healing process may be accompanied by a progression of the stenosis. If, on the other hand, the ulceration of the atheroma is partially covered by thrombus, the patient may develop the clinical syndrome of unstable angina. If the thrombus continues to grow and occludes the artery, the patient can develop myocardial infarction. Due to spontaneous lysis or medical (interventional) thrombolysis the occluded vessel may be recanalized; the lesion then heals, and the patient may again develop a stable smooth atheroma.

These results have been confirmed by our own group in 41 patients studied intraoperatively or in the catheterization laboratory. In none of the 18 patients with stable angina was a complication of the atheroma seen, whereas in six out of eight patients with unstable angina ulceration or thrombus formation was observed at the site of the atheroma during coronary endoscopy (Fig. 1). These differences were statistically significant [18]. Therefore, at present it seems evident that the coronary atherosclerotic process is a continuous and progressive process presenting with smooth atheroma, dissections, ulcerations, and partial or occluding thrombus. This does not rule out that neurohumoral control of the coronary artery tone plays another significant role in modulating the clinical picture of the angina pectoris syndrome. A dissected and ulcerated atheroma accounts for more localized or sometimes diffuse endothelial damage, resulting in liberation of vasoactive substances such as thromboxane A_2. Thus, coronary vasoconstriction and acceleration of thrombus formation may be induced by these endothelial factors. Emotional stress, exercise, and smoking may also modulate coronary vascular tone and thus aggravate the anginal syndrome of the patient [18].

Table 3. Characterization of the coronary atherosclerotic lesion: angioscopic criteria

Pattern
– Local
– Diffuse
Shape
– Eccentric (regular, irregular)
– Concentric (regular, irregular)
Structure
– Smooth atheroma
– Thrombus
– Calcified lesion
Complication of the atheroma
– Fissure
– Dissection
– Ulcer
– Thrombus at the surface

These results demonstrate the importance of angioscopic characterization of the coronary atherosclerotic lesion (Table 3). They also appear to justify present therapeutic policy in patients with unstable angina and acute myocardial infarction, i.e., prevention of coronary vasoconstriction by the administration of coronary dilatory drugs such as nitrates and calcium antagonists, prevention of thrombus formation by the administration of platelet inhibitors, and diminution of coronary thrombi by intravenous administration of thrombolytic agents [8, 36, 37, 40].

Control of Coronary Angioplasty

Worldwide experiences with balloon angioplasty indicates that coronary stenoses can be successfully dilated in 80%–90% of patients. There has been a long debate as to the mechanism of balloon angioplasty. The idea during the earliest stages of the development of percutaneous TCA was that the atheromatous material would be compressed by the inflated balloon. Later pathoanatomical studies have shown that this is not the only mechanism; dissection and disruption of the plaque with compression of the atheromatous material into the media of the arterial wall is a frequent mechanism in balloon angioplasty. Serious complications at the site of balloon inflation such as dissections followed by thrombotic occlusions occur in 2%–5% of cases, and in successfully treated patients the atherosclerotic lesions appear relatively smooth on angiographic imaging. It seems worthwhile to visualize directly the effect of balloon angioplasty as well as that of newer angioplasty techniques such as radiofrequency angioplasty [16, 19], laser thermal angioplasty [31], and laser angioplasty [23, 24].

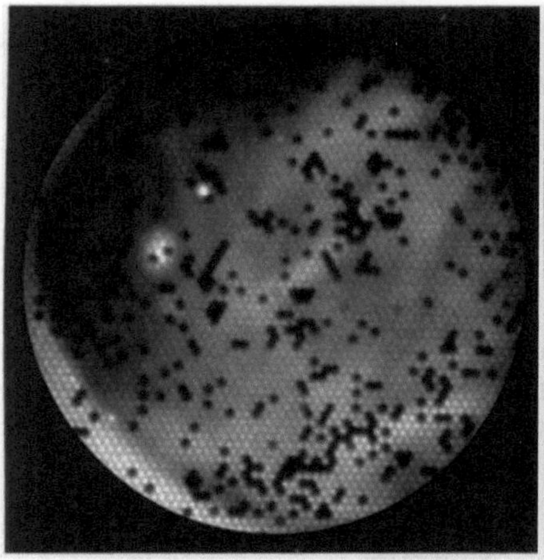

1

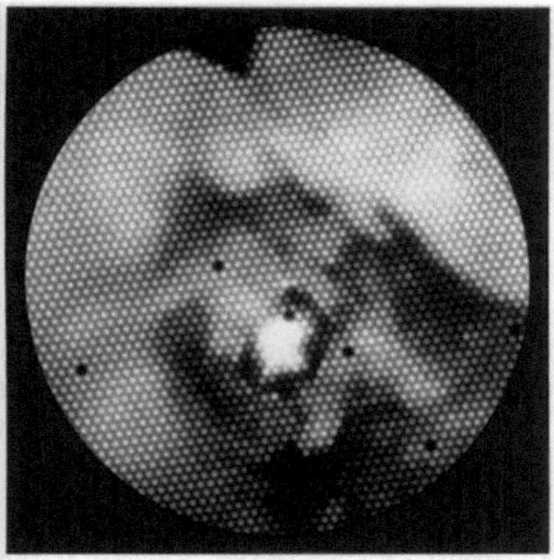

3

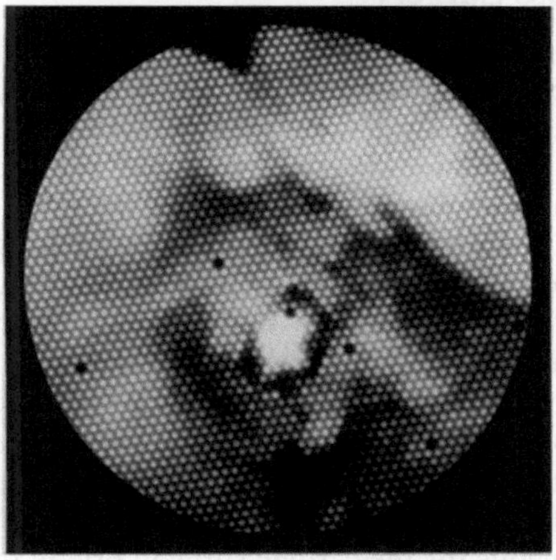

2

Fig. 1. Angioscopic view of a flat and extended thrombus covering an atherosclerotic coronary artery lesion of 80% stenosis (area reduction) in a patient with unstable angina. Note the numerous broken fibers of the angioscope

Fig. 2. Angioscopic control of recanalization in a thrombotically occluded vessel by radiofrequency angioplasty. Note the spherelike tip of the radiofrequency catheter, the broken parts of the thrombus around the catheter tip, and some slight thermal damage of the vascular endothelium (*darker areas*)

Fig. 3. Angioscopic view on the distal anastomosis of an LAD vein graft showing the sutures, and a severe atheromatous plaque at the insertion site of the saphenous vein graft (*right*)

In our series of 45 angioscopic studies in humans, eight angioscopic procedures were performed following balloon angioplasty. In six of eight studies good visualization was achieved, and in three of the six patients intimal disruptions with small flaps were seen through the angioscope, while the coronary vessel appeared angiographically smooth at the site of balloon inflation. There has as yet been no study of a large series of patients following angioplasty who were examined by both angiography and angioscopy. Therefore the diagnostic and prognostic significance of these initial findings is presently unclear. There is no doubt that particularly with the development and application of newer angioplasty techniques coronary angioscopy will play a major role in evaluating the in vivo effects of these techniques on coronary arteries (Fig. 2). Another question is whether coronary angioscopy may help before hand to determine the best interventional method, depending on the different types of lesions, for example, smooth atheroma for application of balloon angioplasty, complicated lesions with dissection and thrombus formation treated by radiofrequency angioplasty, laser thermal angioplasty, or laser angioplasty, and calcific stenoses by laser angioplasty. The results of angioplasty may there by be improved and the risk of to patients minimized.

Control of Coronary Artery Bypass Surgery

Another potential application of coronary angioscopy is in coronary artery bypass surgery. Generally, it is possible for the cardiac surgeon to visualize the proximal and distal anastomoses and the native coronary vessel beyond the site of the distal anastomosis. Sanborn and colleagues [32] reported on visualization in 10 of 11 proximal and in all 10 distal veingraft anastomoses during open-heart bypass surgery. These authors did not comment on the angioscopic appearance of the anastomoses but rather reported on small platelet-fibrin thrombi adherent to a valve in a saphenous vein. Our group has studied nine patients in whom angioscopy was performed intraoperatively. In eight of these good visualization of the distal anastomoses was achieved, and in all but one the anastomosis was free of atherosclerotic lesions. In only one patient was the distal anastomosis sutured within an atherosclerotic segment of the LAD graft (Fig. 3). Therefore, it may be advantageous for the cardiac surgeon briefly to visualize the native coronary artery at the site where the distal anastomosis is to be sutured. This may help to avoid misplacement, which may occur when the anastomosis site cannot be controlled sufficiently by external palpation or endoluminal probing.

Recently Grundfest and coworkers [10] have reported on the application of intraoperative angioscopy for deliniation of peripheral vascular anatomy. These authors obtained sufficient images in 73/86 procedures (85%). Changes in intraoperative management based on angioscopic findings included revision of 5/37 anastomoses, deletion of 4/31 completion angiograms, revision of 8/17 in situ venous valves, and repetition of thrombectomy in 6/7 cases. In 22/73 peripheral angioscopies potential causes of graft occlusion were recognized. These authors concluded that intraoperative angioscopy provides the potential for visual assessment of lumen patency and the quality of anastomotic surgery in preventing secondary occlusions of the bypass graft. It can be expected in the future that endovascular angioscopy both in the coronary and in the peripheral arteries will be performed routinely for improvement of the surgical procedure.

Visual Guidance of Newer Angioplastic Techniques

There are several reasons why alternative techniques are now being developed to complement or displace balloon angioplasty in some patients. These include the restenosis rate of 20%–30% in balloon angioplasties, traumatization of the coronary vessel by balloon inflation, and production of intimal dissections of the dilated vessel. Up to now these new angioplastic techniques (see above) have generally been controlled by coronary angiography. Only one group has evaluated lesions after laser application by performing coronary angioscopy [24]. The use of radiofrequency or laser energies on coronary atherosclerotic lesions could perhaps be controlled and directed by simultaneous angioscopic inspection. At present none of the groups performing angioplasty has reported on simultaneous application of angioscopy and angioplasty in humans. In the future, however, complex catheters will probably be developed that offer angulation, endoscopic visualization, and energy delivery facilities, so that local energy application can be directly controlled by angioscopy.

Limitations of Coronary Angioscopy

There are a number of limitations of coronary angioscopy when applied in the catheterization laboratory (Table 4). A major limitation is that the angioscope can not be guided and angulated intraluminally. Flushing facilities are unsatisfactory by the present method, which is to be improved by our group. A special guiding and flushing catheter has been developed that can be advanced selectively into the affected coronary artery. The thin coronary angioscope can be placed endoluminally into the region of interest. The lumen of the regional guiding catheter is sufficiently large to remove the blood completely without complete obstruction of the main stem of the left or right coronary arteries by the coronary angiography catheter. Moreover, the examination time is limited to 10–30 s. This means that in some patients two or more approaches must be performed in the catheterization laboratory to obtain sufficient visualization of the stenosed coronary artery. Another limitation is the fragility of the angioscopes, which requires careful handling during the entire angioscopic procedure.

Table 4. Limitations of coronary angioscopy

- Poor intraluminal guidance of the angioscope
- No facility of active rotation or angulation of the angioscope tip
- Difficult flushing facilities in the area of interest
- Exact quantification of stenoses impossible
- Examination time limited to 10–30 s
- Fragility of the angioscope

Perspectives of Coronary Angioscopy

In the future several technical improvements can be expected, and we are confident that coronary angioscopy will become a very important additional diagnostic tool for determining the true nature of atherosclerotic lesions, the status of the atherosclerotic process, the selection of angioplasty-technique, and the control of the mechanism of these techniques, and that they will permit the direct visual guidance of newer angioplasty techniques such as radiofrequency and laser angioplasty.

References

1. Ambrose JA, Winters SL, Arora RR, Eng A, Riccio A, Gorlin R, Furster V (1986) Angiographic evolution of coronary artery morphology in unstable angina. J Am Coll Cardiol 7:472–478
2. Brown BG, Petersen RB, Piece DC, Bolson EL, Dodge HT (1983) Arteriographic assessment of coronary disease: advantages, limitations, and clinical uses of a computer-assisted method. In: Rapaport E (ed) Cardiology update, reviews for physicians. Elsevier, New York, p 67
3. Davies MJ, Thomas AC (1985) Plaque fissuring – the cause of acute myocardial infarction, sudden ischaemic death, and crescendo angina. Br Heart J 53:363–373
4. Falk E (1983) Plaque rupture with severe pre-existing stenoses precipitating coronary thrombosis. Br Heart J 50:127–334
5. Forrester JS, Litvack F, Grundfest W, Hickey A (1987) A perspective of coronary disease seen through the arteries of living man. Circulation 75:505–513
6. Friedman M (1967) The coronary canalized thrombus: prevalence, structure, function and relationship to death due to coronary artery disease. Br J Exp Pathol 48:556
7. Fulton WFM (1987) Koronaratherosklerose, Fissurbildung der Plaque und Thrombose. In: De Bono DP, Brochier ML, Hugenholtz PG, Kübler W, Verstraete M (eds) Thrombolytische Therapie des akuten Herzinfarkts. Springer, Berlin Heidelberg New York, pp 9–39
8. Gold HK, Johns JA, Leinbach RC, Yasuda T, Collen D (1987) Thrombolytic therapy for unstable angina pectoris: rationale and results. J Am Coll Cardiol 10:91B–95B
9. Greenstone SM, Shore JM, Heringman EC, Massel TB (1966) Arterial endoscopy (arterioscopy). Arch Surg 93:811–812
10. Grundfest WS, Litvack F, Glick D, Segalowitz J, Treiman R, Cohen L, Foran R, Levin P, Cossman D, Carroll R, Spigelman A, Forrester JS (1988) Intraoperative decisions based on angioscopy in peripheral vascular surgery. Circulation [Suppl I] 78:I–13–17
11. Höher M, Behrenbeck DW, Winter UJ, Hombach V, Hilger HH (1985) Perkutane Gefäßendoskopie mittels ultradünner Fiberendoskope. Z Kardiol 74 [Suppl 3]:99
12. Höher M, Hombach V, Höpp HW, Eggeling T, Kochs M, Arnold G, Hannekum A, Hügel W (1988) Diagnostic potential of angioscopy in patients with coronary heart disease. Z Kardiol 77:152–159
13. Höher M, Hombach V, Hannekum A, Hügel W, Höpp HW, Hirche H (1988) Coronary angioscopy during cardiac catheterization and cardiac surgery. Int J Cardiol Imag 3:153–157
14. Holmes Dr Jr, Hartzler GO, Smith HC, Fuster V (1981) Coronary artery thrombosis in patients with unstable angina. Br Heart J 45:411–416
15. Hombach V, Höher M, Hannekum A, Hügel W, Buran B, Höpp HW, Hirche H (1986) First clinical experiences with coronary endoscopy. Dtsch Med Wochenschr 111:1135
16. Hombach V, Höher M, Arnold G, Osypka P, Kochs M, Eggeling T, Höpp HW, Hirche H, Hilger HH (1987) High frequency angioplasty – a new method for recanalization of occluded arterial vessels. Cor Vas 2:67

17. Hombach V, Höher M, Höpp HW, Kochs M, Eggeling T, Hannekum A, Hügel W, Hilger HH (1988) The clinical significance of coronary angioscopy in patients with coronary heart disease. Surg Endosc 2:1–4
18. Hombach V, Höher M, Kochs M, Eggeling T, Schmidt A, Höpp HW, Hilger HH (1988) Pathophysiology of unstable angina pectoris – correlation with coronary angioscopic imaging. Eur Heart J 9 [Suppl N]:40–45
19. Hombach V, Höher M, Höpp HW, Kochs M, Eggeling T, Osypka P, Hilger HH (1988) High-frequency current angioplasty in coronary heart disease preliminary results. Dtsch Med Wochenschr 113:801–805
20. Jakubowski A, Hickey A, Glick D, Litvack F, Grundfest W, Forrester JS (1989) Angioscopy. In: Issner J, Clarke R (ed) Cardiovascular laser therapy. Raven, New York, pp 201–212
21. Kakkar VV (1985) Atheroma and thrombosis. Pitman, London
22. Lee G, Garcia JM, Corso PJ, Chan MC, Rink JL, Pichard A, Lee KK, Reis RL, Mason DT (1986) Correlation of coronary angioscopic to angiographic findings in coronary artery disease. Am J Cardiol 58:238–241
23. Lee G, Ikeda RM, Chan MC, Lee MH, Rink JL, Reis RL, Theis JH, Low R, Bommer WJ, Kung AH, Hanna FS, Mason DT (1985) Limitations, risks and complications of laser recanalization. A cautious approach warranted. Am J Cardiol 56:181–185
24. Lee G, Ikeda RM, Stobbe D, Ogata C, Theis J, Hussein H, Mason DT (1983) Laser irradiation of human atherosclerotic obstructive disease. Simultaneous visualization and vaporisation achieved by a dual fiberoptic catheter. Am Heart J 105:163–164
25. Lichtlen PR (ed) (1979) Koronarangiographie. Perimed, Erlangen
26. Litvack F, Grundfest WS, Lee ME, Carroll RM, Foran R, Chaux A, Berci G, Rose HB, Matloff JM, Forrester JS (1985) Angioscopic visualization of blood vessel interior in animals and humans. Clin Cardiol 8:65–70
27. Litvack F, Hickey A, Grundfest W, Lee M, Sherman T, Doyle L, Chaux A, Blanche C, Kass R, Matloff J, Swan JHC, Forrester J (1986) Angioscopy is superior to angiography for detecting complex atheroma. Circulation [Suppl II] 74:II–362
28. Maseri A (1980) Pathogenetic mechanisms of angina pectoris: expanding views. Br Heart J 43:648–660
29. McGill HC Jr (1984) Persistent problems in the pathogenesis of atherosclerosis. Arteriosclerosis 4:443
30. Mizmo K, Arai T, Satomura K, Shibuya T, Arakawa K, Okamoto Y, Miyamoto A, Kurita A, Kikuchi M, Nakamura H, Utsumi A, Takendu K (1985) New percutaneous transluminal angioscope. J Am Coll Cardiol 13:363–368
31. Sanborn TA, Haudenschild CC, Garber GR, Ryan TJ, Faxon DP (1987) Angiographic and histologic consequences of laser and thermal angioplasty: comparison with balloon angioplasty. Circulation 75:1281–1286
32. Sanborn TA, Rygaard JA, Westbrook BM, Lazar HL, McCormick JR, Roberts AJ (1986) Intraoperative angioscopy of saphenous vein and coronary arteries. J Thorac Cardiovasc Surg 91:339–343
33. Sherman CT, Litvack F, Grundfest WS, Lee M, Hickey A, Chaux A, Kass R, Blanche C, Matloff J, Morgenstern L, Ganz W, Swan JHC, Forrester JS (1986) Demonstration of thrombus and complex atheroma by in-vivo angioscopy in patient with unstable angina pectoris. N Engl J Med 315:913–919
34. Spears JR, Marais JH, Serur JR, Pomerance O, Geyer RP, Sipzener RS, Weintraub R, Thurer R, Paulin S, Gerstin R, Grossman W (1983) In vivo coronary angioscopy. J Am Coll Cardiol 5:1311–1314
35. Spears JR, Spokojny Am, Marais JH (1985) Coronary angioscopy during cardiac catheterization. J Am Coll Cardiol 6:93–97
36. Vetrovec GW, Cowley MJ, Overton H, Richardson DW (1981) Intracoronary thrombus in syndromes of unstable myocardial ischemia. Am Heart J 102:1202–1208
37. Vetrovec GW, Leinbach RC, Gold HK, Cowley MJ (1982) Intracoronary thrombolysis in syndromes of unstable ischemia: angiographic and clinical results. Am Heart J 104:946–952
38. Vollmar JF, Storz LW (1974) Vascular endoscopy. Possibilities and limits of its clinical application. Surg Clin North Am 54:111–122

39. Wendt T, Müller T, Eckel L, Krause E, Rauber K, Riemann H, Sarai C, Satter P, Sievert H, Stauder M, Vallbracht C, Kober G, Kaltenbach M (1987) In-vivo-Angioskopie: Technik, Indikationen und Ergebnisse beim Menschen. Z Kardiol 76 [Suppl 1]: 51 (abstr)
40. van der Giessen WJ, Mooi W, Rutteman AM, van Vliet HHDM, Slager CJ, Verduow PD (1983) An new model for coronary thrombosis in the pig: preliminary results with thrombolysis. Eur Heart J4 [Suppl C]: 69–76

The Role of Coronary Vasomotion in the Pathophysiology of Unstable Angina

S. CHIERCHIA [1]

Introduction

In patients with unstable angina, selection of the most appropriate treatment is often difficult, as this syndrome encompasses a whole spectrum of clinical conditions whose pathophysiology may vary greatly.

The lack of "specificity" of the clinical diagnosis of unstable angina also applies to a large proportion of pathophysiological studies conducted in patients with this syndrome and to the majority of large scale clinical trials aimed at assessing the prognostic effects of various therapeutical interventions. Obviously, the prevalence of a given pathophysiological mechanism will depend upon the criteria used for patients' selection: the stricter and the more defined the latter and the more homogeneous the study population, the more prevalent a specific pathophysiological mechanism. As a direct consequence, the chance of a given therapeutical intervention to be effective will also increase.

The inherent bias related to the fact that the diagnosis of "unstable angina" bears no mechanistic implications and only carries clinical and, sometimes, prognostic significance, has so far limited our understanding of the factors responsible for the clinical forms grouped under the same denomination. This consideration should be kept well in mind when designing new pathophysiological studies, while interpreting clinical observations and, most importantly, when selecting patients for testing specific therapeutic hypotheses.

So far, the majority of pathophysiological studies conducted in patients with unstable angina have mainly focussed on four major aspects: 1. rapid progression of coronary atheroma; 2. increased tendency (localized or systemic) to develop thrombosis; 3. occurrence of mechanical complications of the atherosclerotic plaque (rupture or fissuring) and 4. abnormal vasomotor responses of the coronary circulation.

Although some or all of these factors may coexist in the same patient and may be difficult to separate in the clinical setting, their relative role is likely to be different in individual cases. Accordingly, an effort should be made in trying to identify the prevailing one(s) in an attempt to tailor therapeutic interventions to the specific needs of the individual patient rather than applying generalized, undiscriminating recipes.

[1] Divisione di Cardiologia, Ospedale San Raffaele, Via Olgettina, 60, 20132 Milano, Italy

W. Bleifeld et al. (Eds.)
Unstable Angina

The specific role of atheroma, thrombosis and plaque fissuring are discussed elsewhere in this book. In this chapter we will mainly concentrate on summarizing the evidence, derived from the literature and from our own experience, supporting the role of coronary vasomotion in the pathophysiology of unstable angina.

Coronary Vasomotor Tone in Epicardial Coronary Arteries

The notion that epicardial coronary arteries behave like passive, rigid conduits is no longer tenable. A large body of evidence now indicates that coronary arterial lumen and tone both result from the complex interplay of distending forces, elastic recoil, vasoconstrictor and vasodilator factors that, in turn, are all subject to a variety of haemodynamic, neural, humoral and intrinsic conditions. In particular, a host of physiological [1–3], pharmacological [4–7] and pathological [8, 9] stimuli, may all influence in a very dynamic fashion, medial smooth muscle tone and affect, sometimes dramatically, vascular cross-sectional area.

The consequences of changes in coronary smooth muscle tone on lumen diameter are, obviously, more important when involving arterial segments already narrowed by severe atherosclerotic obstructions and a tight pathophysiological relationship certainly exists, between excentric atheroma and occurrence of critical vasoconstriction [10].

The amount of coronary vasoconstriction sufficient to impair flow could be minimal if a vessel lumen were critically reduced by a severe subintimal lesion. Conversely, the increase in smooth muscle tone should be considerable, to impair flow in a normal vascular segment. On the basis of these considerations McAlpin suggested that occlusive "spasm" may actually result from normal, physiological changes in vasomotor tone when superimposed upon severe atheromatous lesions, whereas frankly abnormal vasoconstriction would be responsible for transient critical reductions in lumen size of normal arteries [11]. McAlpin's "geometric theory" has been contradicted by objective measurements [12] and, with the possible exception of patients with extremely severe, excentric lesions appears untenable for several other reasons.

First, in most patients with variant angina the disease alternates quiescent and active periods of activity: remissions and exacerbations are usually mirrored by a variable sensitivity to vasoconstrictors such as ergonovine and occur without detectable changes in the severity of coronary lesions. Second, episodes of variant angina usually exhibit a peculiar diurnal distribution with a peak in the early morning hours, and a trough during the daytime [13, 14]. That the distribution is similar in patients with angiographically normal coronary arteries and in those with severe disease suggests a similar pathophysiological mechanism, for both groups. Third, within the same patient, coronary spasm is not necessarily superimposed on the most severe lesion; and, in the presence of similar degrees of coronary atherosclerosis, some patients have spasm, but the majority do not. If coronary spasm resulted from normal increase in vasomotor tone, one would expect variant angina to be much more common in the whole population of patients with critical coronary disease [15].

All these considerations have led us to believe that, in the pathophysiological workout of all clinical manifestations of ischaemic heart disease, including unstable angina, "spasm" should be defined as an abnormal vasomotor response [10–16] resulting from supersensitivity of coronary smooth muscle to a variety of vasoconstrictor stimuli [7] and should be kept well separated from "vasoconstriction", a response which is still within the normal physiological range. While the former is encountered in a limited number of patients, typically those presenting with Prinzmetal's "variant" form, the latter is likely to play a relevant pathophysiological role in a much larger proportion of anginal patients, especially those exhibiting severe, excentric lesions in the ischaemia-related vessel(s).

Objective demonstration of our contention is provided by quantitative measurements obtained at coronary arteriography in patients with coronary artery disease of variable severity, who received increasing doses of intracoronary ergonovine [17]. Whilst the majority responded with only minor changes in coronary diameter, only a minority exhibited supersensitivity to the vasoconstrictor, that was localized to one vascular segment and resulted in total or near-total vessel occlusion.

Prevalence of Abnormal Epicardial Vasomotor Responses in Unstable Angina

The results of several studies based on continuous haemodynamic monitoring performed in patients with unstable angina during coronary care unit (CCU) admission, have consistently shown that the majority of their ischaemic attacks are not preceded by an increase of the major determinants of myocardial oxygen consumption [18–22]. Typically, the haemodynamic pattern observed during such events is characterized by a dramatic impairment of both contraction and relaxation dP/dt, followed by an increase in left ventricular filling pressures [21]. This pattern is strikingly reminescent of that observed in the experimental animal following acute coronary ligation and, in man, after brief coronary occlusions during PTCA. Although these observations indicate that, in these patients, ischaemic events are caused by reduction in regional myocardial perfusion rather than by increased metabolic demand, they do not allow discrimination between coronary vasoconstriction and reversible thrombosis as potential causes.

Apart from anecdotal reports and observations obtained in small series of patients undergoing cardiac catheterization during an acute unstable phase, very few studies have addressed the issue of the prevalence of abnormal epicardial constriction in patients with unstable angina.

Bertrand and coworkers studied a large series of patients with unstable angina and recent myocardial infarction and gave an intravenous bolus of 400 µg of metylergometrine at the time of coronary arteriography [23]. For the two populations, the authors reported, respectively, a 21% and 22% prevalence of occlusive spasm that was promptly reversed by the intracoronary administration of isosorbide dinitrate. Although they concluded that exaggerated coronary vasoconstriction may play a key pathophysiological role in a large proportion of patients (more than one fifth, in their experience) with active unstable angina, extrapolation of their results and conclusions to a general patients' population appears to be difficult for a number of reasons.

First, the French group used a standard, considerably high dose of ergometrine in all patients, rather than trying to assess individual susceptibility to vasoconstrictor stimuli by giving incremental doses. When such high doses are administered, it is hard to discriminate normal pharmacological responses to an extremely powerful agent from frankly abnormal supersensitivity to vasoconstrictor stimuli. This limitation appears particularly pertinent to patients with extremely severe, excentric atheromatous lesions in whom even minimal changes in residual cross-sectional area caused by medial smooth muscle contraction would result in total or subtotal occlusion. Second, the authors give no information as to which inclusion criteria they used, how was the diagnosis of unstable angina established and, most importantly, how many of their patients presented with "variant" angina, a condition which is notoriously associated with a very high prevalence of coronary vasospasm.

Therefore, although certainly remarkable for the large number of patients enrolled and for representing the first systematic attempt to assess the prevalence of coronary vasospasm in a variety of cardiac ischaemic conditions, this study is hampered by serious methodological drawbacks and certainly represents a good example of how critical selection criteria and patients' characterization can be when pathophysiological issues relevant to grossly inhomogeneous syndromes are addressed (see introduction of this chapter).

We recently tried to circumvent some of the methodological problems encountered by the French authors by studying a somewhat smaller group of 31 highly characterized, carefully selected consecutive patients with unstable angina. Those with Prinzmetal and worsening angina with a typical "crescendo" pattern were excluded. We elected to study only patients with frequent, recurrent episodes of angina at rest (>1 episode/day) associated with ST segment depression on the 12 lead ECG and invariably relieved by sublingual or intravenous nitroglycerin, as we felt that the prevalence of abnormal epicardial coronary vasoconstriction could be expected to be high in such a population. The frequency and duration of asymptomatic ischaemic events was also evaluated by continuous ECG monitoring in CCU. All patients underwent diagnostic coronary arteriography after coronary vasodilators had been discontinued for at least 12 hours. Selective contrast injections were performed in several views in control conditions and after prolonged (5 minutes) hyperventilation. Angiograms were assessed, in blind, by quantitative angiography. After hyperventilation 5 patients exhibited a localized focal reduction of coronary diameter of 90% or more that resulted in total (4 patients) or subtotal (1 patient) vessel occlusion. The change in lumen diameter was associated with transient ST segment depression in 3 patients and was promptly reversed by intracoronary nitroglycerin in all. In one case spasm occurred in vessels that appeared "angiographically normal" or only exhibited minor wall irregularities and in 4 it was superimposed on haemodynamically significant (>50% diameter reduction) lesions. In the remaining 26 patients hyperventilation either caused diffuse reduction in coronary diameter of 30% or less or had no measurable effect.

The reasons for choosing hyperventilation rather than administration of ergot-derivatives as a provocative manoeuver were not only dictated by ethical and safety considerations. It was also felt that, if the rationale of the study was to discriminate "normal" and "abnormal" coronary vasomotor responses in patients with unstable angina at rest, a somewhat less potent constrictor such as alcalinization would have been more an appropriate stimulus.

It would therefore appear that, in approximately one sixth of patients undergoing an unstable ischaemic phase and presenting predominantly with recurrent symptoms at rest, coronary supersensitivity to vasoconstrictor stimuli plays a central pathophysiological role. With rare exceptions, objective documentation of abnormal vasoconstriction (and of its ability to cause ischaemia) can only be obtained by provocative testing during angiography and only when pharmacological agents capable of interfering with coronary reactivity have been discontinued. Ideally, the correlation between the phenomena induced in the catheterization laboratory and those that are supposed to occur spontaneously should be obtained in order to extrapolate meaningful conclusions and to direct treatment. Unfortunately, all these conditions are not easy to obtain in the clinical setting.

Whether and how frequently more subtle changes in coronary smooth muscle tone contribute to the pathophysiology of unstable angina is difficult to establish. However difficult to visualize and quantify, vasomotor phenomena occur, almost continuously, in both healthy and diseased vessels. Nevertheless, physiological changes in coronary vasomotor tone are unlikely to account, per se, for the critical recurrent changes in regional myocardial perfusion that are observed in patients with unstable angina. In fact, whilst symptoms in these patients are typically episodic and sudden in onset, normal vasomotion takes place day by day and hour by hour, even in the presence of severe coronary atheroma, without causing unstable symptoms. Whatever the etiology of unstable angina and of myocardial infarction, it must be recognized that these conditions are frequently unheralded and probably result from sudden pathological events in the vessel wall.

The functional or anatomical alterations in the vessel wall that determine abnormal vasomotor responses are also likely to shift the local clotting equilibrium towards a procoagulant tendency. A vicious circle can therefore originate where vasoconstriction, by favouring blood stagnation, can foster further thrombosis. This, in turn, enhances vasoconstriction by releasing powerful vasoactive substances such as serotonin and thromboxane A_2 (TxA_2).

Relationship Between Vessel Wall Abnormalities, Vasoconstriction and Thrombosis

A host of experimental and clinical studies indicate that interactions between the functionally or anatomically abnormal vessel wall and blood constituents play a relevant role in the pathophysiology of unstable angina. Flow turbulence and stagnation at the site of a critical lesion or disruption of intimal or endothelial continuity can create favourable conditions for platelet adhesion and aggregation, with release of powerful vasoactive agents such as thrombin, thromboxane A_2 and serotonin. Spontaneous, cyclic reductions in blood flow have been consistently observed in experimental animals after application of an external constrictor [24, 25]. The pattern of these flow changes is reminescent of that observed in patients with angina at rest undergoing continuous monitoring of great cardiac vein flow. They have been attributed by different authors either to platelet aggregation [24] or to changes in coronary smooth muscle tone at the site of the stricture [25]. Given the tight inter-relation among vessel wall abnormalities, platelet aggregation and vasoconstriction, conclusive interpretation of this findings is difficult because thrombus formation can be both the initiating event and its consequence.

Endothelial cells are protected against platelet deposition by prostacyclin [26], an arachidonic acid derivative that, by stimulating platelet and smooth muscle adenylate-cyclase, inhibits aggregation and causes vasodilatation. Imbalance of the prostacyclin-thromboxane A_2 system, resulting from loss of endothelial function or continuity, was proposed as a potential mechanism of abnormal coronary vasoconstriction [27]. The hypothesis found some support in the observation that both peripheral and coronary sinus levels of thromboxane B_2 (TxB_2) one of the stable metabolites of the parent compound TxA_2, are increased during episodes of vasospastic angina [28, 29]. However, measurements of TxB_2 plasma levels are of questionable value for this substance does not circulate in measurable concentrations and the measured levels may simply reflect platelet activation induced in the sampling system. Moreover, it is not possible to ascertain from these studies whether the increase in TxA_2 is the primary cause of coronary vasoconstriction or merely its consequence.

In two independent studies, conducted simultaneously by our group and by Robertson and coworkers, inhibition of thromboxane A_2 synthesis by either low dose aspirin or by indomethacin failed to affect the number, severity and duration of transient ischaemic attacks caused by coronary spasm [30, 31].

More recently, Vejar and co-authors studied the relationship between TxA_2 production and ischaemia in a group of patients with unstable angina and frequent ischaemic attacks documented by continuous ECG monitoring in the CCU [32]. All patients were started on full conventional anti-ischaemic therapy with nitrates, calcium-antagonists and beta-blockers. They were then randomized to a seven days treatment with either placebo or low-dose aspirin (2 mg/kg i.v.). TxA_2 production was assessed by measuring the urinary levels of the stable metabolite II dehydro TxB_2. In all patients, TxB_2 urinary levels frequently exceeded by more than two standard deviations the mean upper limit of normal. However, in the majority of instances, phasic activation of thromboxane production occurred in isolation, in the absence of ST segment changes and/or symptoms indicative of transient myocardial ischaemia. Furthermore, administration of aspirin consistently reduced the number and magnitude of episodes of increased TxA_2 release without affecting significantly the number, severity and duration of ischaemic attacks.

The study is interesting and certainly raises several intriguing questions. If thromboxane release is, indeed, a reliable marker of intracoronary platelet aggregation, then intravascular plugging appears, per se, an insufficient stimulus to cause ischaemia in most instances. By the same token, episodic increases of thromboxane A_2 do not seem to cause sufficient coronary vasoconstriction to impair perfusion. Indirect support to this hypothesis is also provided by the absence of significant effects of Aspirin on the number, severity and duration of ischaemic attacks in spite of the marked reduction of TxB_2 urinary levels. In this respect, patients with unstable angina resemble those with the "variant" form, whose episodes are also unaffected by cyclo-oxygenase blockade [30, 31].

The observations of Vejar apparently deny a direct causal relationship between thrombotic and ischaemic events in patients with unstable angina. They suggest that the beneficial effects of aspirin on the long term prognosis of these patients are probably attributable to inhibition of thrombus growth and, possibly, to prevention of sudden cardiac death, rather than to reduction of transient ischaemic events. Although this interpretation is certainly tenable on theoretical grounds, it is hard to understand how prevention of thrombus growth and intravascular occlusion should not be accompanied by a parallel reduction of transient ischaemic events.

The alternative hypothesis that the beneficial effects of aspirin on long term prognosis of patients with unstable angina could be unrelated to antithrombotic activity, is contradicted by the observation that other antiplatelet agents, such as ticlopidine also appear to exert a protective effect in spite of lacking cyclo-oxygenase blocking activity.

Endothelial Regulation of Coronary Smooth Muscle Tone

Prostacyclin is only one of the many compounds produced by the vascular endothelium that contribute to the regulation of smooth muscle tone. Initially perceived as a relatively inert physical interface between the vessel wall and the blood stream, the endothelium has been recently identified as a true "organ", capable of a number of functions including production of several substances endowed with vasoactive and anticoagulant properties [33]. Among these, EDRF (Endothelium derived relaxing factor) is a labile, highly diffusible vasodilator that is released when the endothelial cells monolayer is stimulated by a variety of substances such as ADP and ATP, acetylcholine, serotonin, thrombin and neurotransmitters [34, 35].

EDRF, that appears to be nitric oxide [36], is also produced when the normal endothelium is stimulated by the shear stress of flowing blood, thereby providing a fine tuning system that controls arterial and arteriolar lumen when flow changes. EDRF stimulates soluble guanylate cyclase which promotes cyclic GMP formation and vasodilatation. Thus, the intracellular action of EDRF is the same as that of nitrovasodilators with nitric oxide being produced by hydrolysis of L-arginine. In several blood vessels, the endothelium also produces a different factor which hyperpolarizes vascular smooth muscle (endothelium-derived hyperpolarizing factor: EDHF) and also causes, by a different mechanism, vasodilation [37]. The release of more than one relaxing factor has been demonstrated in various bioassays: from cultured endothelial cells and intact blood vessels. The relative importance of the production of nitric-oxyde and the other relaxing factors probably varies in different arteries and between arteries and veins [38].

Loss of endothelial continuity and/or function may impair the production of relaxing factors, thereby favouring vasoconstriction. Subtle changes in endothelial function such those occurring in hypertension, hyperlipidemia, postischaemic reperfusion and in the regenerating process after mechanical injury all lead to defective production of relaxing factors [39]. Inability of releasing relaxing factors by endothelial cells, particularly in response to serotonin and ADP, occurs at an early stage of the disease process and, in these conditions, various circulating products will activate vascular smooth muscle directly. Furthermore, defective production of endothelial relaxing factors will also result in increased local procoagulant activity, for these products also inhibit platelet adhesion and aggregation particularly if released together with prostacyclin, whose effects are synergistic.

Indirect evidence of endothelial damage of dysfunction was gathered by the observation that, in various subsets of patients with ischaemic heart disease, intracoronary administration of low molar doses of acetylcholine, the first endothelium-dependent vasodilator identified, induced paradoxical vasoconstriction and, in some cases, occlusive spasm [8, 40]. Although it was concluded that the abnormal vasomotor response to acetylcholine represented a specific marker of endothelial dysruption or dysfunction, it must be recognized that, especially for higher doses, this agonist produces direct vasoconstrictor effects that are more prominent in the mid and distal segments of epicardial coronary arteries [41].

That acetylcholine has the potential for causing direct vasoconstriction, also implies that susceptible patients may respond "paradoxically" even to low doses of the agent, independently of the absence of a "healthy" endothelium, but simply as a result of generalized smooth muscle supersensitivity to different vasoconstrictor stimuli. Therefore, unless patients undergoing acetylcholine challenging are carefully characterized clinically, and unless the specificity of their response to this agonist is checked against other vasoconstrictors, etiological inferences on the role of endothelial dysfunction in causing abnormal vasomotor responses appear largely unjustified.

Furthermore, even if accepting the idea that vascular responsiveness to acetylcholine can be taken as a relatively simple, clinically relevant marker of endothelial integrity, the fact has to be remembered that this agonist does not circulate in measurable amounts, for it is released, in the media, by adventitial nerves and is rapidly metabolized locally and in the lungs. Therefore, observations obtained by exogenous intravascular administration of pharmacological doses of the agent cannot be assumed to mimic physiological effects and be used to formulate pathophysiological hypotheses.

The endothelium also releases at least two vasoconstrictors, one a product of cyclo-oxygenase activity that appears to be responsible for hypoxia-induced vascular contraction [42]. The other, a 21-aminoacid peptide named endothelin, was isolated from porcine endothelial cells and is endowed with extremely powerful vasoconstrictor activity in various vascular districts, including the coronary circulation [43].

The expression of the pre-proendothelin gene is regulated by a variety of stimuli being inhibited, for instance, by the shear stress of flowing blood, and stimulated by post-ischaemic reperfusion. Unlike for many other naturally occurring vasoconstrictors, the vasoactive effects of endothelin are extremely prolonged [43], they are probably mediated by a non voltage-dependent Ca^{++} current [44] and predominate in smaller, resistive arteries [41].

Imbalance of the EDRF-endothelin system, in the context of an abnormal or perturbed endothelium, has been suggested to play a relevant role in a variety of vascular conditions, including unstable angina. Increased endothelin production, in the face of the impaired endothelial capacity of releasing relaxing factors, may shift the local balance towards vasoconstriction and promote thrombosis. Furthermore, endothelial dysfunction may also affect the binding capacity of thrombomodulin, the endothelial receptor for thrombin, and its ability to antagonize the conversion of fibrinogen to fibrin by thrombin. Defective production of thrombin-thrombomodulin complexes can also result in decreased local levels of activated Protein C, a vitamin K-dependent hepatic protein, that also promotes anticoagulant activity.

Human mind is not short of simplistic analogies and, in this respect, the hypothesis discussed above is reminiscent of an older one, suggesting that imbalance of the prostacyclin-thromboxane A_2 system could have been crucial for the pathogenesis of unstable angina. However, at least in the context of atheromatous disease, endothelial dysfunction is likely to develop progressively, over prolonged periods of time, whilst acute coronary events are typically episodic and usually occur abruptly. This may suggest that endothelial dysfunction is, per se, an unlikely primary candidate for the etiology of unstable coronary syndromes.

Time and experience have thought clinicians that many exciting ideas and hypotheses hardly sustain the challenge of careful scientific scrutiny. The intrinsic complexity and interplay of the innumerous factors that contribute to the regulation of vascular smooth muscle tone in health and disease still makes the mechanisms that, in the individual patient, are specifically responsible for abnormal vasomotor responses, to remain elusive.

References

1. Yasue H et al. (1974) Role of autonomic nervous system in the pathogenesis of Prinzmetal's variant form of angina. Circulation 50:534
2. Yasue H et al. (1976) Prinzmetal's variant form of angina as a manifestation of alpha-adrenergic receptor-mediated coronary artery spasm: documentation by coronary arteriography. Am Heart J 91:148
3. Raizner AE, Chahine RA, Ishimori T (1980) Provocation of coronary artery spasm by the cold pressure test: hemodynamic, arteriographic and quantitative angiographic observations. Circulation 62:925
4. Curry RC et al. (1977) Effects of ergonovine in patients with or without coronary artery disease. Circulation 56:803
5. Yasue H et al. (1978) Coronary arterial spasm and Prinzmetal's variant angina induced by hyperventilation and Tris-buffer infusion. Circulation 58:56
6. Crea F, Davies GJD, Romeo F, Chierchia S, Bugiardini R, Kaski JC, Freedman SB, Maseri A (1984) Myocardial ischemia during ergonovine testing: different susceptibility to coronary vasoconstriction in patients with exertional and variant angina. Circulation 69:690
7. Kaski JC, Crea F, Meran D, Chierchia S, Araujo L, Rodriguez Plaza L, Maseri A (1987) A localised hypersensitivity of epicardial coronary smooth muscle, is responsible for coronary spasm in active variant angina. Circulation 74:1255
8. Ludmer PL, Selwyn AP, Shook TL, Wayne RR, Mudge GH, Wayne Alexander R, Ganz P (1986) Paradoxical vasoconstriction induced by acetylcholine in atherosclerotic coronary arteries. N Engl J Med 31:1046
9. Zeiher AM, Drexler H, Wollschlaeger H, Saurbier B, Just H (1989) Coronary vasomotion in response to sympathetic stimulation in humans: importance of the functional integrity of the endothelium. JACC 14:1181
10. Maseri A, Chierchia S (1982) Coronary artery spasm: demonstration, definition, diagnosis and consequences. Prog Cardiovasc Dis 15:169
11. McAlpin RM (1980) Contribution of dynamic vascular wall thickening to luminal narrowing during coronary arterial constriction. Circulation 61:296
12. Freedman SB, Richmond DR, Kelly DT (1982) Pathophysiology of coronary artery spasm. Circulation 66:705
13. Chierchia S et al. (1981) Holter monitoring in classical and variant angina: a clue to different pathogenetic mechanisms. Am J Cardiol 47:399
14. Chierchia S et al. (1984) Alpha-adrenergic receptors and coronary spasm: an elusive link. Circulation 69:8
15. Chierchia S (1982) Pathogenetic mechanisms of coronary vasospasm. Acta Med Scand 660:49
16. Maseri A, Chierchia S, L'Abbate A (1980) Pathogenetic mechanisms underlying the clinical events associated with atherosclerotic heart disease. Circulation 62 (suppl. 5):3
17. Hackett D, Larkin S, Chierchia S, Davies GJ, Maseri A (1987) Intracoronary ergonovine for the provocation of coronary spasm. Circulation 75:577
18. Chierchia S, Marchesi C, Maseri A (1978) Evidence of angina not caused by increased metabolic demand and patterns of electrocardiographic and hemodynamic alterations during "primary" angina. In Maseri A, Klassen GA, Lesch M (eds) Primary and secondary angina pectoris. New York, Grune and Stratton, p 145
19. Figueras J et al. (1979) Mechanisms of rest and nocturnal angina: observations during continuous hemodynamic and electrocardiographic monitoring. Circulation 59:955

20. Chierchia S et al. (1980) Hemodynamic monitoring in angina at rest. Herz 5:189
21. Chierchia S et al. (1980) Sequence of events in angina at rest: primary reduction in coronary flow. Circulation 61:759
22. Chierchia S et al. (1983) Impairment of myocardial perfusion and function during painless myocardial ischemia. JACC 1:924
23. Bertrand ME, LaBlanche JM, Tilmant PY, Thieuleux FA, Delforge MR, Carre AG, Asseman P, Berzin B, Libersa C, Laurent JM (1989) Frequency of provoked coronary arterial spasm in 1089 consecutive patients undergoing coronary arteriography. Circulation 65:1299
24. Folts JD, Crowell EB, Rowe CG (1976) Platelet aggregation in partially obstructed vessels and its elimination with aspirin. Circulation 54:365
25. Uchida Y et al. (1975) Cyclical reduction in coronary blood pressure and flow induced by coronary artery constriction. Jpn Heart J 16:454
26. Gryglewsky R et al. (1976) Arterial wall are protected against deposition of thrombi by a substance (prostaglandin X) which prevent platelet aggregation. Prostaglandins 12:685
27. Dunsting GJ, Moncada S, Vane JR (1979) Prostaglandins, their intermediates and precursors: cardiovascular actions and regulatory roles in normal and abnormal circulatory systems. Prog Cardiovasc Dis 21:405
28. Lewy RI et al. (1979) Comparison of plasma concentrations of thromboxane B_2 in Prinzmetal's variant angina and classical angina pectoris. Clin Cardiol 2:404
29. Sobel M et al. (1981) Circulating platelet products in unstable angina pectoris. Circulation 69:300
30. Chierchia S et al. (1982) Failure of thromboxane A_2 blockade to prevent attacks of vasospastic angina. Circulation 66:4
31. Robertson RM et al. (1980) Thromboxane A_2 in vasotonic angina pectoris: evidence from direct measurements and inhibitory trials. N Engl J Med 304:998
32. Vejar M, Fragasso G, Hackett D, Lipkin D, Maseri A, Burn GVR, Ciabattoni G, Patrono C (1990) Dissociation of platelet activation and spontaneous myocardial ischaemia in unstable angina. Thromb Haemos
33. Furchgott RF, VanHoutte PM (1987) Endothelium derived relaxing and contracting factors. FASEB J 3:2007
34. Furchgott RF, Zawadzki JV (1980) The obligatory role of endothelial cells in the relaxation of arterial smooth muscle by acetylcholine. Nature 288:373
35. Furchgott RF (1983) Role of endothelium in responses of vascular smooth muscle. Circ Res 53:557
36. Palmer RMJ, Ashton DS, Moncada S (1988) Vascular endothelial cells synthetize nitric oxyde from L-Arginine. Nature 333:664
37. VanHoutte PM (ed) (1988) Vasodilatation. Vascular smooth muscle, peptides, autonomic nerves and endothelium. Raven Press, New York
38. VanHoutte PM (1988) The endothelium modulation of vascular smooth muscle tone. N Eng J Med 319:512
39. VanHoutte PM (1989) Endothelium, platelets and vsospasm. In: Meyer P, Marche P (eds) Blood cells in hypertension. Raven Press, New York, p 1
40. Kugiyama K, Yasue H, Horio Y, Morikami Y, Fujii H, Kimura T (1986) Possible role of parasympathetic nervous system in the pathogenesis of exercise-induced coronary artery spasm. Am Heart J 112:605
41. Newman C, Hackett D, El-Tamimi H, Maseri A, Davies G (1988) Acetylcholine has dose-dependent bimodal effects of coronary blood flow in man. Clin Sci 74:45P
42. Vanhoutte PM, Katusic ZS (1988) Endothelium-derived contracting factor: endothelin and/or superoxide anion? Trends Pharmacol Sci 9:229
43. Yanagisawa M, Kurihara H, Kimura S, Tomobe Y, Kobayashi M, Mitsui Y, Yazaki Y, Goto K, Masaki T (1988) A novel potent vasoconstrictor peptide produced by vascular endothelial cells. Nature 332:411
44. Lauer MR, Gunn MD, Clusin W (1989) Effect of endothelin on cytosolic calcium and membrane current in single ventricular myocytes. Circulation 80:II-194

Findings in Myocardial Ischemia by Metabolic Imaging with Positron Emission Tomography*

H. R. SCHELBERT [1]

Introduction

The development of positron emission tomography and its application in patients with coronary artery disease offer the possibility to noninvasively demonstrate metabolic consequences of ischemia in human myocardium. Investigations performed with this new imaging modality have reported a segmental augmentation in glucose utilization in myocardial regions with either decreased blood flow or impaired contractile function or both [1–6]. Interventional restoration of blood flow to such myocardial regions can result in a significant improvement or even normalization of contractile function [2, 5]. The noninvasively demonstrated segmental augmentation of exogenous glucose utilization relative either to regional myocardial blood flow or to glucose utilization in normal myocardium has therefore been referred to as a metabolic correlate of "hibernating myocardium." Rahimtoola was first to call attention to this particular state of altered myocardium [7]. Hibernating myocardium, according to Rahimtoola [7, 8] and Braunwald and Rutherford [9], is a state in which chronically reduced myocardial blood flow as a consequence of severe coronary artery disease is associated with an impairment in segmental contractile function. Presumably, a new steady state is attained in which demand adapts to the chronically diminished supply of blood flow and oxygen. Indeed, Braunwald and Rutherford [9] postulated that the impairment or loss of contractile function drastically reduces the energy requirements for contractile work and thus might exert a protective effect. Lastly and importantly, therapeutic restoration of coronary blood flow reverses this abnormal state and invariably results in an improvement of contractile function.

While clinically useful, the term hibernation implies the existence of a true steady state of diminished demand and diminished supply. The question

* Operated for the U.S. Department of Energy by the University of California under Contract DE-FC03-87ER60615. This work was supported in part by the Director of the Office of Energy Research, Office of Health and Environmental Research, Washington, D.C., by Research Grants HL 29845 and HL 33177, National Institutes of Health, Bethesda, MD, and by an Investigative Group Award by the Greater Los Angeles Affiliate of the American Heart Association, Los Angeles, CA.

[1] Division of Nuclear Medicine and Biophysics, UCLA School of Medicine, Los Angeles, CA 90024, USA

W. Bleifeld et al. (Eds.)
Unstable Angina

whether such new steady state can indeed be achieved in human myocardium and be maintained for prolonged time periods remains, however, unanswered. It is therefore possible that hibernation and its metabolic expression in human myocardium does in fact represent at least in some patients an imbalance between demand and supply and, thus, reflects the metabolic counterpart of unstable angina.

Metabolic Consequences of Ischemia and Their Demonstration with Positron-Emitting Tracers of Substrate Metabolism

A reduction in oxygen supply in absolute terms or an inadequate response to increased demand as, for example, during increased cardiac work is associated with an almost instantaneous decline or loss of contractile function. The inadequate supply of oxygen or supply-demand balance causes, as demonstrated in animal experimental studies, profound metabolic alterations. Oxidation of fatty acid becomes impaired, while deposition of fatty acid in the endogenous lipid pool increases [10, 11]. Flux of glucose through the glycolytic pathway increases. The higher glucose demand is met initially by increased catabolism of endogenous glycogen and subsequently through increased glucose uptake from plasma. During mild states of ischemia, glucose appears to be metabolized oxidatively. However, more severe reductions in blood flow and thus in oxygen supply lead to an impairment in overall oxidative metabolism. A disproportionately greater fraction of high-energy phosphate in the form of ATP is generated anaerobically through glycolysis. It is associated with increased production of hydrogen ions and lactate. Because these metabolites inhibit glycolysis, they must be removed from tissue if glycolysis and thus residual high-enery phosphate production are to continue. Thus, some residual blood flow is essential in order to maintain some degree of energy production. Further decreases in blood flow lead to a rise in tissue concentrations of lactate and of hydrogen ions which inhibit glycolysis and therefore deprive the cell of one of its last resources of production of high-energy phosphate. Loss of high-energy phosphate combined with an inability to consume ATP ultimately lead to a loss of transmembraneous ion concentration gradients, cell membrane disruption, and cell death followed by scar tissue formation.

Several of these metabolic alterations can be demonstrated noninvasively with positron emission tomography and positron-emitting tracers of specific segments of substrate metabolism. The rate of tricarboxylic acid (TCA) cycle activity can now be assessed quantitatively with ^{11}C-labeled acetate [12–19]. This agent readily crosses the sarcolemmal membrane, is activated to acetyl-CoA and oxidized in the TCA cycle. The radiolabel leaves the myocardium in the form of $[^{11}C]CO_2$. The rate of $[^{11}C]CO_2$ release is proportional to the rate of clearance of ^{11}C activity from myocardium and therefore corresponds to the rate of oxidation of acetate by the TCA cycle and, further, because of its close linkage to oxidative phosphorylation, to regional myocardial oxygen consumption. Therefore, an index of myocardial oxygen consumption can be derived noninvasively from myocardial tissue time-activity curves obtained by rapid serial imaging with positron emission tomography of the uptake and subsequent clearance of [^{11}C]acetate in human myocardium. Consistent with the impairment in oxidative metabolism during ischemia, the rate of clearance of ^{11}C activity from myocardium is reduced in proportion to the lower oxygen consumption.

Evaluation of myocardial fatty acid metabolism similarly requires dynamic imaging with positron emission tomography of the uptake and subsequent clearance of [^{11}C]palmitate in myocardium [20–27]. Myocardium extracts and metabolizes this ^{11}C-labeled tracer in a fashion that is identical to its natural unlabeled parent. ^{11}C activity characteristically clears from myocardium in a biexponential fashion, which reflects the major metabolic fate of fatty acid. The slow clearance phase corresponds to the fraction of free fatty acid that is deposited in the endogenous lipid pools and their turnover rate, whereas the rapid clearance phase corresponds to the fraction of fatty acid that is immediately transferred into mitochondria and catabolized via beta-oxidation and the TCA cycle to [^{11}C]CO_2. Again, because the slope of this clearance curve component is related to the rate of oxidation of fatty acid, it is decreased in myocardial ischemia as a sign of suppressed oxidation of free fatty acid.

Utilization of exogenous glucose can be demonstrated noninvasively with [^{18}F]2-fluoro-2-deoxyglucose [28–30]. This fluorinated glucose analog exchanges across the capillary and sarcolemmal membranes in proportion to its natural counterpart and competes with glucose for hexokinase, the enzyme which mediates phosphorylation of glucose to glucose-6-phosphate [31–33]. In contrast to its natural counterpart, glucose-6-phosphate, the phosphorylated [^{18}F]2-fluoro-2-deoxyglucose is a poor substrate for glycogen formation, glycolysis, and the pentose-fructose shunt. Moreover, it is impermeable to the cell membrane. The tracer label thus becomes effectively sequestered into myocardium. Regional myocardial ^{18}F tissue concentrations are therefore proportional to regional rates of exogenous glucose utilization. Segmental increases in tracer activity in ischemic myocardium are therefore consistent with the augmented flux of glucose through the glycolytic pathway.

Segmentally Increased [^{18}F]2-Fluoro-2-Deoxyglucose: A Metabolic Correlate of Hibernating Myocardium?

Although additional positron-emitting tracers are available, the three tracers, [^{11}C]acetate, [^{11}C]palmitate, and [^{18}F]2-fluoro-2-deoxyglucose alone have proven useful for demonstrating noninvasively key metabolic features of ischemia in human myocardium. Rates of [^{11}C]acetate clearance from ischemic myocardium are prolonged and reflect the impairment of oxidative metabolism and reduced oxygen consumption [34, 35]. The impairment of fatty acid oxidation is reflected by a decrease in the relative size and clearance slope of the rapid clearance curve component on the regional myocardial [^{11}C]palmitate time-activity curve, whereas the increase in the relative size of the slow clearance phase reflects the increased fatty acid deposition in the endogenous lipid pool [21, 23, 24, 27]. Clinically most useful has been [^{18}F]2-fluoro-2-deoxyglucose. This tracer characteristically accumulates in ischemic but viable myocardium in excess of regional myocardial blood flow and more intensely than in normal myocardium and thus reflects the increased glycolytic flux as observed in mild to moderate states of myocardial ischemia (Figs. 1–3).

In patients with stable coronary artery disease, the segmentally enhanced [^{18}F]2-fluoro-2-deoxyglucose uptake most frequently occurs in myocardial regions with impaired wall motion. The increased tracer uptake is observed in patients with and without antecedent myocardial infarction [1–6, 36] and occurs in the absence or presence of stress-induced as well as apparently unprovoked angina. Furthermore, its presence does not depend on clinical evidence of symptoms of acute myocardial ischemia prior to or at the time of the imaging study. Therefore, the segmentally enhanced glucose uptake in myocardial regions with impaired contractile function has been referred to as a metabolic correlate of myocardial hibernation. Indeed, observations of improved segmental contractile function after surgical revascularization [2, 5] or after percutaneous transluminal coronary angioplasty [37] strongly support this contention. Thus, from a clinical point of view, the augmented glucose utilization as demonstrated noninvasively with positron emission tomography and [^{18}F]2-fluoro-2-deoxyglucose accurately identifies potential reversibility of segmental myocardial dysfunction.

From a physiologic point of view, however, the question whether a true steady state at levels of diminished supply and demand can indeed be maintained chronically, and perhaps indefinitely, remains unanswered. Although an impairment or loss of contractile function reduces energy expenditures, so that all residual-energy phosphate can be spent for sustaining critical cellular processes, it nevertheless would appear that the persistence of residual metabolic activity and energy production and, consequently, preservation of cellular integrity depends upon a precarious supply-demand balance or a critical balance between glycolytic production of lactate and hydrogen ions and their removal by residual blood flow. Therefore, even moderate increases in glycolytic rates and thus production of lactate or inhibitory metabolites, while residual blood flow remains unchanged or, conversely, additional decreases of an already critically low flow at constant rates of glycolysis and lactate production could upset this precarious balance and cause a further decline in high-energy production.

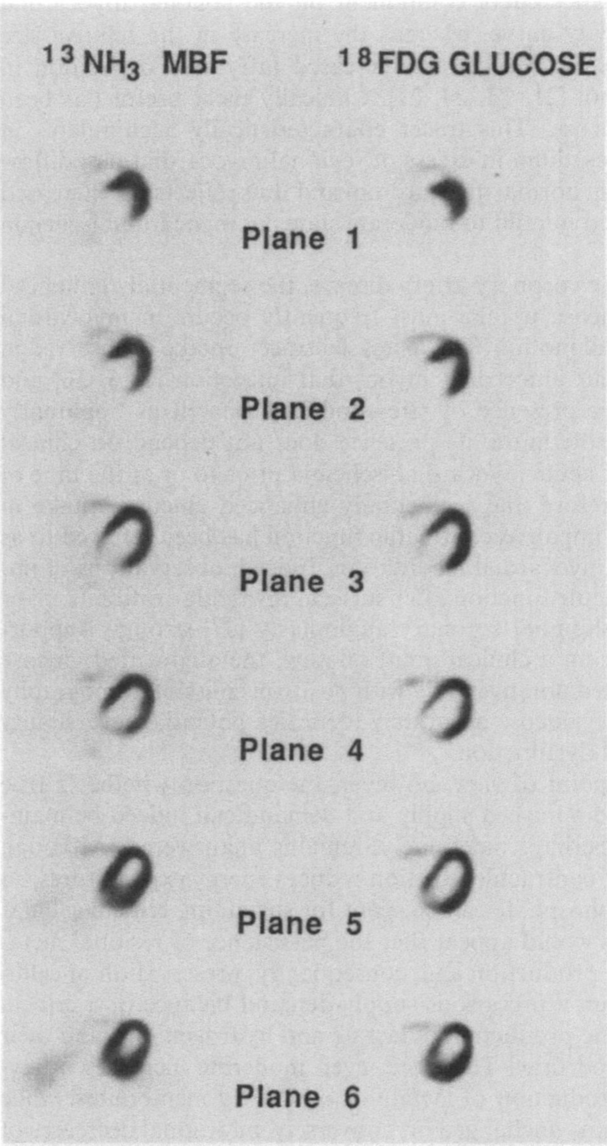

Fig. 1. Myocardial blood flow and glucose metabolism in a normal volunteer. Six contiguous cross-sectional images are shown, acquired after intravenous administration of [^{13}N] ammonia ($^{13}NH_3$) and after intravenous [^{18}F]2-fluoro-2-deoxyglucose (^{18}FDG). The images proceed from the base to the inferoapical region of the left ventricle and are viewed from the subject's feet. Note the homogeneously distributed ^{13}N and ^{18}F activity concentrations throughout the left ventricular myocardium, consistent with homogeneous myocardial blood flow and glucose metabolism in this normal volunteer

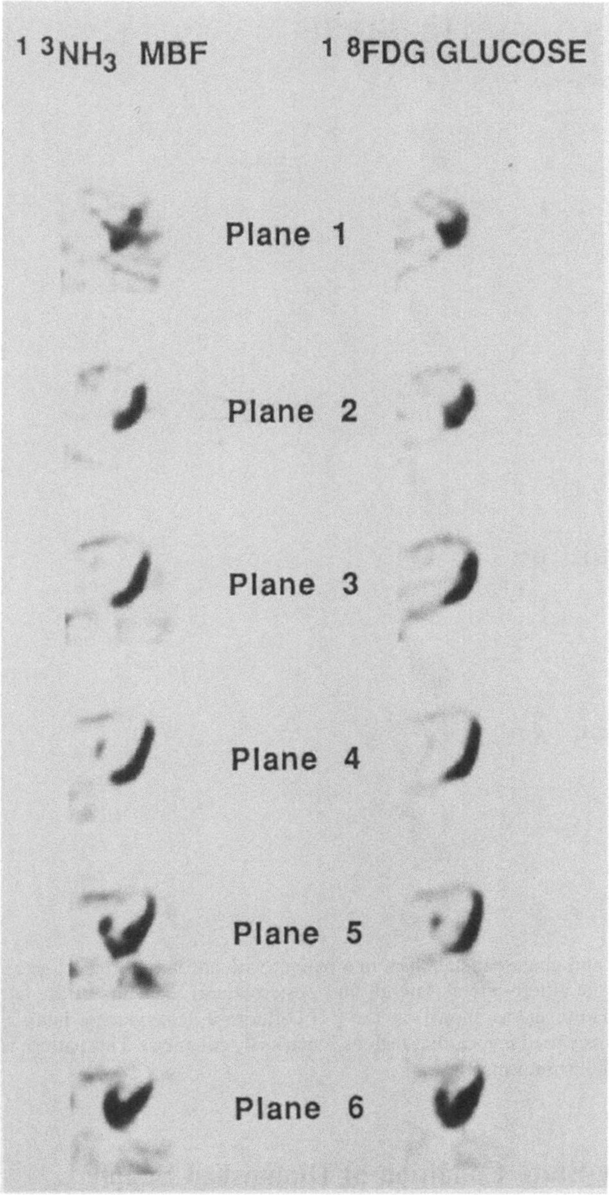

Fig. 2. Myocardial blood flow and glucose metabolism in a patient with coronary artery disease. The cross-sectional images are displayed in the same fashion as in Fig. 1. Note on the myocardial perfusion images the decreased blood flow to the anterior and anteroseptal wall, the left ventricular apex, and the interventricular septum. The [^{18}F]2-fluoro-2-deoxyglucose images reveal a similar abnormal distribution of glucose metabolism, which is severely reduced in the hypoperfused myocardial regions. This concordant reduction in blood flow and glucose metabolism is referred to as blood flow metabolism match

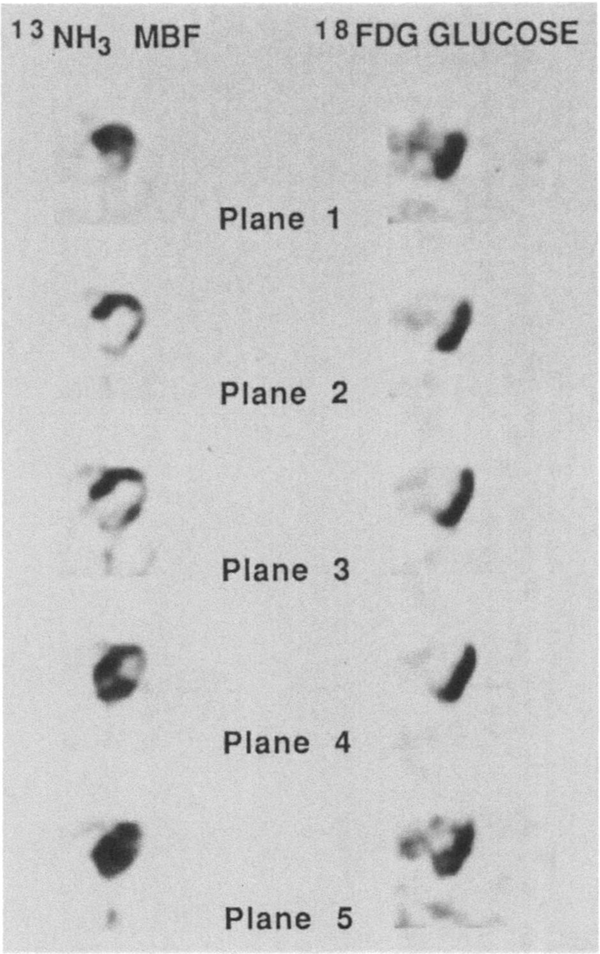

Fig. 3. Myocardial blood flow and glucose metabolism in a patient with coronary artery disease. In this patient, blood flow to the antero-lateral, lateral, and posterolateral segments of the left ventricle is severely reduced. However, as shown on the [^{18}F]2-fluoro-2-deoxyglucose images, glucose utilization in these hypoperfused myocardial regions is markedly enhanced. This pattern is referred to as blood flow metabolism mismatch

Evidence for a Steady-State Condition of Diminished Supply and Demand

Several pieces of evidence, obtained from animal experiments, appear to support the notion that a steady-state condition of diminished supply and demand can indeed be maintained for some time. Matsuzaki et al. [38], for example, attained in dog experiments an equilibrium state between decreased blood flow and impaired contractile function over a 5-h period. A sustained 66% reduction in blood flow to the endocardium was associated with a sustained 38% reduction in systolic wall thickening. Other animal experimental studies appear consistent with the possibility of a new steady state between diminished supply and demand. Of interest are the observations by Fedele et al. [39], who demonstrated in dog experiments that substrate metabolism during such apparently balanced states of reduced supply and demand were maintained oxidatively. This metabolic steady state was achieved after a transient increase in myocardial lactate release and thus a transient increase in anaerobic glycolysis. Because these investigators did not determine substrate levels and substrate usage, it remains uncertain whether substrate selection in these experiments shifted from preferential utilization of free fatty acid to preferential utilization of the more oxygen efficient glucose. Such measurements would have provided an explanation for the increase in [^{18}F]2-fluoro-2-deoxyglucose uptake and thus for the observations of a relative or absolute increase in glucose utilization in patients with chronic stable coronary artery disease. On the other hand, Opie et al. [40] observed during sustained though moderate reductions in blood flow to small regions of canine myocardium an increase in extraction of glucose and augmented release of lactate, although a substantial fraction of glucose continued to be metabolized oxidatively.

Can a Steady State Be Maintained in Human Coronary Artery Disease?

To what extent these findings in animals can be extrapolated to human coronary artery disease remains uncertain. In the controlled animal experimental environment, hemodynamic parameters and thus demand and supply can be maintained relatively constant. Further, steady-state conditions of lower demand and lower supply were imposed on myocardium over only relatively short time periods. Different from these dog experiments, the impairment or loss of contractile function together with the reduced blood flow exists chronically in human coronary artery disease. Importantly, both demand and supply are likely to change constantly in human myocardium in response to normal daily activities. Even if physical activity were minimized or restrained, mental and emotional stress and thus changes in the neural and humoral control of the heart and cirulation would still be sufficient to alter heart rate, venous and arterial pressures and thus ventricular loading conditions and cardiac work. Furthermore, changes in the neurohumoral milieu are followed by changes in the myocardial inotropic state and thus changes in cardiac work and oxygen demand. Conversely, other studies have described an increased vasoreactivity in patients with advanced coronary artery disease which would lower blood flow and thus further diminish the already compromised supply of oxygen as well as reduce tissue perfusion and result in a rise of tissue concentrations of inhibitory metabolites.

Physical stress in coronary artery disease patients induces segmental myocardial blood flow defects or can cause an increase in the extent and severity of already existing perfusion abnormalities at rest. These changes can occur even in the absence of angina [41]. Emotional stress similarly can induce acute ischemic episodes [42] or, as demonstrated by Deanfield et al. [43], a transient reduction in segmental reduction in segmental blood flow. Even normal daily activity without considerable physical exertion induce frequent and often asymptomatic ischemic electrocardiographic changes which were found to be associated with transient reductions in blood flow [44, 45]. These reductions may occur even in the absence of hemodynamic changes or evidence of increased cardiac demand and thus were ascribed to transient reductions in coronary flow due to changes in coronary vasomotor tone [44]. Thus, frequent changes in both demand and supply raise the question whether at least in some patients with advanced coronary artery disease, hibernation in a true physiologic sense can indeed exist, or whether the impairment of regional wall motion, though reversible, together with augmented glucose utilization does in fact invariably represent hibernating myocardium.

If the segmentally enhanced [^{18}F]2-fluoro-2-deoxyglucose uptake is to be specific for hibernating myocardium, it then must exist only in segments with both decreased blood flow and impaired contractile function. However, in the study by Tillisch et al. [2], who selected patients according to resting wall motion abnormalities, blood flow was reduced in only 16 (39%) of the 41 dysfunctional segments with augmented glucose utilization. The remaining 25 (61%) segments with enhanced [^{18}F]2-fluoro-2-deoxyglucose uptake and impaired wall motion revealed normal blood flow by quantitative analysis of the [^{13}N]ammonia perfusion images. Similar findings were reported by Yonekura et al. [4]. These investigators evaluated in 26 patients with angiographically documented coronary artery disease regional myocardial blood flow at rest and during supine bicycle exercise with [^{13}N]ammonia and positron emission tomography. Regional myocardial glucose utilization was examined during a separate study session remote from the blood flow study but performed within 1 week. Supine bicycle exercise induced new flow defects in myocardial regions with normal resting blood flow. Six of these regions (46%) exhibited on remote study with [^{18}F]2-fluoro-2-deoxyglucose at rest segmental enhancements of glucose utilization. These findings would argue against the notion that the observed augmented glucose utilization is confined to segments with resting perfusion abnormalities or chronically reduced blood flow. The pattern therefore does not appear to be specific for hibernating myocardium. The fact that it occurred in the study by Yonekura et al. [4] in regions with only stress-induced perfusion abnormalities, as was observed in the study by Tillisch et al. [2] in myocardial regions with impaired contractile function, suggests the possibility that a similar segmental augmentation of glucose utilization is associated also with "stunned myocardium" [46].

Observations in animal experiments as well as clinical observations do in fact support the existence of enhanced glucose utilization in stunned or postischemic myocardium. Camici et al. [47], for example, submitted patients with coronary artery disease to supine bicycle exercise and monitored segmental myocardial blood flow by serial imaging with the ultrashort-lived positron-emitting flow tracer ^{82}Rb. Administration of [^{18}F]2-fluoro-2-deoxyglucose was delayed until the exercise-induced perfusion abnormality had resolved. Tracer uptake was consistently elevated in postischemic myocardial regions. Although these investigators did not evaluate regional wall motion, the observation of augmented tracer uptake following stress-induced ischemia suggests that myocardial stunning similar to myocardial hibernation characteristically exhibits augmented glucose utilization. This possibility was subsequently confirmed in animal experimental studies. Reperfusion after transient coronary occlusions was found to be invariably associated with reduced fatty acid oxidation and TCA cycle activity and, importantly, with augmented glucose utilization [35, 48–50]. The augmented glucose utilization was readily demonstrated by an often dramatic elevation of segmental [^{18}F]2-fluoro-2-deoxyglucose uptake.

Camici et al. [47] initially ascribed and subsequently confirmed in isolated arterially perfused hearts that the augmented glucose utilization may, at least in part, reflect the replenishment of glycogen stores which had been depleted during ischemia [51]. Subsequent experiments in chronically instrumented dogs, however, suggested additional mechanisms. Buxton et al. [35] for example, demonstrated that TCA cycle activity and thus overall oxidative metabolism remained initially depressed after reperfusion, whereas Schwaiger et al. found evidence for a prolonged abnormality in fatty acid oxidation [48]. Furthermore, serial studies over a 4-week period in chronic dog experiments demonstrated a transient surge in glycolytic flux [49]. While glucose utilization within hours of reperfusion appeared to be reduced in proportion to the residual blood flow deficit, it was markedly increased at 24 h of perfusion and persisted for as long as 1 week. Furthermore, this increase in glycolytic flux was associated with persistently decreased glycogen stores and an increase in the fraction of exogenous glucose that entered glycolysis and an increase in lactate release [50]. These observations suggest that replenishment of glycogen stores alone are unlikely to account for the augmented glucose utilization, but that additional mechanisms as, for example, mitochondrial dysfunction associated with an increase in anaerobic glycolytic activity may be in involved.

More recent observations suggest that similar changes occur in human myocardium. For example, Tamaki et al. [5] reported that despite adequate surgical revascularization and normalization of resting and stress-induced perfusion abnormalities, glucose utilization remained elevated in 32% of segments with presurgical mismatches. Despite this persistent metabolic abnormality, regional wall motion had improved in 50% of such segments with persistently elevated glucose utilization. Nienaber et al. [37] similarly observed an initial persistence of augmented glucose utilization in myocardial territories that were supplied by severely stenosed coronary arteries, but which were successfully treated with angioplasty. Despite a marked improvement in myocardial blood flow, glucose utilization remained elevated when examined within 2–3 days after angioplasty. Interestingly, there is some anecdotal evidence that the augmented glucose utilization may persist even longer after successful angioplasty and despite an apparent normalization of regional myocardial blood flow both at rest and during exercise. For example, Hashimoto et al. [52] reported two patients in whom glucose utilization remained elevated as late as 7 months following angioplasty and despite an apparent normalization of rest and stress blood flow. Thus, there is considerable evidence in both animal experiments as well as in human myocardium for the augmented glucose utilization as a metabolic abnormality for postischemic or stunned myocardium.

Glucose utilization further is segmentally increased in a third condition, acute myocardial ischemia. Schelbert et al. [53] for example demonstrated an absolute (relative to control myocardium) or relative (to blood flow) increase in [^{18}F]2-fluoro-2-deoxyglucose uptake in dogs during acute, pacing induced myocardial ischemia. Similarly, Camici et al. [47] observed an increase in segmental glucose utilization in patients during stress induced myocardial ischemia. These investigators administered [^{18}F]2-fluoro-2-deoxyglucose in some of their coronary artery disease patients during supine bicycle exercise. Glucose uptake was maintained normal in ischemic segments despite marked reductions in blood flow. Tracer uptake was therefore increased in ischemic myocardium relative to regional myocardial blood flow.

Segmental Increases in Glucose Utilization as a Sign of Unstable Angina

Thus, animal experimental studies as well as clinical investigations have provided considerable evidence for the segmental increase in glucose utilization or the "blood flow metabolism mismatch pattern" on positron emission tomography as the operational term for the increase in glucose utilization relative to blood flow as a sign of different types of altered myocardial states, acute ischemia, stunned and hibernating myocardium.

The blood flow metabolism mismatch as demonstrated with positron emission tomography possibly reflects in many patients a true state of myocardial hibernation. This appears to be particularly true for those patients with decreased regional blood flow and segmentally impaired contractile function at rest. Although demand and supply frequently change in these patients, the magnitude of these changes might be relatively small and thus is unlikely to profoundly modify or disturb this new steady state. On the other hand, the blood flow metabolism mismatch may reflect in other patients a state of metabolic unstable angina. In these patients, periods of severe reductions of blood flow or of imbalances between supply and demand may alternate with periods of relative normal flows or reperfusion. Observations in animal experimental studies are consistent with this notion [54]. Repetitive coronary occlusions alternating with periods of reperfusion were shown to result in a progressive deterioration and ultimately loss of contractile function despite the fact that blood flow and supply of oxygen had returned to near normal levels or were markedly in excess of the decreased demand. Although the term angina per se implies clinical or symptomatic evidence of myocardial ischemia, ischemic episodes as documented by long term electrocardiographic monitoring, evaluation of blood flow at rest or during mental or physical stress can occur entirely without symptoms. Therefore, the absence of anginal episodes in many patients prior to or during the metabolic studies with positron emission tomography does not argue against the possibility that the blood flow metabolism mismatch does in fact reflect an unstable condition between supply and demand.

This might in fact explain the segmental increases in [^{18}F]2-fluoro-2-deoxyglucose in patients with dysfunctional but normally perfused myocardial regions. This possibility of an unstable steady state might also apply to patients with resting perfusion abnormalities in whom abnormal coronary vasoreactivity or a marked increase in demand lead to profound though temporary imbalances between lactate production and lactate removal or residual tissue perfusion and in whom transient imbalances superimpose acute ischemic as well as post-ischemic metabolic disturbances on an already chronically abnormal metabolic state.

Recent evidence suggests that this metabolic pattern may indeed be associated with different pathophysiologic substrates. Preliminary investigations into the rates of recovery of blood flow, glucose metabolism, and segmental contractile function demonstrated that both metabolism and function rapidly improve after therapeutic revascularization in patients with stable angina [37]. In contrast, the recovery of blood flow and, more markedly, of regional contractile function was delayed in those patients who clinically presented with evidence of unstable angina. Although larger perfusion defects and areas of mismatches in these patients were present and suggested that the slower recovery rates may have depended upon a more severe ischemic injury, the findings also support the notion of differences in the pathophysiology underlying the blood flow metabolism mismatch.

Obviously, the possibility of the blood flow metabolism mismatch as the reflection of unstable angina requires further investigations. If confirmed, it would raise several important questions. For example, do acute ischemic episodes, if superimposed on an already compromised metabolic state, cause a more severe depression or loss of glycolytic activity, and if so, is this followed by a transient rise in glycolytic flux [2]. Furthermore, do repeated ischemic episodes ultimately cause cessation of glycolytic activity, and do they therefore accelerate the progression of ischemia to necrosis and scar formation [2]? Furthermore, can the blood flow metabolism mismatch pattern be utilized to distinguish between stable and unstable angina and thus be used clinically for predicting rapid deterioration of ischemia [2]? The latter would be useful for deciding between conservative and aggressive treatment strategies. Finally, can the metabolic pattern on positron emission tomography be used for monitoring the efficacy of pharmacologic interventional strategies in the treatment of stable and unstable angina?

Summary and Conclusions

Ischemic but viable human myocardium can accurately be identified by metabolic imaging with positron emission tomography. The segmentally enhanced utilization of exogenous glucose as demonstrated with [^{18}F]2-fluoro-2-deoxyglucose has indeed become a hallmark of myocardial viability and of hibernating myocardium. While clinically useful, the term mechanistically implies a new steady state between diminished blood flow and reduced oxygen demand. Given the constant changes in supply and energy demand in human myocardium, it is unlikely that such steady state can always be attained. Thus, it is possible that the blood flow metabolism mismatch reflects in many patients an unstable metabolic condition between supply and demand. These changes may occur over a relatively small range, so that the metabolic pattern resembles a state of hibernation in a true sense. In contrast, these changes in supply and demand may occur in many patients over a much larger range associated with marked although transient decreases in blood flow or increases in energy demand. In these patients, the blood flow metabolism mismatch is then likely to represent unstable metabolic ischemia, where acute ischemic episodes alternate with periods of relatively normal supply and demand. Whether true hibernation and unstable metabolic ischemia are associated with different physiologic substrates remains uncertain at present. Preliminary observations do suggest this possibility. The introduction of new tracers of specific segments of myocardial substrate metabolism with positron emission tomography, together with newly developed quantitative approaches for determining rates of blood flow and metabolism are, however, likely to provide new insights into such possible mechanisms and to clarify differences between true hibernation and unstable metabolic ischemia.

Acknowledgements. The author wishes to thank Wendy Wilson for preparing the illustrations and Kerry Engber for her skillful secretarial assistance.

References

1. Marshall RC, Tillisch JH, Phelps ME, Huang SC, Carson RC, Henze E, Schelbert HR (1983) Identification and differentiation of resting myocardial ischemia and infarction in man with positron computed tomography ^{18}F-labeled fluorodeoxyglucose and N-13 ammonia. Circulation 67:766–778
2. Tillisch J, Brunken R, Marshall R, Schwaiger M, Mandelkern M, Phelps M, Schelbert HR (1986) Reversibility of cardiac wall motion abnormalities predicted by positron tomography. New Engl J Med 314:884–888
3. Brunken R, Tillisch J, Schwaiger M, Child JS, Marshall R, Mandelkern M, Phelps ME, Schelbert HR (1986) Regional perfusion, glucose metabolism and wall motion in chronic electrocardiographic Q-wave infarctions. Evidence for persistence of viable tissue in some infarct regions by positron emission tomography. Circulation 73:951–963
4. Yonekura Y, Tamaki N, Kambara H, Senda M, Saji H, Ban T, Kawai C, Konishi J (1988) Detection of metabolic alterations in ischemic myocardium by F-18 fluorodeoxyglucose uptake with positron emission tomography. Am J Cardiac Imaging 2:122–132

5. Tamaki N, Yonekura Y, Yamashita K, Saji H, Magata Y, Senda M, Konishi Y, Hirata K, Ban T, Konishi J (1989) Positron emission tomography using fluorine-18 deoxyglucose in evaluation of coronary artery bypass grafting. Am J Cardiol 64:860–865
6. De Landsheere CM, Raets D, Pierard LA, Materne P, Del Fiore G, Lemaire C, Quaglia L, Guilaume M, Peters JM, Lamotte D, Kulbertus HE, Rigo P (1985) Fibrinolysis and viable myocardium after an acute infarction: A study of regional perfusion and glucose utilization with positron emission tomography. Circulation 72:III-393
7. Rahmitoola SH (1985) A perspective on the three large multicenter randomized clinical trials of coronary bypass surgery for chronic stable angina. Circulation 72:V-123
8. Rahimtoola SH (1989) The hibernating myocardium. Am Heart J 117:211–221
9. Braunwald E, Rutherford JD (1986) Reversible ischemic left ventricular dysfunction: Evidence for "hibernating myocardium." J Am Coll Cardiol 8:1467–1470
10. Liedtke AJ (1981) Alterations of carbohydrate and lipid metabolism in the acutely ischemic heart. Progr Cardiovasc Dis 23:321–336
11. Opie LH (1976) Effects of regional ischemia on metabolism of glucose and fatty acids. Circ Res 38:152–174
12. Pike VW, Eakins MN, Allan RM, Selwyn AP (1982) Preparation of [l-^{11}C] acetate – an agent for the study of myocardial metabolism by positron emission tomography. Int J Appl Radiat 33:505–512
13. Buxton DB, Schwaiger M, Nguyen A, Phelps ME, Schelbert HR (1988) Radiolabeled acetate as a tracer of myocardial tricarboxylic acid cycle flux. Circ Res 63:628–634
14. Buxton DB, Nienaber CA, Luxen A, Ratib O, Hansen H, Phelps ME, Schelbert HR (1989) Noninvasive quantitation of regional myocardial oxygen consumption in vivo with [l-^{11}C] acetate and dynamic positron emission tomography. Circulation 79:134–142
15. Brown M, Marshall DR, Burton BS, Sobel BE, Bergmann SR (1987) Delineation of myocardial oxygen utilization with carbon-11-labeled acetate. Circulation 76:687–696
16. Brown MA, Myears DW, Bergmann SR (1988) Noninvasive assessment of canine myocardial oxidative metabolism with ^{11}C-acetate and positron emission tomography. J Am Coll Cardiol 12:1054–1063
17. Armbrecht JJ, Buxton DB, Schelbert HR (1990) Validation of [l-^{11}C] acetate as a tracer for noninvasive assessment of oxidative metabolism with positron emission tomography in normal, ischemic, post-ischemic and hyperemic canine myocardium. Circulation
18. Henes CG, S.R. B, Walsh MN, Sobel BE, Geltman EM (1989) Assessment of myocardial oxidative metabolic reserve with positron emission tomography and carbon-11 acetate. J Nucl Med 30:1489–1499
19. Armbrecht JJ, Buxton DB, Brunken RC, Phelps ME, Schelbert HR (1990) Regional myocardial oxygen consumption determined noninvasively in humans with [l-^{11}C] acetate and dynamic positron tomography. Circulation
20. Lerch RA, Bergmann SA, Ambos HD, Welch MJ, Ter-Pogossian MM, Sobel BE (1982) Effect of flow-independent reduction of metabolism on regional myocardial clearance of ^{11}C palmitate. Circulation 65:731–738
21. Lerch RA, Ambos HD, Bergmann SR, Welch MJ, Ter-Pogossian MM, Sobel BE (1981) Localization of viable, ischemic myocardium by positron-emission tomography with ^{11}C palmitate. Circulation 64:689–699
22. Schön HR, Schelbert HR, Najafi A, Robinson G, Huang SC, Barrio J, Phelps ME (1982) C-11 labeled palmitic acid for the noninvasive evaluation of regional myocardial fatty acid metabolism with positron computed tomography. I. Kinetics of C-11 palmitic acid in normal myocardium. Am Heart J 103:532–547
23. Schön HR, Schelbert HR, Najafi A, Hansen H, Robinson GR, Huang SC, Barrio J, Phelps ME (1982) C-11 labeled palmitic acid for the noninvasive evaluation of regional myocardial fatty acid metabolism with positron computed tomography. II. Kinetics of C-11 palmitic acid in acutely ischemic myocardium. Am Heart J 103:548–561
24. Schelbert HR, Henze E, Schön HR, Najafi A, Hansen H, Huang SC, Barrio JR, Phelps ME (1983) C-11 palmitic acid for the noninvasive evaluation of regional myocardial fatty acid metabolism with positron computed tomography. IV. In vivo demonstration of impaired fatty acid oxidation in acute myocardial ischemia. Am Heart J 106:736–750

25. Schelbert HR, Henze E, Schön HR, Keen R, Hansen HW, Selin C, Huang SC, Barrio JR, Phelps ME (1983) C-11 palmitate for the noninvasive evaluation of regional myocardial fatty acid metabolism with positron computed tomography. III. In vivo demonstration of the effects of substrate availability on myocardial metabolism. Am Heart J 105:492–504
26. Schelbert HR, Henze E, Sochor H, Grossman RG, Huang SC, Barrio JR, Schwaiger M, Phelps ME (1986) Effects of substrate availability on myocardial C-11 palmitate kinetics by positron emission tomography in normal subjects and patients with ventricular dysfunction. Am Heart J 111:1055–1064
27. Grover-McKay M, Schelbert HR, Schwaiger M, Sochor H, Guzy PM, Krivokapich J, Child JS, Phelps ME (1986) Identification of impaired metabolic reserve by atrial pacing in patients with significant coronary artery stenosis. Circulation 74:281–292
28. Phelps ME, Hoffman EJ, Selin CE, Huang SC, Robinson G, MacDonald N, Schelbert H, Kuhl DE (1978) Investigation of [^{18}F]2-fluoro-2-deoxyglucose for the measure of myocardial glucose metabolism. J Nucl Med 19:1311–1319
29. Ratib O, Phelps ME, Huang SC, Henze E, Selin CE, Schelbert HR (1982) Positron tomography with deoxyglucose for estimating local myocardial glucose metabolism. J Nucl Med 23:577–586
30. Gambhir SS, Schwaiger M, Huang SC, Krivokapich J, Schelbert HR, Nienaber CA, Phelps ME (1989) Simple noninvasive quantification method for measuring myocardial glucose utilization in humans employing positron emission tomography and Fluorine-18 deoxyglucose. J Nucl Med 30:359–366
31. Sokoloff L, Reivich M, Kennedy C, Des Rosiers MH, Patlak CS, Pettigrew KD, Sakurada O, Shinohara M (1977) The [^{14}C]-deoxyglucose method for the measurement of local cerebral glucose utilization: Theory, procedure and normal values in the conscious and anesthetized albino rat. J Neurochem 28:897–916
32. Phelps ME, Huang SC, Hoffman EJ, Selin C, Sokoloff L, Kuhl DE (1979) Tomographic measurement of local cerebral glucose metabolic rate in humans with (F-18) 2-fluoro-2-deoxy-D-glucose: Validation of method. Ann Neurol 6:371–388
33. Huang SC, Phelps ME, Hoffman EJ, Sideris K, Selin CJ, Kuhl DE (1980) Non-invasive determination of local cerebral metabolic rate of glucose in man. Am J Physiol 238:E69–E82
34. Brunken R, Schwaiger M, Tillisch J, Marshall R, Phelps M, Schelbert H (1986) Severity of segmental myocardial blood flow reduction and persistence of metabolic activity in patients with chronic ischemic heart disease. J Nucl Med 27:891
35. Buxton DB, Schwaiger M, Vaghaiwalla Mody F, Krivokapich J, Nienaber C, Armbrecht J, Luxen A, Ratib O, Phelps ME, Schelbert HR (1989) Regional abnormality of oxygen consumption in reperfusion assessed with [l-^{11}C] acetate and positron emission tomography. Am J Cardiac Imaging 3:1–12
36. Fudo T, Kambara H, Hayashi M, Hashimoto T, Nohara R, Tamaki N, Yamashita K, Konishi J, Kawai C (1989) Significance of exercise-induced ST-segment elevation in patients with Q wave anterior myocardial infarction: Evaluation by positron emission tomography. J Am Coll Cardiol 13:203A
37. Nienaber C, Brunken R, Sherman T, Yeatman L, Gambhir SS, Krivokapich J, Demer L, Child J, Schelbert H (1989) Recovery of myocardial metabolism by PET precedes improvement of ischemic wall motion after PTCA. J Am Coll Cardiol 13:28A
38. Matsuzaki M, Gallagher KP, Kemper WS, White F, Ross J Jr (1983) Sustained regional dysfunction produced by prolonged coronary stenosis: gradual recovery after reperfusion. Circulation 68:170–182
39. Fedele FA, Gewortz J, Capone RJ, Sharaf B, Most AS (1988) Metabolic response to prolonged reduction of myocardial blood flow distal to a severe coronary artery stenosis. Circulation 78:729–735
40. Opie LH, Owen P, Riemersma RA (1973) Relative rates of oxidation of glucose and free fatty acids by ischemic and non-ischemic myocardium after coronary artery ligation in the dog. Eur J Clin Invest 3:419–435
41. Weiner DA et al. (1987) Significance of SMI during exercise testing in patients with coronary artery disease. Am J Cardiol 59:725

42. Rozanski A, Bairey CN, Krantz DS, Friedman J, Resser KJ, Morell M, Hilton-Chalfen S, Hestrin L, Bietendorf J, Berman DS (1988) Mental stress and the induction of silent myocardial ischemia in patients with coronary artery disease. New Engl J Med 318:1005–1012
43. Deanfield JE, Selwyn AP, Chierchia S, Maseri A, Ribeiro P, Krikler S, Morgan M (1983) Myocardial ischemia during daily life in patients with stable angina: Its relation to symptoms and heart rate changes. Lancet 2:753–758
44. Deanfield JE, Kensett M, Wilson RA, Seha M, Horlock P, De Landsheere CM, Selwyn AP (1984) Silent myocardial ischaemia due to mental stress. Lancet 2:1001–1005
45. Deanfield JE, Shea MJ, Wilson RA, Horlock P, de Landsheere CM, Selwyn AP (1986) Direct effects of smoking on the heart: Silent ischemic disturbances of coronary flow. Am J Cardiol 57:1005–1009
46. Braunwald E, Kloner RA (1982) The stunned myocardium: Prolonged, postischemic ventricular dysfunction. Circulation 66:1146–1149
47. Camici P, Araujo LI, Spinks T, Lammertsma AA, Kaski JC, Shea MJ, Selwyn AP, Jones T, Maseri A (1986) Increased uptake of ^{18}F-fluordeoxyglucose in postischemic myocardium of patients with exercise-induced angina. Circulation 74:81–88
48. Schwaiger M, Schelbert HR, Keen R, Vinten-Johansen J, Hansen H, Selin C, Barrio J, Huang SC, Phelps ME (1985) Retention and clearance of C-11 palmitic acid in ischemic and reperfused canine myocardium. J Am Coll Cardiol 6:311–320
49. Schwaiger M, Schelbert HR, Ellison D, Hansen H, Yeatman L, Vinten-Johansen J, Selin C, Barrio J, Phelps ME (1985) Sustained regional abnormalities in cardiac metabolism after transient ischemia in the chronic dog model. J Am Coll Cardiol 6:336–347
50. Schwaiger M, Neese RA, Araujo L, Wyns W, Wisneski JA, Sochor H, Swank S, Kulber D, Selin C, Phelps M, Schelbert HR, Fishbein MC, Gertz EW, Hansen H (1989) Sustained nonoxidative glucose utilization and depletion of glycogen in reperfused canine myocardium. J Am Coll Cardiol 13:745–754
51. Camici P, Bailey IA (1984) Time course of myocardial glycogen repletion following acute transient ischemia. Circulation 70:II-85
52. Hashimoto T, Kambara H, Fudo T, Hohara R, Hayashi M, Takatsu Y, Tamaki N, Konishi J, Kawai C (1989) Increased fluorine-18 deoxyglucose uptake after percutaneous transluminal coronary angioplasty in recently infarcted myocardium. Am J Cardiol 63:743–744
53. Schelbert HR, Phelps ME, Selin C, Marshall RC, Hoffman EJ, Kuhl DE (1980) Regional myocardial ischemia assessed by ^{18}Fluoro-2-deoxyglucose and positron emission computed tomography. In: Advances in Clinical Cardiology (Vol. I): Quantification of Myocardial Ischemia. New York: Gerhard Witzstrock: 437–447
54. Nicklas JM, Becker LC, Bulkley BH (1985) Effects of repeated brief coronary occlusion on regional left ventricular function and dimension in dogs. Am J Cardiol 56:473–478

Silent Myocardial Ischemia and Prognosis in Patients with Unstable Angina

P. Ouyang [1], G. Gerstenblith [2], and S.O. Gottlieb [1]

Introduction

Although the clinical syndrome of angina pectoris was first described over 200 years ago [16], it is only over the past one and a half decades that it has become clear that myocardial ischemia is often not accompanied by symptoms. Such asymptomatic or silent episodes of myocardial ischemia appear to result in similar hemodynamic abnormalities as do symptomatic episodes. Several studies have shown that silent ischemia occurs in 10%–90% of patients with coronary artery disease, depending on the clinical subset studied. The highest incidence of silent ischemia of 60%–90% has been found in patients with unstable angina [14, 18, 26]. Although the prognostic significance of silent myocardial ischemia remains under investigation in many subsets of patients with coronary artery disease [4, 9, 12, 13, 25, 29], there is increasing evidence that in patients with unstable angina the presence of continuing silent ischemia does provide prognostic information.

Methods To Detect Silent Ischemia

Exercise treadmill testing is the standard means for screening and identifying patients with coronary artery disease. Although continuous ambulatory electrocardiographic monitoring has been used extensively for detection of arrhythmias over the past 25 years, Holter suggested in his original study that this technology might be useful to detect ST segment changes [17]. Over the past decade or so there has been increasing interest in the use of this technique to detect transient episodes of ST segment shifts. These episodes have been correlated with other indices of abnormalities of myocardial perfusion and function [5, 6, 8, 22]. Thus continuous ambulatory electrocardiographic monitoring can be useful in detecting ongoing ischemia in patients with known coronary artery disease.

[1] Division of Cardiology, Francis Scott Key Medical Center, 4940 Eastern Avenue, Baltimore, MD 21224, USA
[2] Division of Cardiology, Johns Hopkins Hospital, 601 N. Wolfe Street, Baltimore, MD 21205, USA

W. Bleifeld et al. (Eds.)
Unstable Angina

Prognostic Implications of Silent Ischemia

Patients with unstable angina, defined as angina occurring at rest and associated with reversible electrocardiographic changes, can usually be rendered free of chest pain following admission to a coronary care unit when treated with bed rest, antiplatelet or anticoagulant therapy, and aggressive antianginal therapy with nitrates, beta-blockers, and calcium antagonists. However, these patients continue to have a high incidence of recurrent ischemia, myocardial infarction, and death [7, 19]. Pooled data from five studies of unstable angina published between 1982 and 1988 involving 337 patients in whom ambulatory electrocardiographic monitoring of ST segment shifts was performed, show a relative risk of death or infarction that is 2.7–9 times greater than that experienced by patients without transient ST changes on ambulatory electrocardiographic monitoring (Table 1) [14, 18, 26, 27, 31]. Most of the studies were performed before aspirin or heparin were shown to be of significant benefit in patients with unstable angina.

The Johns Hopkins study included 70 patients admitted to the coronary care unit with unstable angina in whom two-lead continuous electrocardiographic monitoring was performed for 48 h following institution of therapy with nitrates, propranolol, and nifedipine [14]. Thirty-seven patients (53%) had at least one episode of silent ischemia. In all there were 205 ischemic episodes and over 90% of the episodes were silent. Over 2 years of follow-up there were two deaths and eight nonfatal myocardial infarctions, and 11 patients in the group with silent ischemia underwent revascularization for continued unstable angina. In contrast, among the patients without silent ischemia there were no deaths and only one nonfatal infarction ($p < .01$, versus silent ischemia group), and five patients underwent revascularization for continued unstable angina ($p < .05$, versus silent ischemia group; Fig. 1). These investigators also investigated the importance of duration of silent ischemia; patients

Table 1. Prognostic implications of ST segment changes on ambulatory monitoring in patients with unstable angina. (Data obtained from six studies published between 1982 and 1988)

Reference	*N*	Follow-up	Outcome	Relative risk
Johnson et al. [18] [a]	92	3 months	Death/MI	2.7
Gottlieb et al. [14]	70 [b]	1 months	Death/MI	5.4
Gottlieb et al. [15]	70 [b]	2 years	Death/MI	9.0
Nademenee et al. [26]	49	3–6 months	Death/MI	3.4
Arnim et al. [31]	38	1 month	Death/MI	3.4
Pozzati et al. [27]	88	1 year	Death/MI	2.7
	337			3.4 (Av.)

MI, Myocardial infarction

[a] Symptomatic or silent ischemia; other studies evaluated silent ST changes only.

[b] Patients in these studies were included only once in the total *n*.

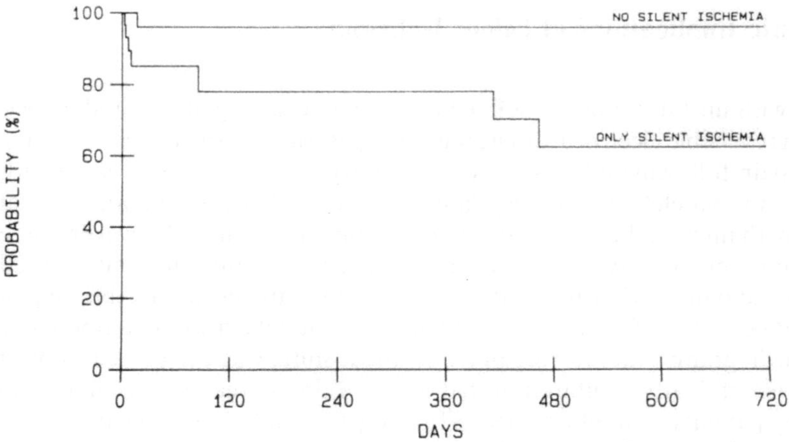

Fig. 1. Kaplan-Meier curves illustrating the probabilities of *not* experiencing death or myocardial infarction over the 2-year follow-up period for 37 patients with and 33 patients without silent ischemic ST changes on initial Holter monitoring. The difference between the two groups is significant at the $p<0.01$ level. (From Gottlieb et al. [15], p 758)

with silent ischemia were grouped as to whether they had under or over 60 min of silent ischemia in 24 h of monitoring. Actuarial Kaplan-Meier analysis at 1-month follow-up showed a significantly greater likelihood of recurrent ischemic outcomes – defined as death, nonfatal infarction, or revascularization for ongoing symptoms – in the group with over 60 min of silent ischemia per 24 h of monitoring (Fig. 2). Multivariate analysis after 2 years of follow-up showed that silent ischemia carried a fivefold relative risk of unfavorable ischemic outcome and was the most important prognostic predictor, even when compared to continued chest pain.

Nademenee et al. [26] also found a greater incidence of ischemic events in patients with unstable angina who had over 60 min of silent ischemia compared to patients without or with under 60 min of silent ischemia. In 3–6 months of follow-up, 18 of 20 (90%) of patients without silent ischemia were alive and well. In contrast, only 1 of 18 (6%) patients with over 60 min of silent ischemia were alive and well. These investigators also demonstrated an association between severity of coronary artery disease and duration of silent ischemia (Fig. 3). In a study of 38 patients, all of whom were receiving intravenous nitroglycerin, beta-blockers, calcium channel blockers, and heparin followed by acetylsalicyclic acid, von Arnim et al. [31] showed transient ischemia on ambulatory monitoring in 42% of the patients; 82% of these episodes were silent. In the group with ischemic episodes on monitoring, 88% had a subsequent ischemic event (death, nonfatal infarction, or revascularization) over 30 days of follow-up compared to only 45% in the group without transient ischemia ($p<.02$).

In patients with stable exertional angina the activity of coronary artery disease is frequently assessed using exercise treadmill testing. This has also

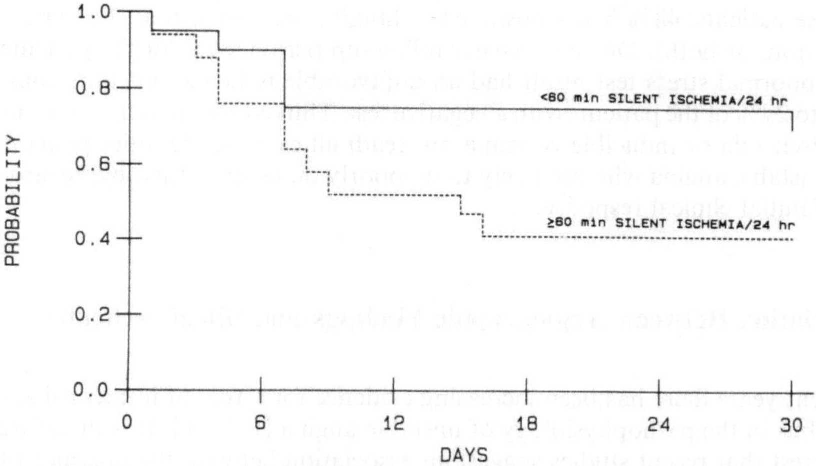

Fig. 2. Kaplan-Meier curves showing the cumulative probabilities of *not* experiencing myocardial infarction or revascularization for recurrent angina during a period of 30 days in the patients with silent ischemia, comparing the patients with less than 60 min of silent ischemia per 24 h and those with more than 60 min per 24 h during the 2 days of electrocardiographic monitoring ($p = 0.04$). (From Gottlieb et al. [14], p 1217)

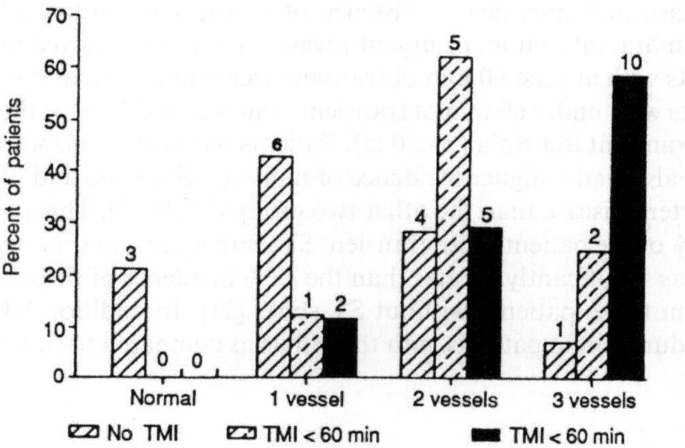

Fig. 3. Relation between the presence and duration of transient myocardial ischemia (*TMI*) found on Holter recording and the number of diseased coronary vessels found at angiography in patients with unstable angina. The numbers on the top of each histogram bar refer to the number of patients. (From Nademenee et al. [26], p 6)

been shown to be safe and to provide useful prognostic information in patients admitted to hospital with unstable angina if performed after the frequency of chest pain has been stabilized following institution of therapy [3, 11, 28]. In a study of 125 patients admitted to hospital with unstable angina, Butman et al. [3] performed exercise testing after a pain-free period of at least 3 days.

Of these patients, 48% had a positive test (angina, at least 1 mm ST segment depression, or both). During a 1-year follow-up period, 87% of the patients with abnormal stress test result had an unfavorable ischemic outcome compared to 29% of the patients with a negative test. Thus either ongoing transient silent ischemia or inducible ischemia on treadmill exercise identifies patients with unstable angina who are likely to do poorly on medical therapy, regardless of initial clinical response.

Association Between Angiographic Findings and Silent Ischemia

In recent years there has been increasing evidence for a role of intracoronary thrombus in the pathophysiology of unstable angina [1, 2, 30]. It is therefore of interest that recent studies suggest an association between the presence of thrombus and silent ischemia. Langer et al. [20] studied 136 patients admitted to the coronary care unit who received 24 h of continuous electrocardiographic monitoring during the first coronary care unit day. Among these patients 90 had at least 1 episode of at least 1 mm ST segment shift, and 89% of the episodes of transient ischemia were asymptomatic. These patients underwent coronary angiography, and the angiograms were evaluated for severity of coronary artery disease and presence or absence of features suggestive of thrombus. Death, nonfatal infarction, or urgent revascularization occurred in 67% of the 46 patients with at least 60 min of transient ischemia, compared to 32% of the 44 patients with under 60 min of transient ischemia and 22% of the 46 patients without transient ischemia ($p < .025$). Patients with more episodes of transient ischemia also had a higher incidence of multivessel disease and of left main coronary artery disease than the other two groups (Table 2). Thrombus was found in 44% of the patients with transient ST changes on continuous monitoring, which was significantly greater than the 22% incidence of thrombus that was found in those patients without ST shifts [21]. In addition ST shifts were of longer duration in patients with thrombus as compared to those without.

Table. 2. Association between angiographic finding and Holter ST changes in 136 patients with unstable angina. (Data from Langer et al. [20])

	No ST change ($n=46$)	ST change ($n=90$)		p
		ST <60 min ($n=44$)	ST >60 min ($n=46$)	
Multivessel disease	22%	32%	67%	<0.025[a]
Left main disease	4%	9%	29%	<0.025[a]
Thrombus	22%	44%		<0.03

[a] Group with ST changes lasting >60 min compared to the other two groups.

Other investigators have found that patients with unstable angina and ST segment shifts on ambulatory electrocardiographic monitoring more often had complex coronary lesions and higher grade of stenosis than those without transient silent ischemia [27]. These findings suggest that silent ischemia occurs more frequently in patients with thrombus and severe multivessel or left main coronary artery disease. These would be the group of patients likely to fare worst.

Circadian Variability of Silent Ischemia

There appears to be a circadian variation to the occurrence of myocardial infarctions [23] and sudden death [24], with a peak occurrence in the early morning hours shortly after waking from sleep. Figueras et al. [10] found circadian variation in the frequency of resting angina in 16 patients with unstable angina treated with nitrates alone, with a late evening peak (Fig. 4). These investigators also demonstrated a decrease in threshold to pacing-induced ischemia at night compared to morning or afternoon. We have also found a similar circadian variation with a late evening peak in the frequency of episodes of ST segment depression on continuous electrocardiographic monitoring in patients with unstable angina treated with nitrates and betablockers, suggesting an intrinsic circadian variation that may be altered by medical therapy.

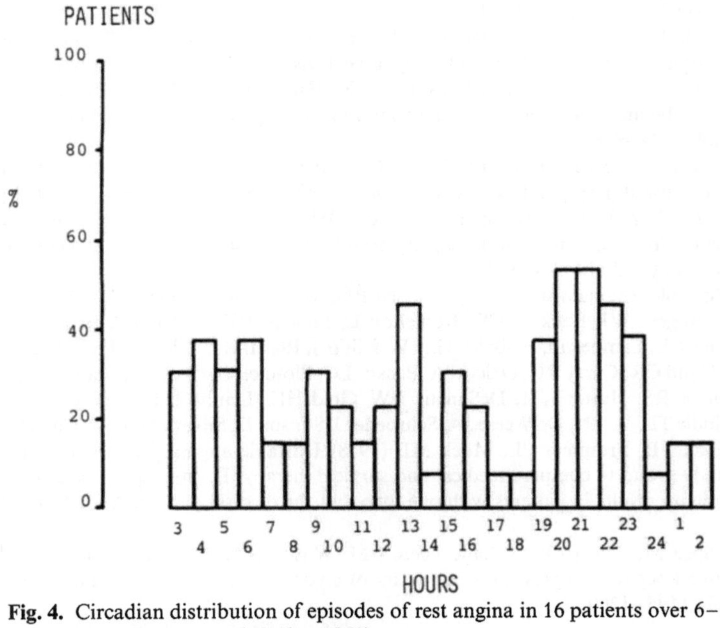

Fig. 4. Circadian distribution of episodes of rest angina in 16 patients over 6–10 days of observation. (From Figueras et al. [10], p 1250)

Summary

There is strong evidence that silent myocardial ischemia is a marker for adverse prognosis in the patient with unstable angina. There is also evidence that silent ischemia, like symptomatic ischemia, is a variable that has a range of severity and intensity. It appears associated with angiographic findings thought to be of importance in the pathophysiology of unstable angina. Current therapy for unstable angina includes aspirin or heparin, beta-blockers, nitrates, and calcium antagonists. If the patient suffers continued pain, angiography and revascularization are indicated. However, in the patient who becomes pain free further evaluation for prognostic risk stratification should include angiography and evaluation of ongoing active ischemic disease with ambulatory electrocardiographic monitoring or exercise stress testing. It is not yet known whether silent ischemia is a marker for high risk of further ischemic events, or whether it is causally related to subsequent death or infarction. Further investigation will be needed to provide these answers.

References

1. Ambrose JA, Winters SL, Stern A, Eng A, Teicholz LD, Gorlin R, Fuster V (1985) Angiographic morphology and the pathogenesis of unstable angina pectoris. J Am Coll Cardiol 5:609–618
2. Ambrose JA, Hjemdahl-Monsen CE, Borric S, Gorlin R, Fuster V (1988) Angiographic demonstration of a common link between unstable angina pectoris and non-Q wave acute myocardial infarction. Am J Cardiol 61:244–247
3. Butman SM, Olson HG, Gardin JM, Piters KM, Hullett M, Butman LK (1984) Submaximal exercise testing after stabilization of unstable angina pectoris. J Am Coll Cardiol 4:667–673
4. Cecchi AC, Dovellini EV, Marchi F, Pucci P, Santoro GM, Fazzini PF (1983) Silent myocardial ischemia during ambulatory electrocardiographic monitoring in patients with effort angina. J Am Coll Cardiol 1:934–939
5. Chierchia S, Lazzari M, Freedman B, Brunelli C, Maseri A (1983) Impairment of myocardial perfusion and function during painless myocardial ischemia. J Am Coll Cardiol 1:924–930
6. Cohn PF, Brown EJ Jr, Wyne J, Holman BL, Atkins HL (1983) Global and regional left ventricular ejection fraction abnormalities during exercise in patients with silent myocardial ischemia. J Am Coll Cardiol 1:931–933
7. Cooperative Unstable Angina Study Group: Russell RO, Moraski RE, Kouchoukos N, Karp R, Mantle JA, Rogers WJ, Rackley CE, Resnekov L, Falicov RE, Al-Sadir J, Brooks H, Anagnostopoulos CE, Lamberti J, Wolk M, Gay W, Killip T, Rosati RA, Oldham HN, Wagner GS, Peter RH, Conti CR, Curry RC, Daicoff A, Becker LC, Plotnick G, Gott VL, Brawley RK, Donahoo JS, Ross RS, Hutter AM, DeSanctis RW, Gold HK, Leinbach RC, Buckley MJ, Austen WG, Biddle TL, Yu PN, De Weese JA, Schroeder J, Stinson D, Silverman J, Kaplan EM, Gilbert JP, Newell JB, Frommer PL, Mock MB (1978) Unstable angina pectoris: national co-operative study group to compare medical and surgical therapy. II. In-hospital experience and initial follow-up results in patients with one, two and three vessel disease. Am J Cardiol 42:839–848
8. Deanfield JE, Shea M, Ribiero P, de Landsheere CM, Wilson RA, Horlock R, Selwyn AP (1984) Transient ST-segment depression as a marker of myocardial ischemia during daily life. Am J Cardiol 54:1195–1200

9. Erikssen H, Thaulow E (1984) Follow-up of patients with asymptomatic myocardial ischemia. In: Rutishausen W, Roskamm H (eds) Silent myocardial ischemia. Springer, Berlin Heidelberg New York, pp 156–164
10. Figueras J, Cinca J, Balda F, Moya A, Rius J (1986) Resting angina with fixed coronary artery stenosis: nocturnal decline in ischemic threshold. Circulation 74:1248–1254
11. Freeman MR, Chisholm RJ, Armstrong PW (1988) Usefulness of exercise electrocardiography and thallium scintigraphy in unstable angina pectoris in predicting the extent and severity of coronary artery disease. Am J Cardiol 62:1164–1170
12. Giagnoni E, Secchi MB, Wu SC, Morabito A, Oltrona L, Mancarella S, Volpin N, Fossa L, Bettazzi L, Arangio G, Sachero A, Folli G (1983) Prognostic value of exercise EKG testing in asymptomatic normotensive subjects: a prospective matched study. N Engl J Med 309:1085–1088
13. Gordon DJ, Ekelund LG, Karon JM, Probstfield JL, Rubenstien C, Sheffield LT, Weissfeld L (1986) Predictive value of the exercise tolerance test for mortality in North American men: the Lipid Research Clinics mortality follow-up study. Circulation 74:252–261
14. Gottlieb SO, Weisfeldt ML, Ouyang P, Mellits ED, Gerstenblith G (1986) Silent ischemia as a marker for early infavorable outcomes in patients with unstable angina. N Engl J Med 314:1213–1219
15. Gottlieb SO, Weisfeldt ML, Ouyang P, Mellits ED, Gerstenblith G (1987) Silent ischemia predicts infarction and death during 2 year follow-up of unstable angina pectoris. J Am Coll Cardiol 10:756–760
16. Heberden W (1772) Some account of a disorder of the breast. Med Trans R Coll Physicians 2:59–67
17. Holter NJ (1961) New method for heart studies. Continuous electrocardiography of active subjects over long periods is now practical. Science 134:1213–1220
18. Johnson SM, Mauritson DR, Winniford MD, Willerson JT, Firth BG, Cary JR, Hillis LD (1982) Continuous electrocardiographic monitoring in patients with unstable angina pectoris: identification of high-risk subgroup with severe coronary artery disease, variant angina, and/or impaired early prognosis. Am Heart J 103:4–12
19. Krauss KR, Hutter AM, DeSanctis RW (1972) Acute coronary insufficiency: course and follow-up. Circulation 45/46 (suppl I): I-66
20. Langer A, Freeman MR, Williams AE, Armstrong PW (1988) The relationship of Holter monitor ST shift and coronary thrombus in unstable angina. Circulation 78: II-421
21. Langer A, Freeman MR, Armstrong PW (1988) Ischemic ST changes on admission ECG and 24 hour Holter predict unfavourable outcome, multivessel disease, and left main stenosis in unstable angina. J Am Coll Cardiol 11:233A
22. Levy RD, Shapiro LM, Wright C, Mockus L, Fox KM (1986) The hemodynamic significance of asymptomatic ST depression assessed by ambulatory pulmonary artery pressure monitoring. Br Heart J 56:526–530
23. Muller JE, Stone PH, Tuti ZG, Rutherford JD, Czeisler CA, Parker C, Poole WK, Passamani E, Roberts R, Robertson T, Sobel BE, Willerson JT, Braunwald E and the MILIS Study Group (1985) Circadian variation in the frequency of onset of acute myocardial infarction. N Engl J Med 1313:1315–1322
24. Muller JE, Ludmer PL, Willich SN, Tofler GH, Aylmer G, Klangos I, Stone PH (1987) Circadian variation in the frequency of sudden cardiac death. Circulation 75:131–138
25. Multiple Risk Factor Intervention Trial Research Group (1985) Exercise electrocardiogram and coronary heart disease mortality in the Multiple Risk Factor Intervention Trial. Am J Cardiol 55:16–24
26. Nademenee K, Intrarachot V, Singh PN, Josephson MA, Rieders D, Mody FV, Bramah SN (1987) Prognostic significance of silent myocardial ischemia in patients with unstable angina. J Am Coll Cardiol 10:1–9
27. Pozzati A, Bugiardini R, Borghi A, Ottani P, Morgagni G, Puddu P (1988) Prognostic significance of myocardial ischemia refractory to maximal medical therapy in unstable angina. Circulation 78: II-421
28. Severi S, Orsini P, Marraccini C, Michelassi C, L'Abbate A (1988) The basal electrocardiogram

and the exercise stress test in assessing prognosis in patients with unstable angina. Eur Heart J 9:441–446
29. Sharma B, Asinger R, Francis GS, Hodges M, Wyeth RP (1987) Demonstration of exercise-induced painless myocardial ischemia in survivors of out-of-hospital ventricular fibrillation. Am J Cardiol 59:740–745
30. Sherman CT, Litvack F, Grundfest W, Lee M, Hickey A, Chaux A, Kass R, Blanche C, Matloff J, Morgenstern L, Ganz W, Swan HJC, Forrester J (1986) Coronary angioscopy in patients with unstable angina pectoris. N Engl J Med 315:913–919
31. von Arnim TH, Gerbig HW, Krawietz W, Hofling B (1988) Prognosic implications of transient – predominantly silent – ischaemia in patients with unstable angina pectoris. Eur Heart J 9:435–440

III. Management of Unstable Angina – Medical and Interventional Therapy

Calcium Antagonists and Beta-Blockers in the Treatment of Unstable Angina

J. LUBSEN [1]

Introduction

Unstable angina is an ill-defined syndrome which in terms of clinical symptoms and signs can be placed between stable effort angina and unequivocal acute myocardial infarction (AMI). Patients recognized clinically as having unstable angina are generally considered to be at high risk of progression to AMI, and the immediate objective of management is therefore both to abate symptoms and to prevent progression to AMI. Unstable angina is generally assumed to have a complex, multifactorial pathophysiology [1]. Apart from thrombosis, obstructive coronary disease and increased vasomotor tone are both thought to contribute to a degree which varies from patient to patient. Various classes of drugs, including calcium antagonists and beta-blockers, are therefore often given together or tried out in sequence.

Relatively few trials assessing medical treatment of unstable angina have been performed. Yusuf et al. [2] have presented an overview of known trials with calcium antagonists, beta-blockers, aspirin, and heparin. A more detailed review of trials with calcium antagonists has only recently been published by Held et al. [3]. Both groups of authors have also pooled the results so as to obtain summary estimates of the effect on total mortality and on the incidence of myocardial infarction. Pooling has recently received a great deal of attention and has even been called a new scientific discipline (meta-analysis) [4]. Here we consider first the pooled results as reported elsewhere [2, 3] and then whether these can be viewed as a sufficient summary of what has been learned from randomized trials about the medical management of unstable angina with calcium antagonists and beta-blockers. In this context, we consider the assumptions that underlie pooling, the question of whether trials of such an ill-defined entity as unstable angina can be pooled, and the clinical relevance of the pooled results. Several trials are discussed in more detail to show where pooling might have led to erroneous conclusions.

[1] Center for Clinical Decision Analysis, Erasmus Universiteit, P.O. Box 1738, 3000 DR Rotterdam, The Netherlands

W. Bleifeld et al. (Eds.)
Unstable Angina

Trials with Calcium Antagonists and Beta-Blockers in Unstable Angina: Pooled Results and Their Interpretation

In their review, Yusuf et al. [2] review three randomized trials [5–7] testing the calcium antagonist nifedipine. None of these reported a reduction in the number of infarctions. Overall, the incidence of myocardial infarctions was 21%, both among 472 treated patients (21%) and among 460 controls (21%). The pooled risk reduction was 4%, with a wide 95% confidence interval ranging from a 30% reduction to a 32% increase. Due to the small number of deaths, mortality data were considered inadequate [2]. The same authors review five trials with beta-blockade including 4700 patients. The pooled myocardial infarction risk reduction was 13%, with a 95% confidence interval ranging from 1% to 23% reduction [2]. As before, mortality data were considered inadequate.

In addition to three small trials with diltiazem [8–10], Held et al. [3] evaluate the same three nifedipine trials as Yusuf et al. [2]. Contrary to the latter, Held et al. distinguish trials with placebo as control separately from trials with standard treatment (i.e., propranolol and/or nitrates in this context) as control. In three trials with placebo as control [5, 7, 8], Held et al. counted 89 infarctions among 409 patients allocated to calcium antagonists and 89 infarctions among 397 patients allocated to control. Mortality was 8 out of 439 and 7 out of 427, respectively. In three trials with standard treatment as control [6, 9, 10], these authors counted 21 infarctions and 6 deaths among 152 patients allocated to calcium antagonists, as opposed to 6 infarctions and 2 deaths among 151 patients allocated to control.

The absence of any positive effect of calcium-antagonists in the above figures is disturbing in the light of their widespread use. It is therefore of considerable interest to ask whether this is perhaps a consequence of pooling rather than a reflection of a general lack of effect.

In answering this question, it is necessary to analyze how Yusuf et al. [2] reached their conclusion from the pooled data. From a statistical point of view, they represent a weighted average of the effect observed in the trials, with the weights depending on the size of each individual trial. The underlying assumption is that in biological reality the effect of a treatment has the same direction across all trials pooled, i.e., one must assume that there is no effect modification and that "like with like" is pooled concerning type of patients and treatment effects.

Thus, there are two reasons why calcium antagonists might have appeared ineffective in the pooled results discussed above. The first is that they have indeed no effect. The second is that there is effect modification, i.e., that they have a positive effect in some patients and a negative in others – effects that have averaged out to zero in pooling trials that study widely different types of patients. From the clinical point of view, it is of considerable importance to distinguish between these explanations. If the first is correct, then calcium antagonists should indeed be avoided. If the second is correct, and if the subgroups of patients in which a calcium antagonist has either a negative or a positive effect can be recognized as distinct clinical entities, then the conclusion is that their use should be limited to those instances in which a positive effect can be expected.

One way of looking at this question is to perform a so-called heterogeneity test in the context of a meta-analysis [11]. The null hypothesis tested is that all trials pooled have a similar effect in the same direction. Yusuf et al. [2] do not mention whether such a test was performed. It would most likely turn out to be not significant. Nonsignificance, however, cannot necessarily be construed off as proof of similarity, and it is therefore necessary also to look closely at the clinical context in which unstable angina trials have been done in the search for which of the two explanations seems best supported by currently available information.

Clinical Context of Unstable Angina Trials

A critical issue in both trial design and generalization of the results to indications that can be recognized in clinical practice is the clinical context in which a trial is done. Since unstable angina is an ill-defined entity, it should be no surprise that different trials have looked at different types of patients.

Two very different types of unstable angina trials must be considered. The first type, which we refer to here as early-entry trials, focuses on patients who are diagnosed at admission to hospital as having unstable angina. The second type, referred to as late-entry trials, focuses on patients who are diagnosed as having unstable angina at some time during hospital stay.

An early-entry trial requires that inclusion and exclusion criteria are phrased only in terms of symptoms and signs that can be recognized by the attending physician at hospital admission. At that moment, a patient is diagnosed as having unstable angina if there is a recent history of chest pain at rest suggesting acute ischemia but not infarction with compatible ECG. Although symptoms and signs do not suggest AMI as such, its presence can be ruled only out on the basis of cardiac enzymes. In cases of infarction, these take time to become positive and the results take time to be returned from the laboratory. Thus early-entry trials, which by definition cannot require enzyme assessments for eligibility, operate in a gray diagnostic zone, and among those randomized there will be patients who later appear to have been developing infarction already at the moment of randomization.

Late-entry trials, on the other hand, focus on patients in whom AMI has been ruled out during hospital stay. The typical patient will have experienced recurrent chest pain attacks combined with ECG patterns suggesting transient ischemia, but infarction has been ruled out on the basis of repeated cardiac enzyme assessments.

Typically, early- and late-entry trials focus also on different time spans. In an early-entry trial, the concern is with the immediate outcome of early treatment in an ill-defined clinical entity, i.e., the recurrence of symptoms and the total short-term occurrence of infarction, including its sequelae. Conceptually, they resemble in this respect trials of AMI treatment. Late-entry trials, on the other hand, focus on the subsequent recurrence of symptoms or the occurrence of symptoms over a somewhat longer time span in a well-defined clinical entity. In this respect they are more akin to secondary prevention trials of AMI.

Another issue relating to the clinical context of unstable angina trials is the treatment that was given shortly before randomization or in addition to experimental treatment thereafter. Patients who become unstable despite being on a certain type of medication are almost by definition failures in terms of that particular treatment. Also, concomitant treatment given in addition to experimental treatment after randomization may modify the effect of the latter. It must be borne in mind that, although trials advertise themselves as looking at the effect of one specific agent, they are often in fact looking at the relative net effects of various types of combination therapy. This applies in particular to unstable angina, where the use of combination therapy is widespread, and where combinations can either improve or impair oxygen balance and thereby prevent or induce myocardial infarction (which is one way of "stabilizing" unstable angina).

It can be concluded that the clinical context in which a particular unstable angina trial was carried out deserves close scrutiny and care must be taken in generalizing the results beyond its specific context, both in terms of the clinical entity which was studied (early versus late) and in terms of medication given before and after randomization. In these terms, it can be questioned whether very different trials can simply be pooled together as a basis for formulating general conclusions and recommendations.

Trials of Calcium Antagonists and Beta-Blockers

Early-Entry Trials

The largest early-entry unstable angina trial known to date is the double-blind, randomized Holland Interuniversity Nifedipine/Metoprolol Trial (HINT). Its main results (Table 1) have been reported elsewhere [7], as has an extensive description of its background, design, and methods [12]. HINT enrolled patients who either had an anginal pain episode in the hospital accompanied by varying ST-T changes suggesting reversible ischemia or had a history of anginal pain at rest (more than 15 min in duration) within 12 h of admission combined with either ST-T abnormalities or a known history of coronary disease. Excluded were patients with ECG signs of acute infarction or pain which did not respond immediately to routine pain relief based on sublingual nitroglycerin (such lack of reaction was considered a sign of infarction). Furthermore, patients were excluded who were already on nifedipine. Eligibility

Table 1. Risk reductions (in percentages) and their 95% confidence intervals as regards recurrent ischemia or myocardial infarction within 48 h in the HINT trial [7]

Treatment	*n*	Risk reduction (relative to placebo)
No previous beta-blockade		
Placebo	84	–
Metoprolol	79	−24% (−51 to +16)
Nifedipine	89	+15% (−17 to +64)
Combination	86	−20% (−47 to +19)
Previous beta-blockade (continued)		
Placebo	81	–
Nifedipine	96	−32% (−53 to −3)

was assessed immediately at CCU admission without waiting for results of enzyme assessments, and 62% of patients were randomized within 3 h after the last attack of pain.

At randomization, two subgroups were distinguished: those patients who had already been treated with a beta-blocker and those who had not. Subjects from the latter subgroup were randomized to either nifedipine (6 × 10 mg/24 h), metoprolol (2 × 100 mg/24 h), the combination of nifedipine and metoprolol in the same dosages, or to double placebo (matching both nifedipine and metoprolol). Subjects from the subgroup who were already on beta-blockade were continued on it (generally on metoprolol) and were randomized to receive in addition either nifedipine (6 × 10 mg/24 h) or matching placebo. The main outcome parameter was recurrence of ischemia or progression to MI within 48 h in all patients in whom baseline enzyme tests were later returned as within normal limits.

Of interest as far as its clinical context is concerned is the short-term clinical course of the 537 HINT patients enrolled. Of these, 4% later appeared to have had elevated enzymes already at the moment of randomization, and 8% were in the process of evolving MI, with an onset that was later in retrospect judged to have been before randomization. A further 9% sustained MI within 48 h but with an onset after randomization, and a further 19% had recurrent chest pain without MI. In total of 60% had an uncomplicated clinical course over 48 h.

These figures underscore the evidence of gray diagnostic zone surrounding unstable angina at hospital admission. Although suspicion of AMI was an exclusion criterion, 12% of HINT patients had nevertheless already sustained MI or were in the process of doing so. In only 9% was there an infarction within 48 h that could possibly have been prevented by the treatments studied.

For reasons to be mentioned below, enrollment was stopped prematurely. The main findings as regards the effects of metoprolol and nifedipine are given in Table 1. In patients not on beta-blockade already at randomization, metoprolol reduced the total incidence of recurrent ischemia or MI within 48 h by

24%, although the 95% confidence interval shows an overlap with no effect. Nifedipine, on the other hand, seemed to increase the incidence of the same endpoint. Although this effect was not significant by conventional standards, the trend was nevertheless considered sufficiently worrisome by the HINT policy advisory board to terminate the trial ahead of schedule, the argument being that it was highly unlikely that the trend would reverse [12].

Regarding the effect of nifedipine, results were strikingly different in patients who were already on beta-blockade at randomization. In these patients, there was strong evidence that the addition of nifedipine to continued beta-blockade reduces the incidence of recurrent ischemia or MI within 48 h (see Table 1).

To adapt to a complex clinical situation, the HINT design was necessarily complex. This complexity is not reflected in pooled results as reported elsewhere [2, 3]. Both Yusuf et al. [2] and Held et al. [3] reviewed all patients randomized together and compared them to all patients not receiving nifedipine as control, disregarding the difference between monotherapy and combination therapy and disregarding the distinction between patients who were already on beta-blockade and those not (it is noted that the figures listed by Held et al. [3] for the HINT trial cannot even be found in the quoted reference [7]). Held et al. [3] might as well have pooled the two nifedipine and metoprolol monotherapy groups (Table 1) together with the other trials with standard treatment as control which were considered. In addition, it would perhaps have been more reasonable to pool only the nifedipine and placebo groups among patients already on beta-blockade with the trial by Gerstenblith et al. [5] in order to pool like with like as far as concomitant therapy with beta-blockade is concerned.

Another early-entry trial was performed by Muller et al. [6]. These researchers randomized 63 patients to conventional treatment (propranolol if not contraindicated and isosorbide dinitrate) and another 63 to nifedipine. Yusuf et al. [2] counted this trial among the trials with nifedipine and Held et al. [3] counted it under the heading of standard treatment as control. Overall, there was no difference as regards recurrence of chest pain. However, these investigators observed that nifedipine seemed to be effective in patients who were already on a beta-blocker before randomization, while patients did not do better under conventional therapy.

Late-Entry Trials

Gerstenblith et al. [5] have assessed the effect of nifedipine (40–80 mg/24 h) when added in randomized double-blind fashion to a standard regimen of propranolol (160 mg/24 h). Patients were required to have chest pain at rest with transient ECG changes and were randomized only when enzymes had remained below twice the upper limit of normal for 24 h beforehand. Follow-up lasted 4 months. During this period there were 44% treatment failures (sudden death, MI, or persistent angina requiring invasive intervention) among 68 patients randomized to nifedipine. Among 70 patients randomized to placebo the failure rate was 61%.

For quite some time, this trial has been quoted as supporting the overall efficacy of nifedipine in unstable angina. Its relevance as a late-entry trial in patients in whom MI was excluded, and who all also received a beta-blocker has perhaps been overlooked. One may question, again, whether like with like is pooled when this trial is taken together with nifedipine-treated subgroups with or without beta-blockade from an early-entry trial such as HINT, as was done by Yusuf et al. [2] and by Held et al. [3].

A trial similar in design to the one of Gerstenblith et al. [5] but assessing the effect of the addition of nifedipine (80 mg/24 h) to propranolol has been reported from the same institution by Gottlieb et al. [13]. Follow-up was shorter however (1 month). The number of patients and events in this trial was too small to allow any conclusions.

Conclusions and Recommendations

Soon after nifedipine was introduced, favorable results in the treatment of unstable angina were reported. In retrospect and in view of later findings quoted above, it seems likely that this early enthusiasm, which was based on results obtained by adding nifedipine to beta-blockade if instability persisted [14], was warranted, but that the relevance of concomitant beta-blockade for the effect of nifedipine was overlooked.

As far as generalization to a specific clinical context is concerned, the findings of HINT [7, 12] apply to a well-defined and important (relatively high short-term risk for recurrent ischemia or infarction) indication occurring in a minority (in the order of 25%) of patients at CCU admission or immediately thereafter. As regards the trial by Muller et al. [6], the report does not explicitly state whether normal enzymes were required for eligibility or not. Also, there was no placebo control group, and interpretation therefore rests entirely on how one rates the efficacy of conventional treatment.

Based on these two trials taken together, however, several conclusions seem clinically relevant with respect to clinical pharmacologic insights [1] but not from pooled results [2, 3]. The following suggestions are drawn regarding early treatment with nifedipine and beta-blockers:

1. In patients who are not already on one, a beta-blocker such as metoprolol can be expected to reduce the incidence of recurrent chest pain and progression to MI. In this context and against the background of the diagnostic uncertainty at hospital admission, findings from AMI trials with beta-blockers provide additional support.
2. Of the calcium-antagonists, only nifedipine has been assessed in randomized trials. Its effect can be either positive or negative and probably depends on the clinical context. The fact that pooled results [2, 3] indicate no

overall effect is probably due to effect modification, with a positive effect confined to those patients who are treated concomitantly with a beta-blocker. In particular, a positive effect suggests itself in patients who become unstable despite being on a beta-blocker. This conclusion is supported by theoretical arguments about the interactions between beta-blockade and calcium antagonists [1].

3. The few late-entry trials with nifedipine and beta-blockers have all been relatively small as far as patient numbers are concerned and no definite conclusions can be drawn.

Regarding recommendations for clinical practice, the following can be stated:

1. For patients who become unstable and are not already treated as such, a beta-blocker should be first choice, provided that there are no contraindications. There is no evidence that this should be combined with a calcium antagonist started at the same time.
2. For patients who become or remain unstable despite beta-blockade, the addition of nifedipine can be recommended.
3. The use of nifedipine as monotherapy should be avoided.

References

1. Packer M (1989) Drug therapy. Combined beta-adrenergic and calcium-entry blockade in angina pectoris. N Engl J Med 320:709–718
2. Yusuf S, Wittes J, Friedman L (1988) Overview of results of randomized clinical trials in heart disease. II. Unstable angina, heart failure, primary prevention with aspirin, and risk factor modification. JAMA 260:2259–2263
3. Held PH, Yusuf S, Furberg D (1989) Calcium channel blockers in acute myocardial infarction and unstable angina: an overview. Br Med J 299:1187–1192
4. Sacks HS, Berrier J, Reitman D et al. (1987) Meta-analyses of randomized controlled trials. N Engl J Med 316:450–455
5. Gerstenblith G, Ouyang P, Aschuff SC et al. (1982) Nifedipine in unstable angina. A double blind randomized trial. N Engl J Med 306:885–889
6. Muller JE, Turi ZG, Pearle DL et al. (1984) Nifedipine and conventional therapy for unstable angina. A randomized, double-blind comparison. Circulation 69:728–739
7. Holland Interuniversity Nifedipine/Metoprolol Trial (HINT) Research Group (1986) Early treatment of unstable angina in the coronary care unit. A randomised, double blind, placebo controlled comparison of recurrent ischemia in patients treated with nifedipine or metoprolol or both. Br Heart J 56:400–413
8. Hagemeijer F, Schelling A, Van Marinissen KMR (1985) Impending myocardial infarction treated intravenously with diltiazem. In: Proceedings of Cardiovascular Therapy Symposium, Geneva, p 314A
9. Theroux P, Taeymans Y, Morrisette D et al. (1985) A randomized study comparing propranolol and diltiazem in the treatment of unstable angina. J Am Coll Cardiol 5:717–722
10. Andre-Fouet X, Usdin JP, Gayet C et al. (1983) Comparison of short-term efficacy of diltiazem and propranolol in unstable angina at rest. A randomized trial in 70 patients. Eur Heart J 4:691–698

11. Yusuf S, Simon R, Ellenberg S (1987) Methodologic aspects of overviews of randomized controlled trials. Proceedings of a workshop conducted at the NIH. Stat Med 6:217–409
12. Holland Interuniversity Nifedipine/metoprolol Trial (HINT) Research Group (1987) Eur Heart J 8 [Suppl H]
13. Gottlieb SO, Weisfeldt ML, Ouyang P et al. (1986) Effect of the addition of propranolol to therapy with nifedipine for unstable angina pectoris: a randomized, double blind, placebo-controlled trial. Circulation 73:331–337
14. Hugenholtz PG, Michels HR, Serruys PW et al. (1981) Nifedipine in the treatment of unstable angina, coronary spasm and myocardial ischemia. Am J Cardiol 47:163–173

Antiplatelet Therapy in Unstable Angina: Rationale, Effectiveness, and Dosage

R. LORENZ [1]

Introduction

Antiplatelet therapy with aspirin in unstable angina is now based on solid evidence gathered by means of very different investigational methods. The ultimate rationale for this therapeutic approach is provided by the important involvement of platelet activation in the pathogenesis of unstable angina. This aspect is covered in detail elsewhere in this volume (Hamm et al.) and is only summarized here. Second, the basic pharmacology of antiplatelet drugs that have been used in controlled trials in unstable angina are reviewed briefly. Then, the structure and main findings of the large controlled trials that have finally established the clinical benefit from aspirin in unstable angina are discussed. The implications drawn here for clinical practice are based on the combined analysis of these trials in unstable angina. Two antiplatelet trials in the closely related condition of acute myocardial infarction also have some practical bearing in this context. Finally, the benefit from antiplatelet therapy in unstable angina is placed into perspective.

Pathophysiologic Rationale for Antiplatelet Therapy in Unstable Angina

Intracoronary thrombosis is a frequent finding at necropsy after death preceded by unstable angina. The thrombi are usually of the platelet-rich type and often exhibit a layered architecture. This has been interpreted as reflecting phasic accretion of platelets onto the growing thrombus. The thrombus frequently appears to originate from a fissure in the fibrous cap of a stenosing atheromatous plaque causing hemorrhage into the plaque and platelet adhesion. Downstream from such thrombotic lesions intramyocardial microemboli of platelet aggregates may be detected [1, 2].

Angiography during the unstable phase frequently reveals a typically eccentric stenosis of the involved coronary vessel. Detailed analysis may detect

[1] Medizinische Klinik Innenstadt der Universität, Ziemssenstraße 1, 8000 München 2, West Germany

W. Bleifeld et al. (Eds.)
Unstable Angina

radiographic signs of the thrombotic nature of the critical stenosis especially if recent angiograms taken before the unstable phase are available for comparison [3–5]. Angioscopy during emergency bypass surgery or, more recently, catheterization has confirmed this interpretation of the angiographic findings by direct visualization of thrombotic material accreted onto an atheromatous stenosing lesion [6]. In some cases rapid progression of atherosclerosis or coronary vasospasm may also play a prominent role in the pathogenesis [7, 8].

Ongoing activity of the thrombotic accretion process during clinical presentation with acute infarction or unstable angina is evidenced by formation of thrombus specific products. Massive increases in intracorporeal thromboxane generation and elevated fibrinopeptide levels may be detected. These increases are reversed upon clinical stabilization. This was interpreted as indicating thrombus formation and thromboxane-supported in vivo platelet activation during the acute phase of unstable angina. The biochemical markers of platelet activation can be linked to angiographic signs of intracoronary thrombus formation and to prolonged clinical disease activity [9–15].

These findings gathered with very different methods implicate platelet activation and thrombus formation in the pathogenesis of unstable angina. Thus, they also differentiate this syndrome from stable angina on the pathogenetic level, whereas previously the differentiation had to be clinical [16]. They have led to the formulation of a widely accepted, although certainly simplified, model of unstable angina (Fig. 1). After plaque fissue, hemorrhage into the atheroma, and immediate platelet adhesion, phasic platelet recruitment from the circulation onto the evolving coronary thrombus and phasic redissolution of the thrombus occurs. Secretion of several platelet active products by the activated platelets themselves maintains this vicious cycle. These compounds may also cause coronary vasoconstriction. Antagonistic mediators such as prostacyclin, EDRF, or adenosin formed by endothelial cells may act as a potent negative feedback loop on the vicious cycle and thus limit the growth or redissolve the thrombus.

Among the known mediators of platelet activation thromboxane A_2 is prominent for several reasons. Its aggregating and vasoconstrictive potency is higher than that of other mediators, for example, serotonin and thrombin. The maximal synthetic capacity for thromboxane A_2 upon stimulation is about 5 orders of magnitude above the basal turnover, and, finally, its suppression is the clinically best established antiplatelet intervention. Growing knowledge of the underlying pathology in unstable angina and the pharmacology of aspirin has stimulated clinical research and helped in optimizing the design of studies.

Pharmacology of Antiplatelet Drugs Used in Unstable Angina

Two antiplatelet drugs have been adequately tested in large scale controlled clinical trials in unstable angina: aspirin and sulfinpyrazone.

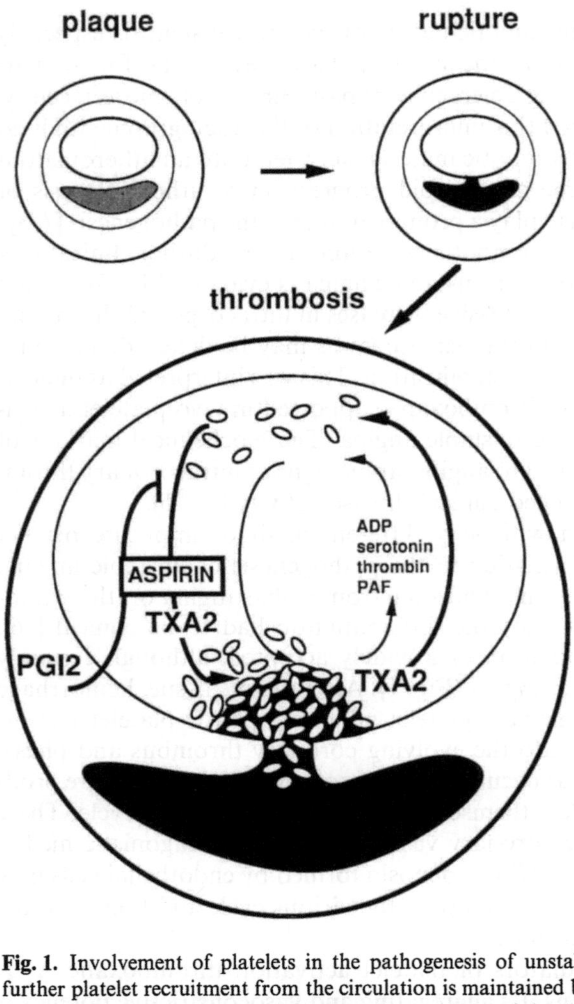

Fig. 1. Involvement of platelets in the pathogenesis of unstable angina. Thrombus growth by further platelet recruitment from the circulation is maintained by secretion of platelet-active compounds. Aspirin may interrupt the thromboxane loop of the vicious cycle, but it may also inhibit the counterregulatory secretion of prostacyclin by the vessel wall

Aspirin

Aspirin irreversibly inhibits cyclooxygenase, the key enzyme of prostanoid formation. The molecular mechanism is covalent transfer of its acetyl moiety onto a serine in the active center of the enzyme [17]. The acetylation reaction of cyclooxygenase is quick and quantitative even at low concentrations of aspirin. The enzyme then can no longer bind a heme group needed for oxygen transfer onto the precursor fatty acids of the prostanoids. Platelets lack de novo synthesis of the enzyme and are therefore permanently deprived their prostanoid pathway after a single exposure to aspirin. The major prostanoid formed by platelets, thromboxane A_2, acts as an important enhancer mechanism of platelet activation and thrombus formation. The antithrombotic effectiveness of aspirin correlates well with its suppression of thromboxane formation. Other putative actions, derived from indirect evidence, have not been clarified on a molecular level, and their clinical relevance has never been substantiated.

However, aspirin inhibits prostanoid formation in all tissues. Therefore, prostacyclin formation in endothelial cells is also reduced. Prostacyclin, the major prostanoid formed in coronary vessels, has an antagonistic profile of actions; it inhibits platelet activation and is a potent vasodilator. Prostacyclin is one important mechanism of endothelial thromboresistance, may limit thrombus propagation over intact endothelium, and may act as an endogenous antagonist to thromboxane A_2. The simultaneous inhibition of prostacyclin by aspirin is therefore unwanted and could be of potential harm. Fortunately, the time course of prostanoid recovery after aspirin exposure is much faster in tissues that can resynthesize new cyclooxygenase, such as endothelium, than in platelets. Lower and less frequent dosing of aspirin therefore offers a pharmacokinetic opportunity to differentiate better the desired effect of aspirin on thromboxane formation in platelets from the unwanted effect on endothelial prostacyclin formation [18].

Aspirin prolongs bleeding time and reduces platelet aggregation but does not normalize shortened platelet survival. By direct comparison with all established antiplatelet regimes we could show that the inhibitory effects on platelet aggregation and thromboxane formation of 100 mg aspirin per day were indeed equal to those of the conventional 1 g dose [19]. The antithrombotic effectiveness of aspirin has meanwhile been well established in a variety of cardiovascular conditions [20].

Sulfinpyrazone

Sulfinpyrazone also inhibits cyclooxygenase. There is at least one active metabolite. However, the inhibition of cyclooxygenase is reversible and less marked than that by aspirin. It therefore continuously requires active levels of the drug, and the time course of the action on platelets is not different from that in other tissues. Sulfinpyrazone may normalize shortened platelet survival in several conditions, but effects on bleeding time and platelet aggregation are only minor compared to aspirin [19]. Sulfinpyrazone has been used in far fewer studies than aspirin. Its usefulness after myocardial infarction and after aortocoronary bypass surgery is questionable [20].

Clinical Trials in Unstable Angina

The clinical benefit from antiplatelet therapy in unstable angina has been evaluated in three large-scale controlled trials. Despite major differences in several aspects of their design their results are similar and complement each other. Considered together, they cover a wide spectrum in the natural history, clinical presentation, and medical management of unstable angina and provide a solid base for current clinical practice.

Basic Structure of the Trials

These well-designed trials have all been conducted during the past 15 years in the United States and Canada. All were prospective, randomized, placebo-controlled, double-blind, and multicenter. The basic features of the protocols are compared in Fig. 2.

The pioneering trial [21] coordinated by the Veterans Administration (VA) was conducted between 1974 and 1981 in 12 centers. It tested the action of antiplatelet therapy with low-dose aspirin (324 mg/day) in unstable angina against placebo. Over 1400 male patients were randomized, including those in

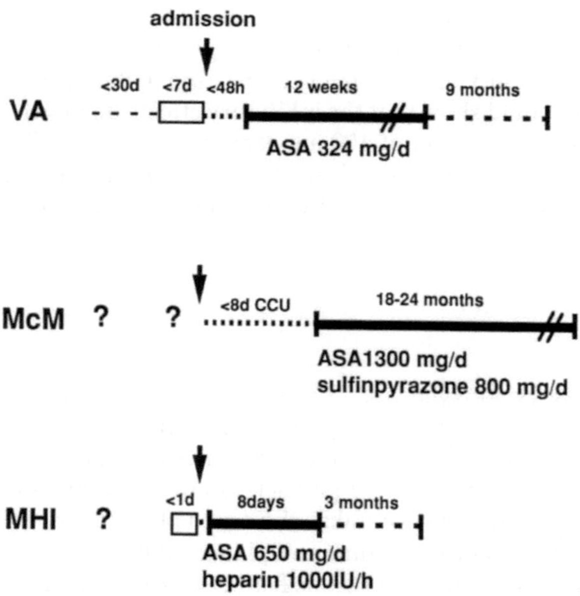

Fig. 2. Study protocol schemes of the three antiplatelet trials in unstable angina synchronized for the time of hospital admission (*arrow*). *From left to right*, time frame accepted for first onset of unstable phase (- - - -), last unstable episode before admission (□), time in hospital before randomization (. . . . . .), scheduled treatment (—), postinterventional observation (- - - -). Maximal duration of each phase of the protocol is printed above time axis or indicated by *?* if unknown. Drug regimes are printed below treatment phase. *ASA*, acetylsalicylic acid

a pilot trial and the segregated group of patients later diagnosed with evolving myocardial infarction at randomization. Inclusion of these patients did not alter the results of the main trial. Treatment was for 3 months. The principal endpoints were death and acute myocardial infarction during that time. However, observational follow-up of vital status at 1 year was nearly complete. Confirmation of coronary artery disease by angiography was very rare in this trial, and invasive cointerventions such as aortocoronary bypass operation or angioplasty were deliberately avoided.

The trial coordinated by the MacMaster University (McM) [22] was conducted between 1979 and 1983 in seven centers. It tested the effects of antiplatelet therapy with either high dose aspirin (4×325 mg/day), sulfinpyrazone (4×200 mg/day) or the combination of both in unstable angina against the respective placebos. About 550 patients were randomized. Treatment and follow-up were long term for up to 24 months. The principal endpoints were nonfatal acute myocardial infarction, cardiac death, and mortality from all causes. Confirmation of coronary artery disease by angiography at any time during the study was available in the majority of patients.

The most recent trial from the Montreal Heart Institute (MHI) [23] was conducted between 1986 and 1988 in two centers. The effects of aspirin (2×325 mg/day), heparin (1000 IE/h), and their combination were tested against the respective placebos. About 480 patients were randomized. Treatment and follow-up were short term for about 1 week only until definite management was decided upon. The principal endpoints were refractory angina, acute myocardial infarction, and death. Early angiography was available in almost all patients and often led to angioplasty or coronary artery bypass graft shortly thereafter. If indicated by persistent instability, the decision for early coronary angiography or intervention was counted under the "soft" first endpoint of refractoriness.

Thus these trials addressed the effects of intermediate, prolonged, and very short treatment with three different antiplatelet regimes. The chainging prevalence of invasive diagnostic procedures and therapeutic cointerventions reflects the new options that have become available during the past two decades and their impact on management of unstable angina. Therefore these trials nicely complement each other both in the time frame of treatment and with respect to the medical and surgical background therapy.

Definition of the Target Condition and Entry Criteria

Exact knowledge of the modalities of patient recruitment in studies is required for the valid extrapolation of results to clinical practice. In the VA trial patients were recruited in general hospitals within 48 h of admission with chest pain suggestive of unstable angina. This was defined as angina of new onset or sudden worsening occurring at least once a day, at rest and lasting over 15 min. It could, however, have started up to 30 days earlier and settled during the previous week. Independent evidence of preexisting coronary artery disease was sought. Acute infarction was excluded by repeat ECG and enzymes at 3 h. Patients with myocardial infarction evolving within 24 h were evaluated as a segregated group.

In the McM trial patients with possibly ischemic pain were recruited within 8 days after admission to the coronary care unit. Unstable angina was defined as either crescendo pain (at least a twofold increase in severity, duration, frequency, or nitroglycerin requirement) or prolonged pain at rest (at least 15 min in duration in a setting of physical and emotional rest). Thus, clinical criteria for unstable angina were quite similar to those used in the VA trial, as was exclusion of acute infarction with a control ECG and enzymes at 24 h. Independent evidence of coronary artery disease was sought too, but documented infarction within the previous year caused exclusion.

In contrast, in the MHI trial patients were recruited immediately at presentation in the emergency room and randomized within 24 h. Unstable angina was defined as an accelerating pattern of chest pain occurring at rest or with minimal exercise or of chest pain lasting 20 min or longer. Objective evidence of coronary artery disease or independent confirmation of the diagnosis by two cardiologists was required. Clinical criteria and exclusion of acute infarction were similar. Recent angiography and bypass surgery also caused exclusion.

Therefore, unstable angina was defined very similarly in all three trials. The typical clinical syndrome, independent evidence of coronary artery disease and best possible exclusion of infarction at entry was required. This corresponds very well to the diagnosic approach in clinical practice. However, the route of patient recruitment and, most importantly, the time frame for recruitment within the natural history of unstable angina was different among the three trials. The VA and McM trials also included patients who had already passed the peak phase of their unstable angina whereas the MHI trial made every effort to restrict entry to patients who currently sought medical treatment with an acute heart attack.

Prerandomization Selection Process and Exclusion Criteria

The filtering process for patients primarily considered for the trial until actual inclusion and randomization is also important for the extrapolation of results into clinical practice. This is compared for the three trials in Fig. 3. As the target condition was defined quite similarly in all three trials, the variable proportion of patients screened who were in fact found to have unstable angina in the definition of the study was principally due to the screening process. Of the initially screened patients approximately 7300 (53%) were found to have unstable angina in the VA trial. The corresponding figures for the McM trial were 4600 (17%) and for the MHI trial 800. No total figure of screened patients was given in the MHI trial.

Despite the clear-cut entry criteria, the further prerandomization selection process of eligible patients was rather extended in the first two trials. For better

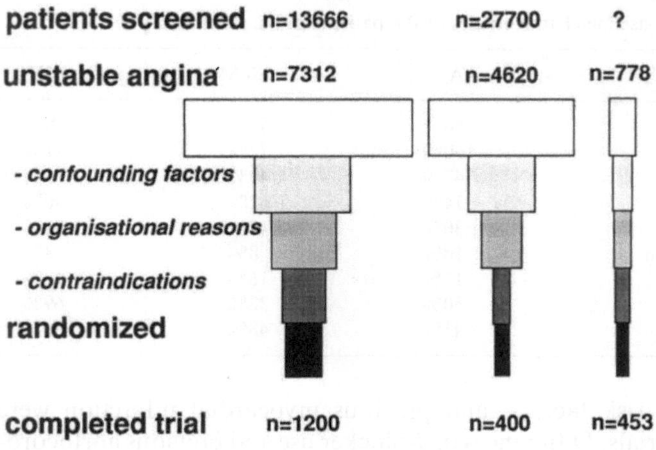

Fig. 3. Comparison of the screening process and prerandomization selection of patients considered for the three trials

comparison, the various exclusion criteria have been roughly grouped into three categories. Most exclusions were due to potentially confounding factors, including interfering medication, preexisting conditions of prognostic relevance, such as recent infarction, aortocronary bypass surgery, or angioplasty, or identifiable factors contributing to angina such as anemia. Inclusion of these patients would have diluted the study population and reduced the power of the study to detect a real therapeutic effect. A second group of exclusions was due to organizational factors such as failure to consent, questionable compliance, or remote residence. These two categories of exclusion criteria generally should not reduce the relevance of the study results for clinical practice. In all three trials the further exclusions due to real contraindications have been relatively small. Contraindications included anticoagulant therapy, history of bleeding, ulcer disease, or allergy. Overall, least exclusions were reported in the MHI trial, which may be due to the recruitment from only two emergency units and to the short-term protocol of this trial. So despite final inclusion of only a minority of patients with unstable angina in the VA and McM trials the results should be reasonably representative for the target condition.

Baseline Characteristics of Patients

It is surprising that with all these differences in recruitment, the patients finally entered were quite similar in the different trials. Some selected data are listed in Table 1. Despite protocol exclusions such as women in the VA trial and age over 70 in the McM trial, the essential demographic and medical data such as

Table 1. Comparison of baseline characteristics of the patients in the three trials

	VA	McM	MHI
Age (years)	56	57	58
Men	100%	72%	71%
Previous MI	47%	40%	35%
>15 min Angina	74%	62%	36%
β-Blockers	30%	?	95%
Previous bypass operation	10%	8%	18%
Diabetes	17%	16%	13%
Smoking	50%	32%	69%
Hypertension	41%	48%	38%

age, cardiovascular risk factors, and previous myocardial infarction were rather similar in all trials. Differences in β-blocker use and previous aortocoronary bypass operation reflect the changing medical response to disease rather than a change in the underlying pathology.

Randomization and Intervention

Stratification as to presence of previous myocardial infarction and previous aspirin use was done only in the VA trial. In the other two smaller trials the factorial design with more than two treatment groups would otherwise have resulted in overstratification. Randomization was done in blocks in all three trials. It generally worked well; no major imbalances occurred that could have influenced the outcome of any of the trials.

Follow-Up, Drug Compliance, and Protocol Adherence

The most important figures related to protocol adherence are summarized in Table 2. Generally, regular completion of protocol and drug compliance was fairly good in all three trials. The figures were lowest in the long-term McM trial. In the short-term MHI trial, carried out among inpatients only, follow-up was virtually complete. Angiographic assessment of coronary morphology has become a standard procedure during work-up in the more recent trials.

Table 2. Protocol adherence and angiographic findings

	VA	McM	MHI
Protocol completed	95%	66%	96%
Vital status known	99%	98%	100%
Drug compliance	85%	89%	100%
Angiography	3.5%	61%	91%
Two- or multivessel disease	–	74%	53%

The prevalance of higher grade coronary artery disease underlying unstable angina is probably only apparently decreasing as coronary angiography is no longer restricted to a subset of patients elected for severity of clinical course. In any event, if a patient is found to meet the study criteria of unstable angina, coronary angiography almost always reveals at least one relevant stenosis. Clinical diagnosis thus proved rather accurate in this setting.

Evaluation of Outcome

All trials tried to exclude myocardial infarctions that had already occurred at the time of randomization. Diagnostic guidelines for later progression to infarction were very similar in all trials and followed generally accepted criteria. The clinical picture with either doubling of enzymes or ECG changes according to the Minnesota code were required. In the VA trial the hardest vital endpoint, all-cause mortality, was predefined. In the other two trials cause-specific mortality rates or combinations with non-fatal myocardial infarction were predefined endpoints. However, the all-cause mortality and separate nonfatal myocardial infarction rates can nevertheless be reconstructed from the figures given. For fair comparison between the trials the same target events were used and always evaluated in the intention to treat approach. The intention-to-treat approach was not strictly maintained in the McM trial, where the (ineffective) treatment with sulfinpyrazone was neglected in the final analysis.

Second, both start of treatment after the clinical manifestation and duration of treatment were different between the trials. This certainly influenced absolute risk within the trial. But no attempts were made to correct the crude risk figures for any of the time intervals. Therefore, for comparison of absolute risks as well as treatment effects the endpoints are reported in Fig. 4 as cumulative risk in trial for both the placebo and aspirin group and the relative risk reduction by the treatment.

Principal Results

The culmination of unstable angina in nonfatal myocardial infarction was significantly reduced by aspirin both in the VA and the MHI trials, but not in the McM trial. The most likely explanation for this failure in the McM trial seems to be the late start of treatment after admission with unstable angina. The figures were low, however, and the apparent increase may well have been a chance phenomenon. In any event, the combination of cardiac death and nonfatal myocardial infarction was significantly reduced also in this trial. As to the control groups, the much higher risk for infarction observed in the short-term MHI trial may be due both to the timing of this trial in the very acute phase of unstable angina and to the increased diagnostic awareness for infarction during a short observation period of an inpatient with multiple enzyme determinations available.

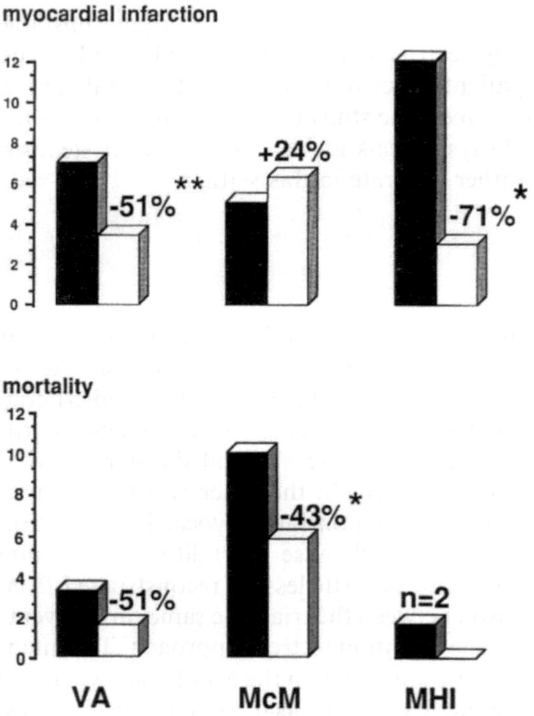

Fig. 4. Frequency (%) of nonfatal myocardial infarction (*upper panel*) and death from any cause (*lower panel*) in the placebo groups (*black columns*) and aspirin groups (*white columns*) of the three trials. Relative risk reduction by aspirin treatment is also indicated in percentages. *, $2p<0.05$; **, $2p<0.01$

Also in the hardest endpoint, total mortality, all trials of aspirin in unstable angina are remarkably consistent. In the VA trial the all-cause mortality after 3 months of treatment was cut by half from over 3%, a result that fell just short of the conventional 5% level of significance. In the McM trial no effect of sulfinpyrazone alone or in combination on any endpoint was seen, and the authors analyzed the benefit of aspirin versus aspirin placebo, irrespective of the simultaneous intake of sulfinpyrazone. Only with this secondary regrouping, the significance limits for the aspirin versus no aspirin contrast were crossed. All-cause mortality at 2 years was significantly reduced by 43%. In the MHI trial the small number of deaths precluded assessment of this end-point. The distribution of deaths was, however, consistent with that in the other trials and even more so at 3-month follow-up evaluation.

This sustained increase of benefit after cessation of treatment was also evident in the VA trial in the 12-month vital status follow-up conducted in over 90% of all patients. The 1.7% absolute reduction in mortality at the end of the 3-month aspirin treatment in this trial even more than doubled during the next

9 months without further treatment. This continued benefit after cessation of aspirin is not easy to explain. With the large numbers in the VA trial it is very unlikely a chance process, as may be said of the same trend in the MHI trial. It is also contrary to the observations with aspirin in acute myocardial infarction. For the aspirin component of the ISIS-2 trial [24] the difference in mortality between the aspirin and placebo groups was largest at the end of treatment at 4 weeks and tended to decline slowly thereafter over the whole 2 years of postinterventional observation. The authors of the VA trial suggested that a subsequently doubled mortality in patients suffering a myocardial infarction during the treatment phase might explain the difference. However, if calculated this can account for only about 0.5% of the 2.5% delayed reduction in mortality by aspirin.

Determinants of Outcome

The different treatment protocols in the three trials allow some considerations on the influence of treatment modalities on the success rate, as shown in Fig. 5.

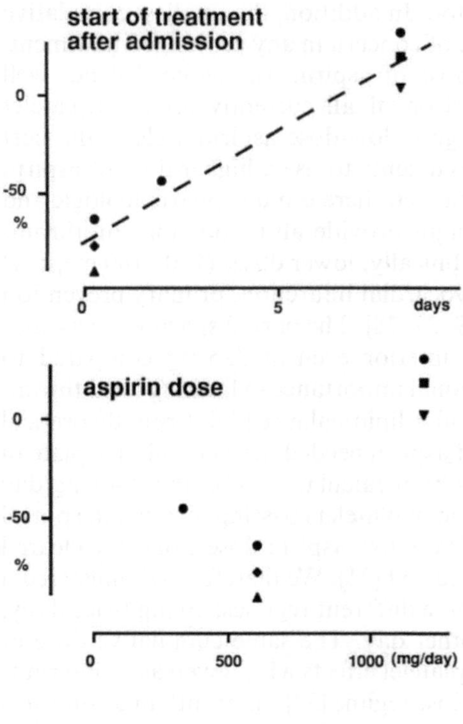

Fig. 5. Relative risk reduction of nonfatal myocardial infarction plotted against start of treatment after hospital admission for unstable angina (*upper panel*) and against aspirin dose used (*lower panel*). Treatment with aspirin only (*closed circles*), sulfinpyrazone (*triangle*), heparin (*pyramid*), and combination of aspirin with sulfinpyrazone (*square*) or heparin (*diamond*)

If reduction of infarction is plotted against start of treatment after hospital admission with unstable angina, an almost linear correlation is evident. A delayed start of treatment may cause the negative selection of patients most prone to early infarction, who then are excluded from randomization. Very early randomization, in turn, includes more patients with evolving infarction. That these profit from aspirin has meanwhile been shown unequivocally in the ISIS-2 trial [24]. Thus, early start of treatment is an important determinant of success.

In contrast, if reduction of infarction is plotted against the aspirin dose used, there is anything but a positive correlation of benefit with dose. This holds not only for the comparison of these three trials in unstable angina but also in the meta-analysis of the much larger number of aspirin trials in secondary prevention [25] and aortocoronary bypass patency [20].

Side Effects of Aspirin Treatment

The gastrointestinal side effects of aspirin are clearly dose dependent [20], and this is likely for the renal side effects, too. In addition, the smallest cumulative dose that is effective should always be of concern in any prolonged treatment. In fact, in the McM trial the high dose of aspirin was reduced if not well tolerated. In the only direct comparison of all currently used antiplatelet regimes in aortocoronary bypass surgery, low-dose aspirin yielded the best result [26]. Thus there are no good arguments to use a higher dose of aspirin than 325 mg/day in unstable angina. In fact, there is much pharmacologic and experimental evidence that aspirin might provide all its possible antithrombotic potential at even lower doses. Clinically, lower doses (100–160 mg/day) have been found effective in acute myocardial infarction, primary prevention and aortocoronary bypass patency [19, 27, 28]. The partial sparing of vascular prostacyclin capacity appears to be inferior even at 325 mg compared to 100 mg, and this may well be of functional importance in limiting local thrombotic propagation and long-term vascular lipid balance [29]. From theoretical pharmacokinetic modeling the dose of aspirin needed for a cumulative plateau effect on thromboxane formation has been calculated to be about 40 mg/day [30]. Furthermore, selective inactivation of platelets passing through the portal circulation during slow resorption of very low aspirin doses, that are cleared by the liver on first pass, has been discussed [31]. We therefore administered a mean dose of 40 mg/day aspirin by three different regimes; 20 mg twice daily, 40 mg every day, and 80 mg every other day. The same cumulative dose of aspirin had significantly superior antiplatelet effects when given as an intermittent pulsed regime rather than a split-dose regime [32]. Intermittent dosing also allows for longer recovery intervals for prostacyclin. Furthermore, the aspirin dose for a plateau effect on platelet function was found higher than 40 mg/day in the range of 100 mg/day [19, 32, 33]. It seems that exposure of platelets to a certain threshold drug level rather than the frequency of exposures is critical for the antiplatelet effect of aspirin. From these findings, ultralow dosing of aspirin and selective presystemic exposure of platelets by very slow release preparations do not appear promising.

Other Considerations

The differential diagnosis of myocardial infarction will remain unclear for some time at clinical presentation in many cases. Fortunately, the complementary ISIS-2 trial has also documented benefit from low-dose aspirin in acute myocardial infarction. Side effects of lysis were not increased intolerably by aspirin treatment [24]. Therefore, the early start of aspirin treatment that is important for maximal benefit in unstable angina should not be delayed until definite exclusion of infarction. In fact, treatment should be continued until definite exclusion of both infarction and unstable angina, as a single dose of aspirin in patients suspected of infarction appeared to provide no benefit but to do no harm either [34]. With the low dosage used in the VA trial, peptic ulcer symptoms were regarded a contraindication only if they had occurred during the previous 3 months. Of course, bleeding conditions and allergic reactions must be ruled out before aspirin administration.

Benefit from Aspirin in Unstable Angina in Relation to Other Conditions

To put the beneficial effects of aspirin in unstable angina into perspective, the figures from representative controlled trials in various conditions, all with low-dose aspirin, are compared in Fig. 6 [35]. The number of deaths prevented per 1000 patients treated is plotted against the time of treatment in the respective trial. It is evident that in unstable angina, as in acute infarction, considerably more lives are saved in a rather short treatment period than will ever be achievable by much longer treatment in less dramatic conditions. But not only in this vital endpoint is antiplatelet therapy especially rewarding in unstable angina, it is also worthwhile in terms of nonfatal myocardial infarction. Here the wide range of benefit from aspirin in terms of prevention of vascular events can be represented only on a logarithmic scale. The number of infarctions prevented by aspirin per 1000 treated in unstable angina is second only to the number of occlusions prevented by aspirin in the elective revascularization procedures of aortocoronary bypass or angioplasty. It is superior to the aspirin effect on nonfatal vascular events in acute infarction, secondary or primary prevention. Therefore the acute phase of coronary artery disease that is marked by the clinical syndrome of unstable angina is very amenable to risk reduction by aspirin.

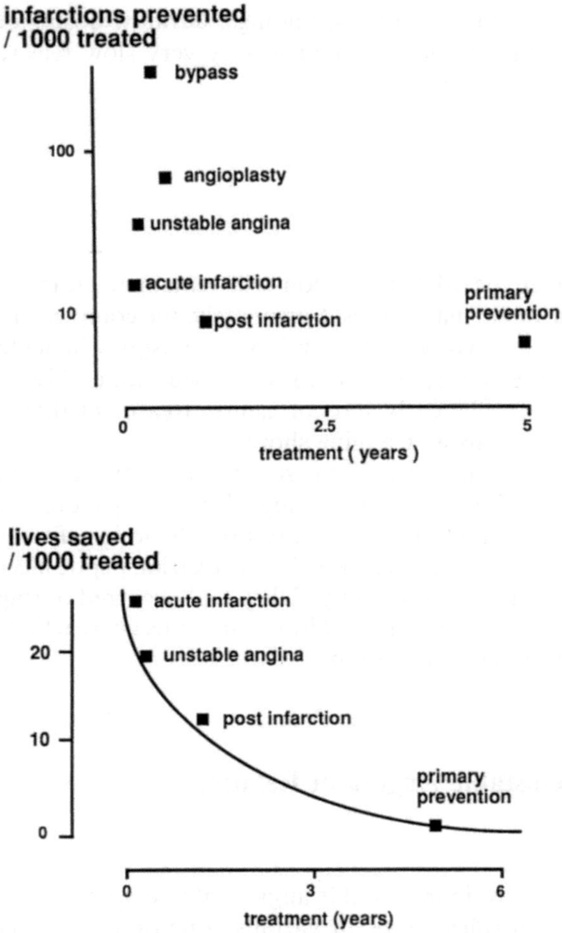

Fig. 6. Relative benefit from antiplatelet treatment with low-dose-aspirin in various cardiovascular conditions plotted against duration of treatment. *Upper panel*, nonfatal vascular occlusions prevented per 1000 patients treated; *lower panel*, lives saved per 1000 patients treated. Data are from representative studies in the conditions indicated

Conclusions

The beneficial effects of antiplatelet therapy with aspirin in unstable angina are now very well established by converging evidence from three carefully controlled trials. Sulfinpyrazone is without effect. Benefit from aspirin has been shown in patients recruited in various ways, general hospital, coronary care unit, or emergency admission and at various times after onset of symptoms. Aspirin is beneficial in very short run treatment as well as in prolonged and even in delayed treatment. The benefit provided is sustained and appears to increase further after termination of drug treatment. The dose of 325 mg aspirin is fully active, and it is very suggestive that even less will suffice and may be preferable in terms of side effects and sparing of protective mechanisms. If the differential diagnosis to infarction is unclear at presentation there is no question that immediate aspirin medication is beneficial in either condition. It does not preclude but rather supplements other measures that may be indicated, for example, lysis or emergency percutaneous TCA. In contrast, many of the other procedures in themselves provide an indication for aspirin. Finally, aspirin is a real frontline intervention for the emergency setting with low cost both in terms of side effects and money. The benefit that aspirin can provide in unstable angina is higher than in many other settings and in the range of much more sophisticated and expensive interventions.

References

1. Falk E (1985) Unstable angina with fatal outcome: dynamic coronary thrombosis leading to infarction and/or sudden death: autopsy evidence of recurrent mural thrombosis with peripheral embolization culminating in total vascular occlusion. Circulation 71:699–708
2. Davies MJ, Thomas AC (1985) Plaque fissuring – the cause of acute myocardial infarction, sudden ischemic death, and crescendo angina. Br Heart J 53:363–373
3. Holmes DR, Hartzler GO, Smith HC, Fuster V (1981) Coronary artery thrombosis in patients with unstable angina. Br Heart J 45:411–416
4. Zack PM, Ischinger T, Aker UT, Dincer B, Kennedy HL (1984) The occurrence of angiographically detected intracoronary thrombus in patients with unstable angina pectoris. Am Heart J 108:1408–1412
5. Ambrose JA, Winters SL, Stern A et al. (1985) Angiographic morphology and the pathogenesis of unstable angina pectoris. J Am Coll Cardiol 5:609–616
6. Sherman CT, Litvak F, Grundfest W et al. (1986) Coronary angioscopy in patients with unstable angina pectoris. N Engl J Med 315:913–919
7. Moise A, Theroux P, Taeymans Y et al. (1983) Unstable angina and progression of coronary atherosclerosis. N Engl J Med 309:685–689
8. Maseri A, L'Abate A, Baroldi G (1978) Coronary vasospasm as a possible cause of myocardial infarction: a conclusion derived from the study of 'preinfarction' angina. N Engl J Med 299:1271–1277
9. Foegh ML, Eliasen K, Johansen S, Helfrich GB, Ramwell PW (1986) Coronary artery thrombosis and elevated urine immunoreactive thromboxane B2. Prostaglandins 32:781–788
10. Henrikson P, Wennmalm A, Edhag O, Vesterquist O, Green K (1986) In vivo production of prostacyclin and thromboxane in patients with acute myocardial infarction. Br Heart J 55:543–548
11. Fitzgerald DJ, Roy L, Catella F, FitzGerald GA (1986) Platelet activation in unstable coronary disease. N Engl J Med 315:983–989
12. Hamm CW, Lorenz RL, Bleifeld W, Kupper W, Wober W, Weber PC (1987) Biochemical evidence of platelet activation in patients with persistent unstable angina. J Am Coll Cardiol 10:998–1004
13. Theroux P, Latour JG, Leger-Gauthier C, De Lara J (1987) Fibrinopeptide A and platelet factor levels in unstable angina pectoris. Circulation 75:156–162
14. Kruskal JB, Commerford PJ, Franks JJ, Kirsch RE (1987) Fibrin and fibrinogen-related antigens in patients with stable and unstable coronary artery disease. N Engl J Med 317:1361–1365
15. Lorenz RL, Hamm CW, Riesner H, Bleifeld W, Weber PC (1990) A prospective study of the diagnostic value of urinary thromboxane in patients presenting with acute chest pain. J Int Med 227:429–434

16. Fuster V, Badimon L, Cohen M, Ambrose JA, Badimon JJ, Chesebro J (1988) Insights into the pathogenesis of acute ischemic syndromes. Circulation 77:1213–1220
17. Roth GJ, Majerus PW (1975) The mechanism of the effect of aspirin on human platelets. I. Acetylation of a particulate fraction protein. J Clin Invest 56:624–632
18. O'Grady J, Moncada S (1978) Aspirin: a paradoxical effect on bleeding time. Lancet ii:780
19. Lorenz R, Siess W, Weber PC (1981) Effects of very low versus standard dose acetyl salicylic acid, dipyridamole and sulfinpyrazone on platelet function and thromboxane formation in man. Eur J Pharmacol 70:511–518
20. Lorenz R (1989) Antiplatelet drugs in the prevention of cardiovascular disease: when, what, to what benefit? Münch Med Wochenschr 131:237–240
21. Lewis HD, Davis JW, Archibald DG, Steinke WE, Smitherman TC, Doherty JE, Schnaper HW, LeWinter MM, Linares E, Pouget JM, Sabharwal SC, Chesler E, DeMots H (1983) Protective effects of aspirin against acute myocardial infarction and death in men with unstable angina. N Engl J Med 309:396–403
22. Cairns JA, Gent M, Singer J, Finnie KJ, Froggatt GM, Holder DA, Jablonsky G, Kostuk WJ, Melendez LJ, Myers MG, Sackett DL, Sealey BJ, Tanser PH (1985) Aspirin, sulfinpyrazone or both in unstable angina. N Engl J Med 313:1369–1375
23. Theroux P, Ouimet H, McCans J, Latour JG, Joly P, Levy G, Pelletier E, Juneau M, Stasiak J, DeGuise P, Pelletier G, Rinzler D, Waters DD (1988) Aspirin, heparin or both to treat acute unstable angina. N Engl J Med 319:1105–1111
24. ISIS-2 (Second International Study of Infarct Survival) Collaborative Group (1988) Randomised trial of intravenous streptokinase, oral aspirin, both, or neither among 17187 cases of suspected acute myocardial infarction: ISIS-2. Lancet ii:349–360
25. Antiplatelet trialists' collaboration (1988) Secondary prevention of vascular disease by prolonged antiplatelet treatment. Br Med J 296:320–331
26. Goldman S, Copeland J, Moritz T, Henderson W, Zadina K, Ovitt T, Doherty J, Read R, Chesler E, Sako Y, Lancaster L, Emery R, Sharma GVRK, Joan M, Pacold I, Montoya A, Parikh D, Sethi G, Holt J, Kirklin J, Shabetai R, Moores W, Aldridge J, Masud Z, DeMots H, Floten S, Haakenson C, Harker LA (1988) Improved early saphenous vein graft patency after coronary artery bypass surgery with antiplatelet therapy: results of a veterans administration cooperative study. Circulation 77:1324–1332
27. Steering committee of the physician's health study research group (1989) Final report on the aspirin component of the ongoing physicians' health study. N Engl J Med 321:129–135
28. Lorenz R, von Schacky C, Weber M, Meister W, Kotzur J, Reichardt B, Theisen K, Weber PC (1984) Improved aortocoronary bypass patency by low-dose aspirin (100 mg daily). Lancet i:1261–1264
29. Boerboom LE, Olinger GN, Kissebah AH, Montgomery RR (1987) Low-dose aspirin protects against lipid accumulation in primate vein bypass grafts. J Thorac Cardiovasc Surg 94:251–258
30. Patrono C, Ciabattoni G, Patrignani P, Pugliese F, Filabozzi P, Batella F, Davi G, Forni L (1985) Clinical pharmacology of platelet cyclooxygenase inhibition. Circulation 72:1177–1184
31. Pederson AK, FitzGerald GA (1984) Dose-related kinetics of aspirin: presystemic acetylation of platelet cyclooxygenase. N Engl J Med 311:1206–1211
32. Lorenz R, Boehlig B, Uedelhoven W, Weber PC (1989) Superior antiplatelet action of alternate day pulsed dosing over split dose administration of aspirin. Am J Cardiol 64:1185–1188
33. Herd CM, Bochner F, Rodgers SE, Duncan EM, Lloyd JV, Turnbridge LJ (1987) A dose-ranging study of the antiplatelet effect of enteric coated aspirin in man. Aust NZ J Med 17:195–200
34. Elwood PC, Wiliams WO (1979) A randomized controlled trial of aspirin in the prevention of early mortality in myocardial infarction. J R Coll Gen Pract 29:413–416
35. Lorenz R (1989) Prophylaxe mit Thrombozytenaggregationshemmern bei kardiovaskulären Indikationen. Internist (Berlin) 30:315–321

Nitrate Therapy in Unstable Angina Pectoris

U. THADANI [1]

Introduction

Unstable angina was until recently considered to result from progression of an atherosclerotic plaque [31], and superimposed coronary artery spasm at the site of the lesion was thought to precipitate ischemic episodes [7, 15]. There is, however, convincing evidence that the culprit lesion in unstable angina is a fissuring of an atherosclerotic plaque which predisposes to platelet deposition and thrombus formation [6, 10, 14, 17, 46]. Plaque progression may also play a role in some patients [31], and in others an increase in myocardial oxygen demand rather than a reduction in flow may be contributory [37, 41]. The emphasis of treatment therefore should be rapid institution of therapy with aspirin or heparin or the combination of the two [5, 26, 49, 58] rather than overzealous use of antianginal drugs, surgery, or angioplasty during the initial phase of unstable angina [11, 32, 43]. Treatment with aspirin, heparin, or both reduces mortality and incidence of myocardial infarction [58] but does not relieve anginal pain or myocardial ischemia immediately. On the other hand, intravenous nitroglycerin relieves ischemic and anginal episodes rapidly and plays an important role in the management of patients with unstable angina. Intravenous nitroglycerin should therefore be used concurrently with aspirin or heparin and other antianginal agents for symptomatic relief of angina and for its antiischemic effects.

Nitrate Therapy

Mechanism of Action of Nitrates in Unstable Angina

Nitrates improve the balance between myocardial oxygen supply and demand (Table 1). This is achieved by their predominant venodilator effects with resultant decrease in venous return and ventricular volumes and end-diastolic pressures [1, 28]. In addition, nitrates reduce afterload and produce dilation of

[1] Cardiovascular Section, Department of Medicine, University of Oklahoma, Health Sciences Center, South Pavillion, Room 5SP300, Oklahoma City, OK 73190, USA

W. Bleifeld et al. (Eds.)
Unstable Angina

Table 1. Mechanism of action of intravenous nitroglycerin in unstable angina

Decreased myocardial oxygen demand	Enhanced myocardial oxygen supply
1. Decreased left ventricular end-diastolic volume (preload) decreases wall stress.	1. Dilatation of coronary arteries: epicardial vessels, eccenteric stenosis and collaterals.
2. Decreased cardiac output decreases arterial pressure.	2. Decreased left ventricular end-diastolic pressure enhances subendocardial blood flow.
3. Decreased arterial compliance and peripheral resistance lowers systolic pressure (afterload).	3. Inhibition of coronary spasm or reduction of coronary vasomotor tone.
	4. Decreased platelet aggregation and deposition prevents coronary artery occlusion and vasospasm (?).

epicardial coronary arteries, collateral channels, and stenotic sites [3, 18, 22, 29, 59, 60]. Nitrates relax vascular smooth muscles through an endothelium-independent mechanism [20, 38] and thereby produce vasodilation at the atherosclerotic site, where the endothelium is either injured or dysfunctional [27]. Nitrates inhibit platelet aggregation in vitro [25, 44, 45] and reduce platelet deposition and vasoconstriction at the site of experimental endothelial injury [24]. Thus, the net effect of nitrates is to improve blood flow to the ischemic regions.

Effects of Nitrates on Morbidity and Mortality in Unstable Angina

Intravenous nitroglycerin producing 10–15 mm Hg reduction in systolic blood pressure reduces infarct size and lowers the incidence of infarct-related complications [4, 16, 21]. Retrospective analysis of published data is suggestive of beneficial effects on mortality [61]. Whether intravenous nitroglycerin and other nitrate preparations reduce the incidence of myocardial infarction or mortality in unstable angina is not known at the present time. Available data are inadequate to answer this important question. Well-designed multicenter studies are urgently required to address this issue.

Effects of Nitrates on Anginal Episodes and Myocardial Ischemia During the Acute Phase of Unstable Angina

There are no adequate data available to show that monotherapy with nitrates is efficacious in patients with unstable angina. In the study reported by Distante et al. [13], many of the patients had variant rather than unstable angina by present definition. Nitrates have been invariably given in addition to other antianginal therapy. The available data (Table 2) support the effectiveness of intravenous nitroglycerin in relieving anginal episodes and myocardial

Table 2. Studies with intravenous nitroglycerin (NTG) in unstable angina

Reference	*n*	NTG dose (μg/min) mean (range)	Reduction (complete relief) of ischemic episodes	Comments
Dauwe et al. [9]	14	47 (30–180)	100	Refractory angina despite beta-blocker and long-acting nitrate therapy
Page et al. [33]	17	40	98	Refractory to beta-blocker and oral nitrates
Brodsky et al. [2]	14	13 (30–350)	36	Refractory angina despite long-acting nitrate therapy Hypotension a major problem during intravenous nitroglycerin
Mikolich et al. [30]	45	55 (5–267)	89 (89)	Refractory to beta-blocker and multiple doses of sublingual nitroglycerin
DePace et al. [12]	20	72 (15–226)	85	Refractory angina despite beta-blocker, oral nitrate and nifedipine therapy
Roubin et al. [40]	16	13	100 (38)	Refractory angina despite beta-blocker, nitrate and calcium blocker therapy
Squire et al. [48]	42	(227–393)	45	Refractory angina despite beta-blocker and long-acting nitrate therapy
Curfman et al. [8]	40	82 (100–200)	70 (36)	Background beta-blocker therapy: fixed-dose nitrate therapy during the study
Kaplan et al. [23]	35	140 (50–350)	94 (71)	Refractory angina despite beta-blocker and long-acting nitrate therapy
Thadani et al. [56]	43	(10–960)	98 (32)	Tolerance development necessitated increase of NTG dose

ischemia in patients who have already failed to respond to treatment with high-dose beta-blockers, oral nitrates, and/or calcium channel blocker therapy [2, 8, 9, 12, 23, 30, 33, 40, 48, 56]. Persisting angina despite therapy with other antianginal agents has necessitated open-label therapy with intravenous nitroglycerin, and it has not been practical or ethical to carry out placebo-controlled studies in this group of patients. Intravenous nitroglycerin has been used in the initial management of these symptomatic patients for 24–72 h, and with the exception of two reports [2, 40], there has been either complete relief or consistent reduction in the number of anginal attacks and ischemic episodes in eight of the ten reported studies (Table 2). In one study, high-dose oral isosorbide dinitrate plus nitroglycerin ointment was shown to be as effective as intravenous nitroglycerin (Fig. 1), but more patients experienced consistent

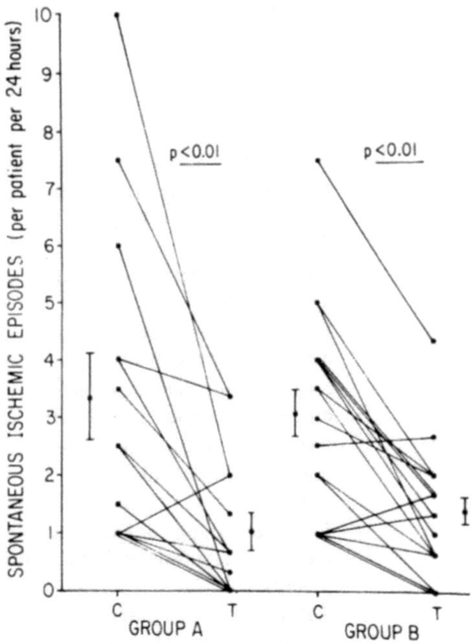

Fig. 1. Individual and group mean (±SD) data for number of spontaneous ischemic episodes (per patient per 24 h) during the control (*C*) and treatment (*T*) periods for intravenous nitroglycerin (*group A*) and oral isosorbide dinitrate plus nitroglycerin ointment (*group B*). The two nitrate regiments produced statistically significant ($p < 0.01$) and equivalent reductions in the frequency of ischemic episodes. (From Curfman et al. [8]; reproduced with permission from the American Heart Association)

relief of angina during intravenous nitroglycerin therapy (Fig. 2) [8]. In this study, recurrence of ischemic episodes necessitated surgical intervention in many of the patients treated with either intravenous nitroglycerin or isosorbide plus nitroglycerin ointment. However, this study was unusual in that the initial dose of the two medications was chosen on the basis of a 15-mm Hg reduction in mean arterial pressure rather than relief of anginal pain, and further dose titration was not permitted during the 72-h period of observation. This is an unusual approach as higher and higher doses of nitrates are often required for the treatment of recurrent angina and myocardial ischemia in this group of patients [56].

Whether nitrates are also effective in patients who are asymptomatic at the time of hospitalization following an episode of unstable angina is not known. Double-blind, placebo-controlled studies have not been performed in this group of patients. It is well established that patients who are symptomatic despite treatment with oral nitrates and other antianginal agents at the time of hospitalization respond rapidly to intravenous nitroglycerin (Table 2). These observations have led to the practice of routine use of intravenous nitroglycerin even in patients who are asymptomatic at the time of hospitalization with the hope of preventing further anginal and ischemic episodes.

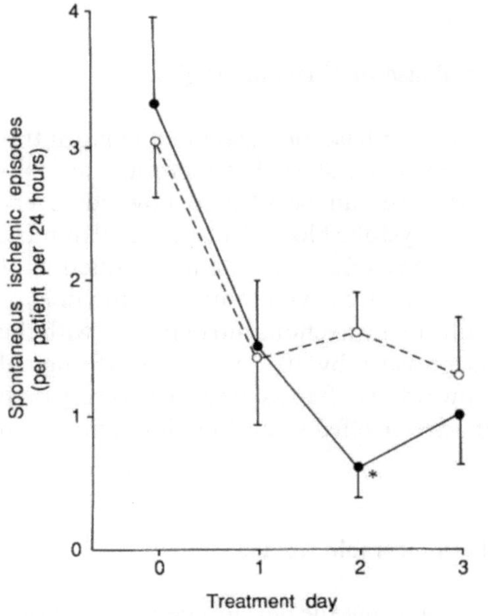

Fig. 2. Number of spontaneous ischemic episodes during the control (*C*) and on each of the 3 successive days of the treatment period. *Filled circles, solid lines,* data for patients receiving intravenous nitroglycerin; *open circles, broken lines,* data for patients receiving isosorbide dinitrate and nitroglycerin ointment. *Bars,* standard deviation. The number of episodes was significantly lower on day 2 in patients receiving intravenous nitroglycerin (*$p < 0.001$). On days 1 and 3, number of ischemic episodes during the two treatments were similar. (From Curfman et al. [8]; reproduced with permission from American Heart Association)

Which Nitrate Preparation to Use in Unstable Angina

Many nitrate preparations and formulations are available for clinical use [51]. From the available data, intravenous nitroglycerin is the formulation of choice; it is effective when therapy with high doses of oral nitrates has been ineffective. It permits immediate delivery and ease of titration [56]. Intravenous isosorbide dinitrate is an alternative [13], but because of its longer duration of action, titration may prove to be a problem in case an adverse reaction develops. Topical formulations, although widely used, do not permit rapid dose titration and absorption is often delayed and unpredictable [50]. Nitroglycerin patches cannot be recommended due to delayed absorption and difficulty in rapid dose titration which is often necessary in patients with unstable angina [50]. Oral formulations of isosorbide dinitrate and isosorbide-5-mononitrate have been used with success [8], but intravenous nitroglycerin is superior in the initial management of patients with unstable angina.

Intravenous Nitroglycerin Therapy

Intravenous Nitroglycerin in the Acute Phase of Unstable Angina

In symptomatic patients during the acute phase of unstable angina, intravenous nitroglycerin (5–10 μg/min) should be started if there are no contraindications to nitrate therapy. The dose can be titrated upwards every 5–10 min until relief of angina or a fall in systolic blood pressure to 90 mm Hg has occurred, or the development of adverse effects necessitates reduction of dosage. On the other hand, in patients who are asymptomatic at the time of hospitalization it is recommended to titrate intravenous nitroglycerin with the aim of reducing mean arterial blood pressure by 10–15 mm Hg. If anginal pain recurs, the dose can be titrated upwards as often as necessary to very high levels (1000 μg/min or higher), and if adverse effects develop, discontinuation of therapy is warranted.

Tolerance to Intravenous Nitroglycein in Unstable Angina

In recent years there has been concern regarding the development of tolerance during long-term nitrate therapy [53, 54, 57]. In patients with stable angina, intravenous nitroglycerin [62] and nitroglycerin patches [34, 39, 50, 55] produce tolerance within 24 h. The study of tolerance to intravenous nitroglycerin in unstable angina is fraught with problems due to the underlying pathophysiologic processes responsible for unstable angina. One is never certain whether recurrence of angina despite intravenous nitroglycerin therapy is due to intermittent platelet deposition or thrombus formation or due to development of true tolerance to nitrate therapy. In a recent open-label study, tolerance was reported to occur in 65% of patients receiving intravenous nitroglycerin, but it was easily overcome in the majority of patients by increasing the dose whenever ischemic chest pain recurred [56]. In this study, 43 hospitalized patients with unstable angina who had continued pain despite treatment with other antianginal agents and aspirin were treated with intravenous nitroglycerin. The starting dose of nitroglycerin was 5 μg/min and was increased progressively until relief of angina or a fall in systolic blood pressure to below 90 mm Hg. This infusion rate was then maintained for up to 36 h. Fourteen of the 43 patients had no recurrence of pain, and nitroglycerin was tapered off and discontinued after 7–24 h without recurrence of pain. One patient experienced no relief of pain despite more than 200 μg/min intravenous nitroglycerin. The remaining 28 patients had recurrence of pain within an average of 8.9 h (range, 1–20 h), which responded to higher doses of nitroglycerin (range, 40–240 μg/min). Further recurrence of pain occurred within an average of 3 h (range, 1–7 h) in 7 of the 28 patients necessitating further increase in intravenous nitroglycerin infusion rate. The majority of the patients were finally weaned off intravenous nitroglycerin and placed on oral intermittent nitrate therapy.

Intermittent Versus Continuous Intravenous Nitroglycerin Nitrate Therapy During the Acute Phase of Unstable Angina

In patients with stable angina it has been recommended to use intermittent nitrate therapy with prolonged nitrate-free intervals in order to prevent nitrate tolerance [35, 42, 47, 57]. This approach cannot, however, be recommended in patients with unstable angina who are at risk of developing a myocardial infarction or even sudden death. Continuous therapy during the first 24–72 h of their initial presentation is therefore recommended. Tolerance does, however, develop but can be overcome by rapidly increasing the dose of intravenous nitroglycerin as often as necessary [52, 56].

Combination of Intravenous Nitroglycerin and Beta-Blockers or Calcium Channel Blockers During the Acute Phase of Unstable Angina

In patients who remain symptomatic despite high-dose intravenous nitrate therapy, addition of a beta-blocker (nonselective or cardioselective) often relieves symptoms and reduces myocardial ischemia [19]. However, beta-blockers with intrinsic sympathomimetic activity should be avoided as this therapy may aggravate anginal episodes in this group of patients [37]. Potent intravenous beta-blockers such as esmolol should be used with caution in combination with intravenous nitroglycerin as hypotensive effects of the two agents may be additive. Routine use of calcium channel blockers, especially the 4-dihydropyridine group of agents cannot be recommended as these agents may increase morbidity and mortality; nifedipine was recently reported to be associated with increased mortality [19].

Adverse Effects of Intravenous Nitroglycerin in Unstable Angina

Headache, although commonly experienced by patients with unstable angina, is sometimes severe and unresponsive to analgesics and may necessitate discontinuation of therapy. In some patients, excessive hypotension may be a problem, especially in patients with unstable angina following an inferior myocardial infarction with right ventricular involvement. Methemoglobinemia is usually not a problem despite treatment with high-dose intravenous nitroglycerin therapy but should be watched for in patients who have concomitant severe obstructive airway disease [51].

Therapy with Long-Acting Nitrates During the Late or the Stable Phase of Unstable Angina

Once the patient with unstable angina has been stabilized for at least 24 h or longer, intravenous therapy should be gradually tapered and oral nitrate therapy two or three times a day started with the first dose of oral therapy prescribed 1–2 h prior to discontinuation of the intravenous infusion for fear of a rebound increase in angina. However, it should be recognized that in this group of patients who have already experienced angina at rest, intermittent nitrate therapy should be used in conjunction with other antianginal agents, i.e., a long-acting beta-blocker or a calcium channel blocker such as diltiazem or verapamil, in order to provide 24-h antianginal and antiischemic effects [57]. Subsequently, patients can be stratified into low- and high-risk groups by performing an exercise test with or without gated pool studies to evaluate left ventricular function or thallium perfusion studies to assess the myocardium at risk.

Summary and Recommendations

The culprit lesion in unstable angina is invariably a fissuring of an atherosclerotic plaque with predisposition to platelet desposition and thrombus formation. In some patients, plaque progression, changes in vasomotor tone, and an increase in myocardial oxygen demand may play a role. The main emphasis of treatment should therefore be institution of aspirin or heparin or the combination of two. However, these agents do not relieve anginal pain or myocardial ischemia rapidly. Although nitrates do not reduce morbidity or mortality in patients with unstable angina, they play an important role in the initial management of these patients. Nitrates by improving the balance between myocardial oxygen supply and demand relieve angina and myocardial ischemia. Patients who fail to respond to high doses of oral nitrates plus beta-blockers and or calcium channel blockers almost always respond to intravenous nitroglcyerin. In symptomatic patients, an initial starting dose of 5–10 μg/min of intravenous nitroglycerin can be rapidly titrated upwards until relief of symptoms or until a fall in systolic blood pressure to 90 mm Hg or the development of adverse effects. In patients who are asymptomatic at the time of hospitalization, the dose can be titrated with the aim of reducing mean arterial blood pressure by 10–15 mm Hg. Intravenous nitroglycerin should be continued for 24–72 h, but higher and higher doses are often required for the treatment of recurrence of symptoms. Tolerance to intravenous nitroglycerin develops rapidly, but it can be overcome by increasing the dose of the medication. There is no role of intermittent nitrate therapy in the initial management of patients with unstable angina. Once the patient is stabilized, intravenous nitroglycerin should be gradually weaned and twice or three times a day therapy with isosorbide dintirate or isosorbide-5-mononitrate substituted prior to discontinuation of the infusion. Intermittent use of nitrates, however, does not provide 24-h antianginal prophylaxis, and this can be achieved only by concomitant beta-blocker or calcium blocker therapy. In stable patients, risk stratification by exercise testing should be performed after 3–7 days, and those with an early positive treadmill test or reduced left ventricular function or those with large perfusion defects on thallium scintigraphy should undergo coronary angiography to define the extent and severity of coronary artery disease. Further management in this group of patients is no different than those with stable angina.

Patients who remain symptomatic despite high-dose intravenous nitroglycerin, beta-blocker, aspirin, and/or heparin therapy need urgent coronary angiography with or without preceding insertion of an intra-aortic balloon pump. Urgent balloon angioplasty or coronary bypass surgery is often necessary in this subgroup of patients, but 10%–13% of these patients may have normal coronary arteries [36], and in this group of patients medical therapy is indicated.

References

1. Bassenge E, Strein K (1986) Dose dependent effects of isosorbide-5-mononitrate on the venous, arterial and coronary arterial system of conscious dogs. Naunyn Schmiedebergo Arch Pharmacol 334:100–104
2. Brodsky SJ, Halperin JL, Klein MD et al. (1980) Intravenous nitroglycerin infusion in unstable angina. Clin Res 28:608 A
3. Brown BG, Bolson E, Petersen RB et al. (1981) The mechanism of nitroglycerin action: stenosis vasodilation as a major component of dosing response. Circulation 64:1089–1097
4. Bussman WD, Passek D, Siedel W et al. (1981) Reduction of CK and CK-MB indexes of infarct size by intravenous nitroglycerin. Circulation 63:615–622
5. Cairns JA, Gent M, Singer J et al. (1985) Aspirin, sulfinpyrazone, or both in unstable angina: results of a Canadian multicenter trial. N Engl J Med 313:1369–1375
6. Capone G, Wolf NM, Meyer B et al. (1985) Frequency of intracoronary filling defects by angiography in angina pectoris at rest. Am J Cardiol 56:403–406
7. Chierchia S, Brunelli C, Simonettti L et al. (1980) A sequence of events in angina at rest: primary reduction in coronary flow. Circulation 61:759–768
8. Curfman GD, Heinsimer JA, Lozner EC et al. (1983) Intravenous nitroglycerin in the treatment of spontaneous angina pectoris: a prospective, randomized trial. Circulation 67:276–283
9. Dauwe F, Affaki G, Waters DD et al. (1979) Intravenous nitroglycerin in refractory unstable angina. Am J Cardiol 43:416 (abstr)
10. Davies MJ, Thomas AC (1985) Plaque fissuring – the cause of acute myocardial infarction, sudden ischemic death, and crescendo angina. Br Heart J 53:363–373
11. DeFeyter PJ, Serruys PW, Soward A et al. (1986) Coronary angioplasty for early post infarction unstable angina. Circulation 74:1365–1370
12. DePace ML, Hering IM, Kotler MN et al. (1982) Intravenous nitroglycerin for rest angina. Potential pathophysiologic mechanisms of action. Arch Intern Med 142:1806–1809
13. Distante A, Maseri A, Severi S et al. (1979) Management of vasospastic angina at rest with continuous infusion of isosorbide dinitrate. Am J Cardiol 44:533–539
14. Falk E (1985) Unstable angina with fatal outcome: dynamic coronary thrombosis leading to infarction and/or sudden death: autopsy evidence of recurrent mural thrombosis with peripheral embolization culminating in total vascular occlusion. Circulation 71:699–708

15. Flaherty JT (1984) Unstable angina: rational approach to management. Am J Cardiol 53:52–57
16. Flaherty JT, Becker LC, Buckley BH et al. (1983) A randomized prospective trial of intravenous nitroglycerin in patients with acute myocardial infarction. Circulation 68:576–588
17. Fuster V, Chesebro JH (1986) Mechanisms of unstable angina. N Engl J Med 315:1023–1025
18. Gorlin R (1983) Dynamic vascular factors in the genesis of myocardial ischemia. J Am Coll Cardiol 1:897–906
19. Holland Interuniversity Nifedipine/Metoprolol Trial (HINT) Research Group (1986) Early treatment of unstable angina in the coronary care unit: a randomized double blind, placebo controlled comparison of recurrent ischemia in patients treated with nifedipine or metoprolol or both. Br Heart J 56:400–413
20. Ignarro LJ, Lippton H, Edwards JC et al. (1981) Mechanism of vascular smooth muscle relaxation by organic nitrates, nitrates, nitroprusside and nitric oxide: evidence for the involvement of S-nitrosothiols as active intermediates. J Pharmacol Exp Ther 218:739
21. Jugdutt BI, Warnica JW (1988) Intravenous nitroglycerin therapy to limit myocardial infarct size, expansion and complications: effect of timing, dosage and infarct size. Circulation 78:906–919
22. Jugdutt BI, Becker LC, Hutchins GM et al. (1981) Effect of intravenous nitroglycerin on collateral flow and infarct size in the conscious dog. Circulation 63:17–28
23. Kaplan K, Davison R, Parker M et al. (1983) Intravenous nitroglycerin for the treatment of angina at rest unresponsive to standard nitrate therapy. Am J Cardiol 51:694–698
24. Lam J YT, Chesebro JH, Fuster V (1988) Platelets, vasoconstriction and nitroglycerin during arterial wall injury: a new antithrombotic role for an old drug. Circulation 78:712–716
25. Levin RI, Jaffe EA, Weksler BB et al. (1981) Nitroglycerin stimulates synthesis of prostacyclin by cultured human endothelial cells. J Clin Invest 67:762
26. Lewis HD Jr, Davis JW, Archibald DG et al. (1983) Protective effects of aspirin against acute myocardial infarction and death in men with unstable angina: results of a Veterans Administration cooperative study. N Engl J Med 309:396–403
27. Ludmer P, Selwyn AP, Shook TL et al. (1986) Paradoxical vasoconstriction induced by acetylcholine in atherosclerotic coronary arteries. N Engl J Med 315:1046–1051
28. McGregor M (1983) Pathogenesis of angina pectoris and role of nitrates in relief of myocardial ischemia. Am J Med 74 [Suppl 6B]:21–27
29. Mehta J, Pepine CJ (1978) Effect of sublingual nitroglycerin on regional flow in patients with and without coronary disease. Circulation 58:803–807
30. Mikolich RJ, Nicoloff NB, Robinson PH et al. (1980) Relief of refractory angina with continuous intravenous infusion of nitroglycerin. Chest 77:375–379
31. Moise A, Theroux P, Taeymans Y et al. (1983) Unstable angina and progression of coronary atherosclerosis. N Engl J Med 309:685–689
32. Muller JE, Turi ZG, Pearle DL et al. (1984) Nifedipine and conventional therapy for unstable angina pectoris: a randomized, double blind comparison. Circulation 69:728–739
33. Page A, Hurtle JF, Roudaut R et al. (1979) Intravenous trinitrin in the treatment of pre-infarctional angina. Nouv Presse Med 8:268–270
34. Parker JO, Fung HL (1984) Transdermal nitroglycerin in angina pectoris. Am J Cardiol 54:471–476
35. Parker JO, Farrel B, Lakey KA et al. (1987) Effect of intervals between doses on the development of tolerance to isosorbide dinitrate. N Engl J Med 316:1440–1444
36. Plotnick GD, Conti CR (1977) Unstable angina: angiography, short and long term morbidity, mortality and symptomatic status of medically treated patients. Am J Med 63:870–873
37. Quyyumi AA, Efthimion J, Quyyumi A et al. (1986) Nocturnal angina: precipitating factors in patients with coronary artery disease and those with variant angina. Br Heart J 56:346–352
38. Rapaport RM, Murad F (1983) Agonist-induced endothelium dependent relaxation in rat thoracic aorta may be mediated through cGMP. Circ Res 52:352–357
39. Reichek N, Priest C, Zimrin D et al. (1984) Antianginal effects of nitroglycerin patches. Am J Cardiol 54:1–7
40. Roubin GS, Harris PJ, Eckhardt L et al. (1982) Intravenous nitroglycerin in refractory unstable angina pectoris. Aust NZ J Med 12:598–602

41. Roughgarden JW (1966) Circulatory changes associated with spontaneous angina pectoris. Am J Med 41:947–961
42. Rudolph W, Blasini R, Reinger G et al. (1983) Tolerance development during isosorbide dinitrate treatment: can it be circumvented? Z Kardiol 72 [Suppl 3]:195–198
43. Russell RO, Rackley CE, Kouchoukos MT (1982) Unstable angina pectoris: management based on available information. Circulation 65 [Suppl II]:II-72
44. Schafer AI, Alexander RW, Handin RI et al. (1980) Inhibition of platelet function by organic nitrate vasodilators. Blood 55:649–654
45. Schror K, Grodzinska DH (1981) Stimulation of coronary vascular prostacyclin and inhibition of human platelet thromboxane A2 after low dose nitroglycerin. Thromb Res 23:59–67
46. Sherman CT, Litvack F, Grundfest W et al. (1986) Coronary angioscopy in patients with unstable angina pectoris. N Engl J Med 315:913–919
47. Silber S, Vogler AC, Krause KH et al. (1987) Induction and circumvention of nitrate tolerance applying different dosage intervals. Am J Med 83:860–870
48. Squire A, Cantor R, Packer M (1982) Limitations of continuous intravenous nitroglycerin prophylaxis in patients with refractory angina at rest. Circulation 66 [Suppl 2]:II-120 (abstr)
49. Telford AM, Wilson C (1981) Trial of heparin versus atenolol in prevention of myocardial infarction in intermediate coronary syndrome. Lancet i:1225–1228
50. Thadani U (1987) The effectiveness of transcutaneous nitrate preparations for angina pectoris. Int J Cardiol 14:9–14
51. Thadani U, Opie LH (1987) Nitrates. In: Opie LH (ed) Drugs for the heart, 2nd edn. Grune and Stratton, Orlando, pp 19–33
52. Thadani U, Whitsett TL (1987) Nitrate therapy. Continuous or pulse dosing. Ration Drug Ther 21:1–6
53. Thadani U, Manyari D, Parker JO et al. (1980) Tolerance to the circulatory effects of oral isosorbide dinitrate: rate of development and cross tolerance to glyceryl trinitrate. Circulation 61:526–535
54. Thadani U, Fung HL, Darke AC et al. (1982) Oral isosorbide dinitrate in angina pectoris: comparison of duration of action and dose response relation during acute and sustained therapy. Am J Cardiol 49:411–419
55. Thadani U, Hamilton SF, Olson E et al. (1986) Transdermal nitroglycerin patches in angina pectoris, duration of effect and rapid tolerance. Ann Intern Med 105:485–492
56. Thadani U, Sharma M, Thompson D et al. (1987) Intravenous nitroglycerin and tolerance in unstable angina. Circulation 76 [Suppl IV]:IV-128 (abstr)
57. Thadani U, Whitsett T, Hamilton SF (1988) Nitrate therapy for myocardial ischemic syndromes: current perspective including tolerance. Curr Probl Cardiol 13:725–784
58. Theroux P, Ouimet H, McCans J et al. (1988) Aspirin, heparin or both to treat acute unstable angina. N Engl J Med 319:1105–1111
59. Winbury MM, Howe BB, Hefner MA (1969) Effect of nitrates and other coronary dilators on large and smaller coronary vessels: a hypothesis for the mechanism action of nitrates. J Pharmacol Exp Ther 168:70–95
60. Winbury WM, Howe BB, Weiss HR (1971) Effect of nitroglycerin and dipyridamole on epicardial and endocardial oxygen tension: further evidence for redistribution of myocardial blood flow. J Pharmacol Exp Ther 176:184–199
61. Yusuf S, Collins R, MacMahon S et al. (1988) Effect of intravenous nitrates on mortality in acute myocardial infarction: an overview of the randomized trial. Lancet i:1088–1092
62. Zimrin D, Reickek M, Bogin KT et al. (1988) Antianginal effects of intravenous nitroglycerin over 24 hours. Circulation 77:1376–1384

Heparin and Aspirin in the Treatment of Unstable Angina

J. L. McCans [1]

Introduction

Since the recognition of unstable angina as a clinical syndrome often leading to acute myocardial infarction, its pathogenesis has remained uncertain. In recent years, however, several lines of investigation have provided evidence for the role of plaque rupture leading to platelet activation and thrombus formation. Visualization of thrombus in the coronary arteries of patients with unstable angina by coronary angiography has been reported by Holmes et al. [1], Zack et al. [2], and Ambrose et al. [3]. Similarly, intracoronary deposits of thrombus material have been observed by means of angioscopy [4]. Plaque fissuring and thrombus formation have been documented at necropsy in patients who died with unstable angina by Falk [5] and Davies and Thomas [6]. Biochemical evidence that platelet activation is important has been provided by Fitzgerald et al. [7] and Hamm et al. [8]. Théroux et al. [9] and Kruskal et al. [10] have reported detection of fibrin and fibrinogen breakdown products in patients with unstable angina implicating ongoing thrombus formation.

A review by Théroux [11] of previously conducted trials indicates that treatment with conventional antianginal drugs (beta-blockers, calcium channel blockers, nitrates) does not provide sufficient protection against the progression of unstable angina to myocardial infarction. Aspirin, which inhibits platelet aggregation, has been shown to be of benefit in the prevention of myocardial infarction and death in the subacute [12] and chronic [13] phases of unstable angina. There have been no reports of the effect of aspirin in the acute phase. Heparin has been studied by several investigators over the past 30 years in the acute phase of unstable angina. Earlier studies suffered from uncontrolled design [14, 15]. More recently, controlled trials have been reported. The results have either been positive but controversial [16, 17] or negative [18].

We have recently reported the initial results of a double-blind randomized study comparing aspirin, heparin, and a combination of the two with placebo [19]. This study was specifically designed to determine the effects of these treatments in the very acute phase of unstable angina, and was thus limited to

[1] Sir Mortimer B. Davis Jewish General Hospital, 3755 Cote Ste-Catherine Rd., Montreal, Quebec H3T 1E2, Canada

W. Bleifeld et al. (Eds.)
Unstable Angina

the period from hospital admission to the initiation of definitive treatment following angiography. The results obtained thus far are presented and their implications discussed.

Methods and Materials

Trial Design. Two tertiary care, university-affiliated hospitals participated in the study. The Montreal Heart Institute and The Sir Mortimer B. Davis Jewish General Hospital. All patients admitted to the two hospitals with a diagnosis of unstable angina or who acquired unstable angina while hospitalized were considered for the study. The diagnosis of unstable angina was based on the following:

1. A clinical history of an accelerating pattern of chest pain occurring at rest or with minimal exercise.
2. Chest pain lasting 20 min or longer with serum levels of creatine kinase less than twice the upper limit of normal on admission.
3. Electrocardiographic changes during pain compatible with ischemia.
4. In the absence of recurrent pain prior to randomization, inclusion in the study required independent confirmation of the diagnosis by two cardiologists.
5. The most recent episode of chest pain had to have occurred within the 24 h preceding the time of randomization.

A log of all hospital admissions was kept during the recruitment phase. Of all the patients admitted for unstable angina, 61.6% were randomized. The most common reason for exclusion was the regular use of aspirin (occasional use of one or two tablets a week was allowed). Of the patients admitted with unstable angina but not enrolled, 48% were excluded on this basis. Another 12% were excluded because of a contraindication to heparin or aspirin use, and 21% were excluded because they had undergone coronary angioplasty within 6 months or bypass surgery within 1 year previously.

Study Protocol. Patients suitable for the study were identified in the emergency rooms. Informed consent was obtained, and patients were randomized as soon after admission as possible. The trial medications were packaged for each patient and coded by the pharmacist associated with the study on a randomized, double-blind basis. The four treatments were balanced within each block of 12 patients. They consisted of:

1. Aspirin 650 mg administered orally, immediately followed by 325 mg twice daily plus placebo bolus and infusion.
2. Placebo capsules plus an intravenous bolus of 5000 IU heparin followed by an infusion of heparin at a rate of 1000 IU per hour.
3. Aspirin and heparin administered at a dosage similar to that given to groups 1 and 2.
4. Placebo capsules and bolus and infusion of placebo.

A partial thromboplastin time was measured 12 h after heparin administration and daily thereafter. The results of the test were known only by the hospital pharmacist who adjusted the infusion rate in order to maintain the coagulation time at 1.5–2 times control values. Adjustments were made according to a predetermined set of rules. A hematologist not otherwise involved in the trial was available to the pharmacist for consultation. The infusion rates of the placebo solutions were also altered from time to time.

Coronary angiography was performed in all but 11 patients who refused it, in 19 who had recently undergone the procedure, in 5 who had an endpoint event, in 4 who had an extracardiac contraindication, and in 4 for indeterminate reasons. Angiography was performed a mean of 4 days after randomization. This delay was in keeping with the current practice of our institutions and was not influenced by the patient's inclusion in the trial. The study was ended when a final therapeutic decision was made, usually within 48 h after coronary angiography. The discontinuation of study medications marked the end of the trial and collection of endpoint data.

A follow-up examination was performed in all patients after 3 months to verify the long-term effect of the early treatment. At that time, more than 90% of the patients were being treated with aspirin; 110 patients had undergone bypass surgery and 121 had undergone coronary angioplasty.

Concomitant Medication. Medications other than antiplatelet and anticoagulant drugs were prescribed during hospitalization at the discretion of the treating physician. The continuation of preadmission medications was recommended; the dose was increased, or another antianginal drug was added whenever chest pain occurred. At the time of admission, 46% were taking nitrates, 56% beta-blockers, and 43% calcium antagonists. An intravenous infusion of nitroglycerin was usually the first choice for additional treatment followed by a beta-blocker or calcium antagonist. During the course of the study, 100% of the patients received nitrates, 96% beta-blockers, and 67% calcium antagonists. Recurrent chest pain despite full therapy was an indication for urgent coronary angiography.

Study Endpoints. There were three major endpoints in this study.

1. *Refractory angina* defined as the presence of recurrent anginal chest pain with ischemic ST-T changes. This must have occurred despite full medical therapy that included at least an infusion of nitroglycerin plus a beta-blocker or calcium antagonist or the need for an urgent intervention (intra-aortic balloon counterpulsation, coronary angiography, coronary angioplasty, or bypass surgery). Occasional angina, chest pain without objective evidence of ischemia, and angina controlled by medical therapy were not considered endpoints.
2. *Myocardial infarction* defined as typical chest pain unrelieved by nitroglycerin and lasting 30 min or more with new ST-T changes or Q waves identified according to the criteria of the Minnesota code [20] and a doubling

of the baseline level of creatine kinase MB levels. The presence of all three criteria was required for diagnosis.

3. *Death*.

Bleeding complications were closely monitored clinically and by serial determinations of hemoglobin and hematocrit. Serious bleeding was defined as a fall in hemoglobin of 2 g or more or the need for transfusion. All endpoints were definitively classified before examination of the data by the policy board.

Protocol Deviations. Protocol deviations were noted in 53 patients. In eight the study medication was started more than 24 h after the most recent episode of chest pain. In 20 retrospective analysis of the clinical presentation and of the levels of cardiac enzymes on admission revealed a clearly evolving myocardial infarction prior to entry into the study; these patients were analyzed with the others with only new events considered as endpoints. Eighteen patients refused further participation in the study. Seven underwent coronary angiography on an outpatient basis after hospital discharge and after the discontinuation of study drugs. Patients with protocol deviations were equally distributed among the four study groups. Only one patient was crossed over to an active treatment while receiving blinded therapy; this was done after the occurrence of a major endpoint.

Statistical Analysis. The projected sample size of 696 patients was based on an anticipated 32% rate of events (2% mortality, 10% myocardial infarction, and 20% refractory angina) sufficient to provide a power of 0.85 to detect a 50% reduction in endpoints. The study was ended early at the policy board's recommendation after the interim analysis of data of the first 479 patients.

Results

Composition of the Study Population. The study population consisted of 61.6% of all patients admitted because of unstable angina with chest pain in the preceding 24 h. It was representative of patients 75 years of age or younger who were not receiving long-term aspirin treatment, and who had not recently undergone angioplasty or bypass surgery. These four factors accounted for nearly 80% of all exclusions. In the placebo group, endpoint events occurred in 33% of the men and 41% of the women ($p=0.52$); in the total population, these figures were 15% and 18% ($p=0.47$), respectively. Cholesterol levels were 6.7 ± 1.8 mmol/l in patients who had an endpoint event as compared with 6.1 ± 1.4 in those who did not ($p=0.06$). Less extensive coronary artery disease was associated with a better outcome ($p=0.03$) favoring the group treated with aspirin plus heparin.

Study Endpoints. The event rates observed in the placebo group corresponded to the predicted event rate, which was based on data from the literature [21–25] and on our previous experience [26]. Two deaths occurred in the study, both patients were in the placebo group. The incidence of myocardial infarction was 11.9% (14/118) in patients receiving placebo (Table 1). The incidence was significantly lower in the three treatment groups: 3.3% (4/121) with aspirin ($p=0.012$), 0.8% (1/118) with heparin ($p=0.0001$), and 1.6% (2/122) with the combination treatment ($p=0.001$). The incidence of refractory angina was 22% (27/118) in the placebo group compared to 8% (10/118) with heparin, 16% (20/121) with aspirin, and 10% (13/122) with the combined therapy. The relative risks compared to placebo for refractory angina for heparin, aspirin and the combined therapy were 0.31 (0.14–0.68), 0.67 (0.35–1.27), and 0.40 (0.20–0.82).

Analysis of the combined endpoints of refractory angina or myocardial infarction, whichever came first, showed benefits relative to placebo reaching the 0.05 significance level in the heparin and the combined treatment groups. Relative risk ±95% was 0.29 (0.14–0.61) and 0.36 (0.18–0.73). There were no statistically significant differences between the three treatment groups with respect to the endpoints of the study. However, trends were observed favoring heparin. As compared with aspirin, heparin was associated with a relative risk of 0.47 for refractory angina (95% confidence limits, 0.21 and 1.05; $p=0.06$), 0.25 for myocardial infarction (0.03 and 2.27; $p=0.18$), and 0.52 for any event (0.24 and 1.14; $p=0.10$). The combination of aspirin and heparin was only slightly superior to aspirin alone but was slightly inferior to heparin alone. Medical treatment was increased during hospitalization because of persistent angina in 44 patients receiving aspirin, 33 receiving heparin, 32 receiving the combined treatment, and 54 receiving placebo ($p=0.0006$, placebo versus heparin). The total duration of the study was similar for the three treatment groups but shorter for the placebo group ($p=0.01$ for the comparison with heparin).

Between the end of the study and the 3-month follow-up visit, myocardial infarction occurred in an additional 14 patients: three in the aspirin group, four in the heparin group, two in the aspirin plus heparin group, and five in the placebo group; the number of deaths in the respective groups was 1, 1, 0, and 4. Bypass surgery or angioplasty had been performed in similar numbers of patients in the four groups: aspirin 57; heparin 66; aspirin plus heparin 56; and placebo 52. Symptoms were the primary indication for surgery in 53% of the patients receiving aspirin, 46% of those receiving heparin, and 69% of those receiving placebo ($p=0.004$ for the comparison with heparin).

Complications. Complications and side effects were relatively infrequent in this study. Bleeding occurred in 20 patients receiving heparin – twice as frequently as in patients not receiving this drug ($p=0.09$). Most of the bleeding complications (77%) occurred at catheterization puncture sites. Serious bleeding, defined as a need for transfusion (six patients) or a fall in hemoglobin of 2 g or more (four patients), was more frequent in the group receiving aspirin plus heparin. Drug discontinuation because of side effects was more frequent among the patients receiving heparin (13 patients) than among those not receiving it (5 patients). The mean time between randomization and the occur-

Table 1. Cardiac endpoints

Events	Placebo ($n=118$)	Aspirin ($n=121$)			Heparin ($n=118$)			Aspirin + heparin ($n=122$)		
	n	*n*	RR	95% CL	*n*	RR	95% CL	*n*	RR	95% CL
Refractory angina	27	20	0.67	0.35–1.27	10	0.31	0.14–0.68	13	0.40	0.20–0.82
Myocardial infarction	14	4	0.29	0.08–0.80	1	0.06	0.01–0.49	2	0.12	0.03–0.56
Death	2	0	–	–	0	–	–	0	–	–
Fatal or nonfatal myocardial infarction	14	4	0.29	0.08–0.80	1	0.06	0.01–0.49	2	0.12	0.03–0.56
Any event	31	20	0.56	0.30–1.05	11	0.29	0.14–0.61	14	0.36	0.18–0.73

RR, Relative risk compared to placebo; 95% CL, 95% confidence limits.

rence of myocardial infarction was 36±30 h (range, 1–112). Myocardial infarction was associated with the appearance of new Q waves in 86% of the patients receiving placebo and 29% of those in the other groups ($p<0.01$). Peak creatine kinase elevations averaged 2369±1932 IU in the placebo group and 1555±2275 IU in the other treatment groups (not significant). The incidence of refractory angina and the total event rate were also significantly reduced with heparin (60%) and with the combination of aspirin and heparin (53%) but not with aspirin alone.

Discussion

In this double-blind, randomized, placebo-controlled study, heparin administered during the acute phase of unstable angina significantly reduced the incidence of all major endpoints. Aspirin also reduced the rate of fatal and nonfatal myocardial infarction. The combination of the two active drugs was not superior to heparin alone and resulted in slightly more complications.

The factors that influence the short-term prognosis of unstable angina are not completely known. Various clinical parameters have been shown to be predictive of outcome in different studies. Studies reported by Krauss et al. [21], Gazes et al. [22], and Mulcahy et al. [25] indicate that one of the most important could be the persistence of recurrent chest pain despite optimal medical treatment. It was more frequent in the placebo group than in the three treatment groups, resulting in a significantly shorter duration of the study in the placebo group despite more intensive medical treatment. Other factors that have been described as predicting a worse prognosis are the clinical presentation of unstable angina [27], a previous history of bypass surgery [28], the use of calcium antagonists [29], the presence of ST-T changes in leads V_1–V_4 [29, 30], involvement of the left main coronary artery [31] or proximal left anterior descending coronary artery [30], and the extent of coronary artery disease [29]. In the current study, multivariate analysis of the effects of these and other selected parameters on outcome showed that aside from study treatment, only age and the number and cumulative duration of chest pain were predictive of development of acute myocardial infarction.

Infarctions occurring in the placebo group were more often Q wave infarctions 12/14 (86%) than in the three treatment groups, 2/7 (29%; $p<0.01$). In addition, there was a trend to higher peak creatine kinase elevation in patients who had an infarction on placebo than on active treatment, 2639±1932 IU versus 1555±2275 IU, respectively. However, this difference did not achieve statistical significance at the 0.05 level [32].

It is noteworthy that despite the strict entry criteria used in this study, 16% of the patients had no coronary stenosis of more than 70%. This percentage corresponds with previous data [33]. However, a completely normal coronary angiogram was obtained in only 5% of the patients.

Previous Studies with Heparin. The results of this study are remarkably similar to those of a study of 214 patients by Telford and Wilson [16]. After 7 days of treatment, these investigators found a 3% incidence of myocardial infarction in the heparin-treated groups as compared to a 15% incidence in the groups not receiving heparin. Although it is widely quoted, this study has not been generally accepted because of problems in its design and analysis [34]. The results of two other randomized studies using smaller samples have been published: in an open trial, heparin infusion for 48 h followed by warfarin therapy was associated with a beneficial effect [17]; in the other study, however, no benefit from heparin could be documented [18]. In the present study, heparin reduced the incidence of refractory angina by 63% as compared with placebo. Heparin reduced the rates of fatal and nonfatal myocardial infarction as compared with placebo administered with or without aspirin by 89%. The sequential method of administering the study drugs (aspirin first, then heparin) was used on the theoretical grounds of possible platelet activation by heparin [35]; clearly, heparin had no such effect in our study since the best results were obtained in the group that received heparin after placebo.

Previous Studies with Aspirin. The beneficial effects of aspirin in unstable angina are discussed by Lorenz (this volume). Our study extends these reported benefits of aspirin to the early phase of unstable angina. The patients started receiving the study drugs 7.9 h (mean) after the most recent episode of pain. Aspirin reduced the combined rate of fatal and nonfatal myocardial infarction by 72% as compared with placebo. The choice of an aspirin dose of 325 mg twice a day was empirical in this study, and recent data suggest that daily doses of 325 mg or less may have a similar beneficial effect [36].

Heparin plus Aspirin in Unstable Angina. The risk that any endpoint events would occur was reduced when the combination therapy was compared with aspirin alone; however, the combination was not superior to heparin alone. Since either drug used alone was very effective, the statistical power of the trial was too low to permit conclusions about the comparative effects of the three treatments. From the data, it can be estimated that an additional 200 patients would be required to document the superiority of the combination therapy over aspirin alone and that an incalculably large number of patients would be needed to show the combination's superiority (if any) to heparin. Therefore, the combination therapy and placebo groups have been discontinued. The ongoing trial now compares treatment with aspirin alone to that with heparin alone.

Our results suggest that platelet and coagulation factors are closely related in the pathogenesis of unstable angina, and that acting on either can control the disease process. The results of the present study, however, do not preclude the use of the combination in other clinical settings or in particular subsets of unstable angina.

Clinical Importance. This study encompassed a typical population of patients hospitalized for unstable angina. It documented a clear benefit of aspirin alone, heparin alone, and both together, with a reduction of serious cardiac events during the acute phase. The benefit of one treatment over the others has not been demonstrated and would require a larger population. The trends favor heparin first, heparin plus aspirin second, and aspirin third. On the basis of our findings and those of other investigators [12, 13, 16], it can be recommended that heparin be administered to all patients who are admitted to the hospital with unstable angina and have no contraindication to its use.

A note of caution must be raised, however, regarding heparin therapy. We observed a significantly greater occurrence of refractory angina and myocardial infarction following the stopping of study medication in patients receiving heparin alone compared to aspirin, heparin and aspirin, or placebo [37]. This observation may be an indication that although heparin can effectively prevent clot formation at the site of a ruptured or fissured plaque in the acute phase of unstable angina, the risk of occlusion remains elevated when heparin is discontinued at 5–7 days. Aspirin appears to prevent this "rebound" and should be started for long-term therapy before heparin is discontinued.

The role of fibrinolysis in unstable angina is still controversial. The success of heparin in this study highlights the critical role of thrombus formation and the rationale for testing fibrinolysis. The relatively late occurrence of complications after hospital admission (mean 36 h) strongly suggests that preventing progressive thrombosis with an antiplatelet or anticoagulant drug should be part of any trial involving fibrinolysis.

References

1. Holmes DR Jr, Hartzler GO, Smith HC, Fuster V (1981) Coronary artery thrombosis in patients with unstable angina. Br Heart J 45:411–416
2. Zack PM, Ischinger T, Aker UT, Dincer B, Kennedy HL (1984) The occurrence of angiographically detected intracoronary thrombus in patients with unstable angina pectoris. Am Heart J 108:1408–1412
3. Ambrose JA, Winters SL, Stern A et al. (1985) Angiographic morphology and the pathogenesis of unstable angina pectoris. J Am Coll Cardiol 5:609–616
4. Sherman CT, Litvack F, Grundfest W et al. (1986) Coronary angioscopy in patients with unstable angina pectoris. N Engl J Med 315:913–919
5. Falk E (1985) Unstable angina with fatal outcome: dynamic coronary thrombosis leading to infarction and/or sudden death: autopsy evidence of recurrent mural thrombosis with peripheral embolization culminating in total vascular occlusion. Circulation 71:699–708
6. Davies MJ, Thomas AC (1985) Plaque fissuring – the cause of acute myocardial infarction, sudden ischaemic death and crescendo angina. Br Heart J 53:363–373
7. Fitzgerald DJ, Roy L, Catella F, FitzGerald GA (1986) Platelet activation in unstable coronary disease. N Engl J Med 315:983–989
8. Hamm CW, Lorenz R, Bleifeld W, Weber PC (1987) Biochemical evidence of platelet activation in patients with persistent unstable angina. J Am Coll Cardiol 5:998–1004
9. Théroux P, Latour JG, Léger-Gauthier C, De Lara J (1987) Fibrinopeptide A and platelet factor levels in unstable angina pectoris. Circulation 75:156–162
10. Kruskal JB, Commeford PJ, Franks JJ, Kirsch RE (1987) Fibrin and fibrinogen-related antigens in patients with stable and unstable coronary artery disease. N Engl J Med 317:1361–1365

11. Théroux P (1987) A pathophysiologic basis for the clinical classification and management of unstable angina. Circulation 75 [Suppl V]:V-103–109
12. Lewis HD Jr, Davis JW, Archibald DG et al. (1983) Protective effects of aspirin against acute myocardial infarction and death in men with unstable angina: results of a Veterans Administration Cooperative study. N Engl J Med 309:396–403
13. Cairns JA, Gent M, Singer J et al. (1985) Aspirin, sulfinpyrazone or both in unstable angina: results of a Canadian multicentre trial. N Engl J Med 313:1369–1375
14. Nichol ES, Phillips WG, Casten GG (1959) Virtue of prompt anticoagulant therapy in impending myocardial infarction: experiences with 318 patients during a 10-year period. Ann Intern Med 50:1158–1173
15. Wood P (1961) Acute and subacute coronary insufficiency. Br Med J 1:1779–1782
16. Telford AM, Wilson C (1981) Trial of heparin versus atenolol in prevention of myocardial infarction in intermediate coronary syndrome. Lancet i:1225–1228
17. Williams DO, Kirby MG, McPherson K, Phear DN (1986) Anticoagulant treatment of unstable angina. Br J Clin Pract 40:114–116
18. Zwerner PL, Gore JM, Corrao JM et al. (1987) Heparin in the treatment of unstable angina: a randomized prospective trial. Circulation 76 [Suppl IV]:IV-180 (abstr)
19. Théroux P, Ouimet H, McCans J, Latour JG, Toly P, Lévy G, Pelletier E, Tuneau M, Stasiak T, De Guise P, Pelletier GB, Rinzler D, Waters DD (1988) Aspirin, heparin, or both to treat acute unstable angina. New Engl J Med 319:1105–1111
20. Rose GA, Blackburn H (1968) Cardiovascular survey methods. WHO Monogr Ser 56:1–188
21. Krauss KR, Hutter AM Jr, De Sanctis RW (1972) Acute coronary insufficiency: course and follow-up. Arch Intern Med 129:808–813
22. Gazes PC, Mobley EM Jr, Faris HM Jr, Duncan RC, Humphries GB (1973) Preinfarctional (unstable) angina – a prospective study – ten year follow-up: prognostic significance of electrocardiographic changes. Circulation 48:331–337
23. Heng MK, Norris RM, Singh BM, Partridge JB (1976) Prognosis in unstable angina. Br Heart J 38:921–925
24. Russell RO Jr, Moraski RE, Kouchoukos N et al. (1978) Unstable angina pectoris: National Cooperative Study Group to compare surgical and medical therapy. II. In-hospital experience and initial follow-up results in patients with one, two and three vessel disease. Am J Cardiol 42:839–848
25. Mulcahy R, Daly L, Graham I et al. (1981) Unstable angina: natural history and determinants of prognosis. Am J Cardiol 48:525–528
26. Théroux P, Taeymans Y, Morrissette D, Bosch X, Pelletier GB, Waters DD (1985) A randomized study comparing propranolol and diltiazem in the treatment of unstable angina. J Am Coll Cardiol 5:712–722
27. Bertolasi CA, Trongé JE, Carreno CA, Jalon J, Vega MR (1974) Unstable angina – prospective and randomized study of its evolution with and without surgery. Am J Cardiol 33:201–208
28. Waters DD, Walling A, Roy D, Théroux P (1986) Previous coronary artery bypass grafting as an adverse prognostic factor in unstable angina pectoris. Am J Cardiol 58:465–469
29. Ouyang P, Brinker JA, Mellits ED, Weisfeldt ML, Gerstenblith G (1984) Variables predictive of successful medical therapy in patients with unstable angina: selection by multivariate analysis from clinical, electrocardiographic and angiographic evaluations. Circulation 70:367–376
30. De Zwaan C, Bar FW, Wellens HJ (1982) Characteristic electrocardiographic pattern indicating a critical stenosis high in left anterior descending coronary artery in patients admitted because of impending myocardial infarction. Am Heart J 103:730–736
31. Takaro T, Hultgren HN, Lipton MJ, Detre KM and participants in the Study Group (1976) The VA cooperative randomized study of surgery for coronary arterial occlusive disease. II. Subgroup with significant left main lesions. Circulation 54 [Suppl III]:III-107–117
32. Théroux P, Ouimet H, Latour JG, McCans J, Pelletier G, Juneau M, Waters D (1989) Prediction and prevention of myocardial infarction during the acute phase of unstable angina. J Am Coll Cardiol 13 (2) [Suppl]:192A
33. Rafflenbeul W, Russell RO, Lichtlen PR (1980) Angiographic anatomy of coronary arteries in unstable angina pectoris. In: Rafflenbeul W, Lichtlen PR, Balcon R (eds) Unstable angina pectoris: International symposium, Hanover 1980. Thieme, Stuttgart, pp 51–57

34. Yusuf S, Sleight P (1981) Atenolol, heparin and the intermediate coronary syndrome. Lancet ii:46
35. Salzman EW, Rosenberg RD, Smith MH, Lindon JN, Favreau L (1980) Effect of heparin and heparin fractions on platelet aggregation. J Clin Invest 65:64–73
36. The Steering Committee of the Physicians' Health Study Research Group (1988) Preliminary report: findings from the aspirin component of the ongoing Physicians' Health Study. N Engl J Med 318:262–264
37. Ouimet H, Théroux P, McCans J, Waters D (1989) Rebound caused by withdrawal of heparin in the acute phase of unstable angina. Circulation 80 (4) [Suppl II]:II-266

Thrombolysis in Patients with Unstable Angina

F. W. BÄR [1]

Introduction

Patients with unstable angina are in a threatening situation: in 10%–30% of them transmural myocardial infarction will develop within a few weeks [1–3]. It is recognized that coronary thrombosis can play a role in this clinical picture. Is the use of thrombolytic therapy helpful in diminishing the risk of myocardial infarction? In order to evaluate the possible value of thrombolytic treatment in patients with unstable angina the following questions should be considered:

- What is the clinical syndrome of unstable angina?
- How frequently does thrombosis play a role in unstable angina?
- How effective is thrombolytic therapy in this syndrome?
- Apart from angiographic changes, are clinical effects also demonstrable after thrombolytic therapy?
- Can the patients be recognized in whom thrombolysis is successful?
- What are the risks of thrombolysis?

Diagnosis of Unstable Angina. In our institution we use the following criteria: angina of recent onset (under 3 weeks), sudden increase in stable angina, postmyocardial infarction angina after a symptom-free period of 3 months, and angina at rest. While one may question whether these criteria are optimal, of more importance is the possible incorrect interpretation of the symptoms. The diagnosis of unstable angina is extremely difficult because it is based on the (subjective) symptoms of the patient and the (subjective) interpretation of the physician.

To decrease the number of incorrect interpretations of complaints, one can require the presence of electrocardiographic abnormalities. The following example illustrates the importance of such an approach. In a prospective study using only clinical history for the diagnosis of unstable angina, three of the four patients with normal coronary arteries did not show electrocardiographic changes; in contrast, 28 of 35 patients with an abnormal electrocardiogram showed coronary abnormalities. There are nonischemic causes such as left ventricular hypertrophy, electrolyte disturbances, and drugs which can result

[1] Cardiologie, Academisch Ziekenhuis Maastricht, Rijksuniversiteit Limburg, Annadal 1, 6201 BX Maastricht, The Netherlands

W. Bleifeld et al. (Eds.)
Unstable Angina

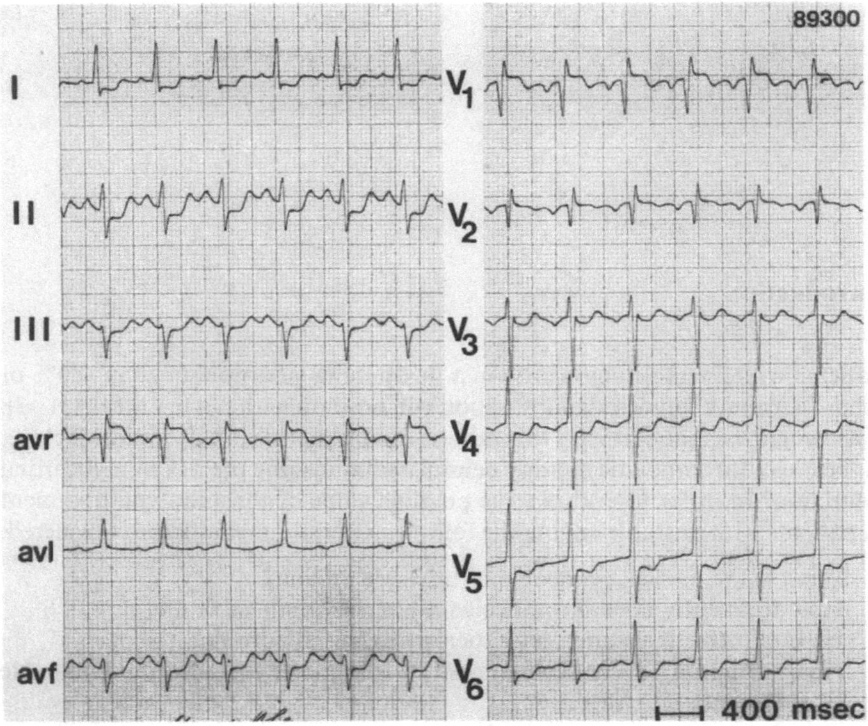

Fig. 1. The 12-lead electrocardiogram during an attack of chest pain in a patient with unstable angina. The ST segment depressions in most leads combined with the ST segment elevation in the leads AVR and V_1 are suggestive of three-vessel disease or a main stem stenosis

in stable ST-T changes. Therefore, transient changes in the electrocardiogram, either during (Fig. 1) or after chest pain (Fig. 2) are the most reliable tools to confirm the diagnosis. However, such strict criteria underestimate the total number of patients with unstable angina, and one should realize that the diagnosis of unstable angina is still valid when limited enzyme release is found. Usually, a small enzyme rise points to a critical obstructive lesion and an extensive amount of still threatened myocardial tissue [4]. In other words, unstable angina and a non-Q-wave myocardial infarction can be two expressions of the same problem.

Importance of Thrombus in Unstable Angina. It is well known that most cases of myocardial infarction result from an acute thrombotic coronary occlusion. When the blockage persists for more than 30 min, myocardial damage appears unless sufficient collateral circulation protects the myocardium. In contrast, in a tightly stenosed but still open vessel with severely diminished flow myocardial injury can appear. Early reperfusion results in infarct size limitation, or an enzyme rise may even be absent. This explains the overlap between myocardial

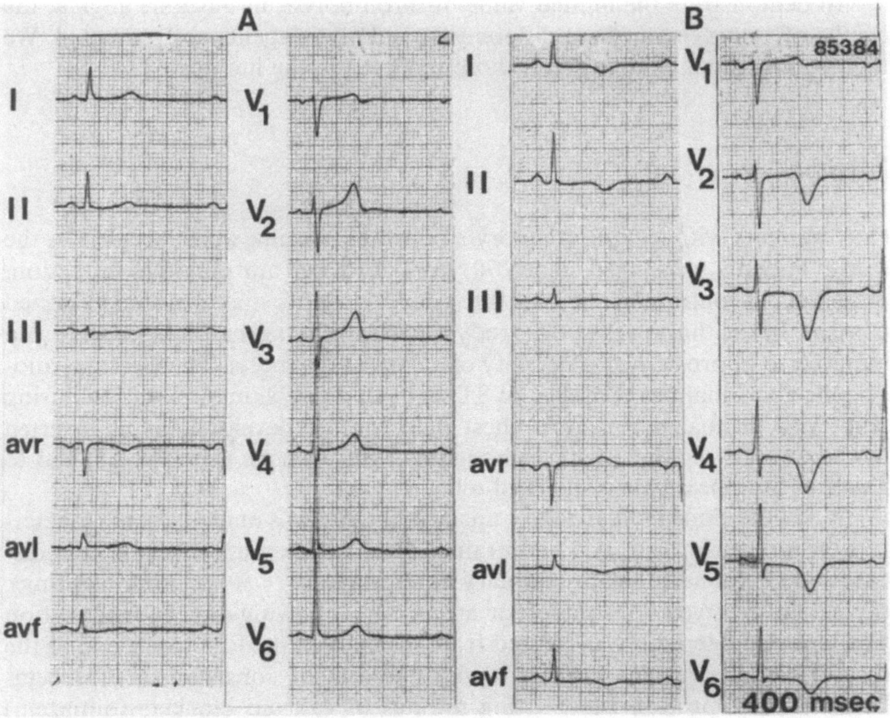

Fig. 2. *Panel A*, the normal 12-lead electrocardiogram on admission of a patient who had suffered angina 1 h earlier. *Panel B*, 2 h later. The patient had no complaints during this period. The inverted T waves in the precordial leads are typical for a lesion high in the left anterior descending artery

infarction and unstable angina. It also demonstrates that thrombosis must play a role in unstable angina. Perfusion problems are not caused solely by thrombus formation but can also appear in severely stenosed atherosclerotic lesions, during spasm of the vessel, or in a rupturing plaque. In such situations thrombolytics are not helpful. Other observations also indicate that thrombus can be present in this syndrome. Autopsy studies [5–7] demonstrated that laminar thrombus formation was present in unstable angina patients who died. These findings were confirmed by coronary angiography [8–14] and angioscopy [15]. An indirect confirmation for the presence of thrombus in patients with unstable angina is the favorable effect of platelet aggregation inhibitors such as aspirin [16, 17]. Also biochemical examinations in these patients suggest that thrombus formation occurs [18, 19].

There is a large variation in the reported incidence of thrombi. A low incidence (1%–12%) is found in patients who had their catheterization 1–3 months after the last attack of angina [8, 9, 11, 13, 20]. The incidence of thrombosis was considerably higher (52%–85%) when patients underwent cardiac catherization within 2 weeks after onset of instability [10, 14, 15].

To demonstrate the limited value of thrombolysis in unstable angina, the results of a study with three different thrombolytic agents are presented. We then compare our findings with those reported in the literature.

Methods

Only patients with a typical history of unstable angina were included in the study. Patients were aged under 70 years, had had no previous infarction, presented no contraindication for thrombolytic agents, and provided informed consent. In the third part of this study electrocardiographic changes were also required to improve the probability of a correct diagnosis. The electrocardiographic abnormalities consisted of ST segment depression or elevation during pain with normalization after chest pain, or the development of inverted T waves following the attack. Sublingual or intravenous nitroglycerin had to result in disappearance or marked relief of pain.

When the clinical diagnosis of unstable angina was made, urgent catheterization was performed. If no contraindications were present (main stem disease >50%, nonsignificant coronary abnormalities; <50%, groin bleeding), the patient received a thrombolytic agent. The following day, catheterization was repeated. Heparin was infused from the start of the first to the end of the second catheterization. Further medical treatment consisted of oral betablockers (metoprolol). Long-acting nitrates or calcium blockers (diltiazem) were added when indicated. All patients received aspirin after the second catheterization. In the first (retrospective) part of the study, 21 unstable patients with a severely narrowed or occluded coronary artery received 250000 U intracoronary streptokinase. Additionally, two prospective studies were carried out. In a single-center study, 20 patients received 100 mg rt-PA intravenously, while in the pilot phase of the multicenter UNASEM trial 25 patients were treated intravenously with 30 mg APSAC (see "Acknowledgements") [21].

Results

Angiographic Results. The results of the three studies were comparable; the combined angiographic data are presented in Fig. 3. A decrease in stenosis between the first and second catheterizations was found in 30 of 66 patients. In the case of multivessel disease, left ventricular wall motion and electrocardiographic abnormalities were used to identify the culprit lesion. Changes in coronary anatomy were most striking in patients with occluded or nearly occluded arteries (99%–100%) and slow or absent flow (TIMI 0 or 1); 22 of 30 patients improved, while only 8 of the 36 patients with TIMI 2 or 3 showed a decrease in severity of the stenosis after thrombolysis. These findings were confirmed by quantitative analysis of the coronary angiograms.

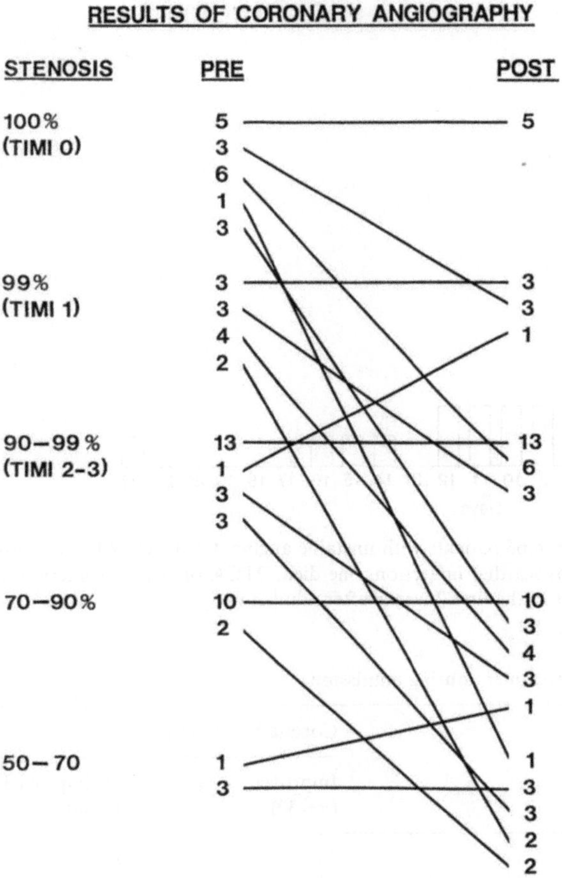

Fig. 3. Severity of the stenosis and flow according to the TIMI grading before and after thrombolytic treatment. Of the 66 patients, 30 showed a decrease in severity of the lesion, 34 no change, and 2 some deterioration. Typically, the 30 patients with no flow (*TIMI 0*) or nearly no flow (*TIMI 1*) did best; 22 of them improved. Only 8 of 36 patients with (nearly) normal flow (*TIMI 2, 3*) showed a diminished stenosis after thrombolytic therapy

Clinical Results. In spite of thrombolytic therapy, approximately 60% of patients had a cardiac event, emphasizing the strict selection criteria of our study (Fig. 4). As could be expected, some patients ($n=8$) had already had myocardial damage prior to thrombolytic therapy, although the electrocardiogram did not show the typical signs of myocardial infarction. An additional six patients suffered a myocardial infarction after treatment. However, in four of these creatine kinase values did not exceed three times the normal value. In spite of thrombolysis 37 patients needed percutaneous TCA or bypass surgery; in 29 of these the intervention was performed during the same admission. One patient died in hospital. At 3-month follow-up, persistent angina (class II according to the New York Heart Association) was present in ten patients.

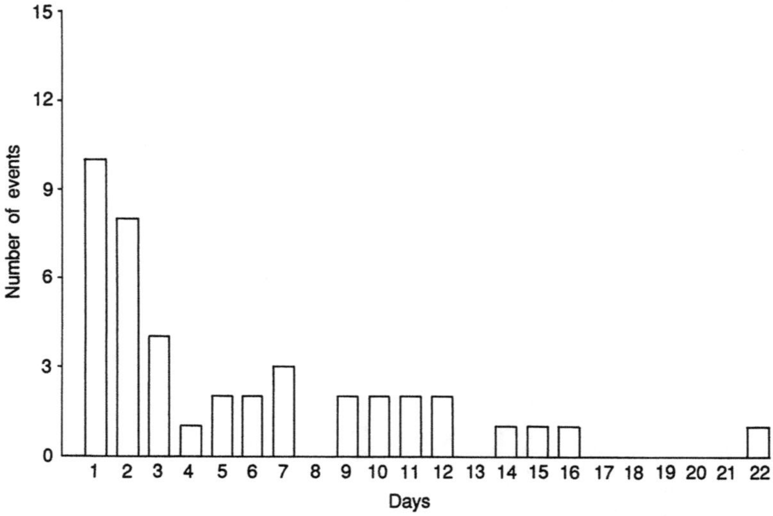

Fig. 4. Cardiac event rate over time in 66 patients with unstable angina. Of these, 42 had at least one event: six patients suffered a myocardial infarction, one died, PTCA or bypass surgery was performed in 37. Risks were highest in the first 2 weeks after admission

Table 1. Outcome of thrombolytic treatment during admission

Outcome	Coronary anatomy	
	Improved ($n=30$)	Not improved ($n=36$)
PTCA/bypass	11	18
Improvement angina	21	27
Myocardial infarction after thrombolysis	1	5

Relationship Between Angiographic and Clinical Findings. Clinical problems were independent of the angiographic results, and were equally distributed between patients who did and patients who did not improve in coronary anatomy (Table 1).

Discussion

Angiographic Data. Only few studies, with a limited number of patients, have reported the effects of thrombolytic agents in unstable angina. The study by Rentrop et al. [22] was the first, treating five patients with impending myocardial infarction with approximately 125000 IU streptokinase ic; no changes in the subtotal lesions were observed. Vectrovec et al. [10] gave 100000–350000 IU streptokinase ic to 12 patients; in ten of these some improvement in coronary anatomy was recorded. Mandelkorn et al. [11] injected 240000 IU streptokinase ic, after which four of nine patients showed angiographic improvement. Ambrose et al. [23] treated 37 unstable patients having nonoccluded arteries, with 100000–300000 IU streptokinase ic and found no difference in severity of the stenosis before and after therapy. Gold et al. [24] were the first to perform a randomized trial in 23 patients with unstable angina: 11 patients received placebo and 12 patients 50 mg rt-PA iv. Coronary angiography was performed after therapy. After the infusion, 8 of 11 placebo patients had signs of thrombi, while none of the 12 patients treated with rt-PA showed intracoronary thrombi. De Zwaan et al. [25] reported on the first two parts of the present study. As emphasized there, they found angiographic improvement after 250000 IU streptokinase ic or 100 mg rt-PA iv in 41 patients. Diameter of stenosis or coronary flow improved in 22 of 41 patients. Gotoh et al. [26] treated 37 patients. Prior to the intervention in 21 patients intracoronary thrombi were diagnosed. After 480000 IU urokinase ic was administered, the angiographic pattern improved in 20 of 21 patients. In 14 patients no thrombus was seen prior to therapy; in none of these patients was coronary anatomy changed. In another placebo-controlled randomized study, Topol et al. [27] studied the effect of 150 g rt-PA iv in 40 patients. Compared to placebo, thrombolysis did not alter the coronary lesions significantly.

The results of these studies are thus inconsistent. Comparison between these studies however, is, very difficult, for the following reasons:

1. The numbers of patients included in the studies were limited.
2. Some studies were retrospective, some prospective, and a few placebo controlled.
3. The inclusion criteria, which are extremely important, varied considerably. For example, de Zwaan et al. [25] described that the best results were found in (nearly) occluded arteries, while Ambrose et al. [23] explicitly excluded this group of patients.
4. Time between onset of unstable angina and angiography or thrombolysis varied considerably. As noted above, this can influence results significantly.
5. It is sometimes difficult to allocate the culprit lesion in patients with multivessel disease, and incorrect judgement results in misleading conclusions. Only few investigators paid attention to this problem. In patients with multivessel disease the electrocardiogram can provide important guidance. For example, negative T-waves after chest pain in precordial leads suggest ischemia in the anterior part of the left ventricle. Also, transient ST segment elevations can reveal the location of the culprit lesion. Left ventricular wall motion (by echocardiography, contrast or nuclear angiography) is another tool to help identify the culprit lesion.
6. Identification of the thrombus was inconsistent. Some investigators only mentioned the presence of thrombi, while others used rather strict criteria. The diagnosis of coronary thrombus is difficult, and in a number of cases it can not be distinguished from an intimal dissection or ulcer.

7. Determination of success of thrombolysis was inconsistent. Some studies used disappearance of the thrombus and others decrease of stenosis.
8. Type, dosage, and route of the drugs were different.

Clinical Effects of Thrombolysis. The clinical effect of thrombolysis in patients with unstable angina has also been evaluated. Nearly all studies show that, in spite of angiographic improvement, stabilizing or improvement of symptoms did not occur regularly. Gold et al. [24] were the only investigators who found thrombolysis to influence morbidity positively. Gotoh et al. [26] demonstrated that inspite of thrombolytic therapy, patients with thrombi still have a higher incidence of persistent angina (71%) than patients without thrombi (36%). Others [24, 25, 27] also described a high chance of cardiac events even after apparently successful thrombolysis (death, myocardial infarction, and percutaneous PTCA or CABG because of instability). In the study of de Zwaan et al. [25] one-third of patients suffered a myocardial infarction before, during, or after treatment. Importantly, most of these patients had only limited infarct size (creatine kinase levels some two or three times normal). Half of the patients in this study needed percutaneous TCA or CABG. De Zwaan et al. [25] suggested that thrombolysis may improve the clinical condition temporarily, which allows the physician to institute the appropriate intervention. Nevertheless, it is still unclear whether thrombolytic therapy is superior to conventional treatment. Even the two small randomized trials [24, 27] were unconclusive.

Can the patients be identified in whom thrombolysis is effective? Especially de Zwaan et al. [25] have tried to identify the patients in whom thrombolytic therapy was effective. They were unable to recognize the patients in whom thrombus formation was the cause of unstable angina when using data gathered prior to catheterization: neither was the clinical history or electrocardiographic findings was helpful for the identification. Gotoh et al. [26] described transient ST segment elevation during pain as suggestive for thrombus formation. In the present study, we were unable to confirm this.

Risks of Thrombolysis. The risks of thrombolytic therapy have been studied mainly in patients with myocardial infarction. Cerebrovascular accidents, not uncommonly leading to death, occur in 0.5–1.5%. Severe bleeding, in particular from the puncture site in the groin but also gastrointestinal bleedings, have been reported in up to 30% [28, 29]. Allergic reactions can develop after streptokinase infusion. In unstable angina, these risks should be balanced against the potential benefits of thrombolysis.

Conclusions

Thrombus is an important factor in unstable angina. The value of thrombolytic therapy in this syndrome, however, is still unknown. Hopefully, the results of large randomized trials will unravel these problems. At the moment, two large placebo-controlled randomized trials are in progress: in Europe the multicenter UNASEM trial [21] and in the United States the TIMI III trial. The results of these studies may indicate whether thrombolysis is a useful alternative for the treatment of patients with unstable angina.

Therefore, at the present time thrombolytic treatment of patients with unstable angina should be discouraged as a routine therapy. The complications of such therapy can be very important and counterbalance the beneficial effects.

Acknowledgements. Some of the work presented in this paper was done by many others; I would like to express my gratitude to: Centre Hospitalier Universitaire, Trousseu, Tours, France (Prof. Raynaud); Centre Hospitalier Universitaire, Angers, France (Prof. Tadei); Centre Hospitalier Universitaire, Beaujon, Clichy, France (Prof. Guerot); Clinique Saint Joseph, Colmar, France (Dr. Monassier); Centre Hospitalier Universitaire, Necker-Enfants-Malades, Paris, France (Prof. Vacheron); Centre Hospitalier de la Timone, Marseille, France (Prof. Serradimigni); Hopital Universitair St. Luc, Brussels, Belgium (Dr. Col); Hopital de la Citadelle, Liege, Belgium (Dr. Materne); Medizinische Klinik, Freiburg, Federal Republic of Germany (Prof. Meinertz); Academic Hospital of the Free University of Amsterdam, Amsterdam, The Netherlands (Prof. Verheugt); Academic Hospital of Maastricht, Maastricht, The Netherlands (Dr. de Zwaan, Dr. Vermeer)

References

1. Neill WA, Ritzmann LW, Selden R (1977) The pathophysiologic basis of acute coronary insufficiency: observations favoring the hypothesis of intermittent reversible coronary obstruction. Am Heart J 94:439–444
2. Neill WA, Whorton TP Jr, Fluri-Lundeen J, Cohen JS (1980) Acute coronary insufficiency-coronary occlusion after intermittent ischemic attacks. N Engl J Med 302:1157–1162
3. Holland Interuniversity Nifedipine/Metoprolol Trial (HINT) Research Group (1986) Early treatment of unstable angina in the coronary care unit: a randomised, double blind, placebo-controlled comparison of recurrent ischaemia in patients treated with nifedipine or metoprolol or both. Br Heart J 56:400–413
4. Plotnick GD, Fisher ML, Lerner B et al. (1982) Collateral circulation in patients with unstable angina. Chest 82:719–725
5. Levin DC, Fallon JT (1982) Significance of the angiographic morphology of localized coronary stenoses: histopathologic correlations. Circulation 66:316–320
6. Falk E (1985) Unstable angina with fatal outcome: Dynamic coronary thrombolysis leading to infarction and/or sudden death: autopsy evidence of recurrent mural thrombosis with peripheral embolization culminating in total vascular occlusion. Circulation 71:699–708
7. Feldman RL (1987) Coronary thrombosis, coronary spasm and speculation on the link between unstable angina and acute myocardial infarction. Am J Cardiol 59:1187–1190
8. Vetrovec GW, Cowley MJ, Overton H, Richardson DW (1981) Intracoronary thrombus in syndromes of unstable myocardial ischemia. Am Heart J 102:1202–1208
9. Holmes DR Jr, Hartzler DO, Smith HC, Fuster V (1981) Coronary artery thrombosis in patients with unstable angina. Br Heart J 45:411–416
10. Vetrovec GW, Leinbach RC, Gold HK, Cowley MJ (1982) Intracoronary thrombolysis in syndromes of unstable ischemia: angiographic and clinical results. Am Heart J 104:946–952

11. Mandelkorn JB, Wolf NM, Singh S et al. (1983) Intracoronary thrombus in nontransmural myocardial infarction and in unstable angina pectoris. Am J Cardiol 52:1–6
12. Ambrose JA, Winters SL, Stern A et al. (1985) Angiographic morphology and the pathogenesis of unstable angina pectoris. J Am Coll Cardiol 5:609–616
13. Bresnahan DR, Davis JL, Holmes DR Jr, Smith HC (1985) Angiographic occurrence of clinical correlates of intraluminal coronary artery thrombus: role of unstable angina. J Am Coll Cardiol 6:285–289
14. Capone G, Wolf NM, Meyer B, Meister SG (1985) Frequency of intracoronary filling defects by angiography in angina pectoris at rest. Am J Cardiol 56:403–406
15. Sherman CT, Litvack F, Grundfest W et al. (1986). Coronary angioscopy in patients with unstable angina pectoris. N Engl J Med 315:913–919
16. Lewis HD, Davis JW, Archibald DA et al. (1983) Protective effect of aspirin against acute myocardial infarction and death in men with unstable angina. N Engl J Med 309:396–403
17. Cairns JA, Gent M, Singer J et al. (1985) Aspirin, sulfinpyrazone, or both in unstable angina: results of a Canadian multicenter trial. N Engl J Med 313:1369–1375
18. Folts JD, Gallagher K, Rowe GG (1982) Blood flow reductions in stenosed canine coronary arteries: vasospasm or platelet aggregation? Circulation 65:248–255
19. Robertson RM, Robertson DM, Roberts LJ et al. (1981) Thromboxane A2 in vasotonic angina pectoris: evidence from direct measurements and inhibition trials. N Engl J Med 304:998–1003
20. Zack PM, Ischinger T, Aker UT, Dincer B, Kennedy HL (1984) The occurrence of angiographically detected intracoronary thrombus in patients with unstable angina pectoris. Am Heart J 108:1408
21. Bär FW, UNASEM collaborative group (1990) Thrombolytic agents in unstable angina. American Heart Association (submitted for publication)
22. Rentrop P, Blanke H, Karsch KR et al. (1981) Selective intracoronary thrombolysis in acute myocardial infarction and unstable angina pectoris. Circulation 63:307–317
23. Ambrose JA, Hjemdahl-Monsen C, Borrico S et al. (1987). Quantitative and qualitative effects of intracoronary streptokinase in unstable angina and non Q-wave infarction. J Am Coll Cardiol 9:1156–1165
24. Gold HK, Johns JA, Leinbach RC et al. (1987) A randomized, blinded placebo-controlled trial of recombinant human tissue-type plasminogen activator in patients with unstable angina pectoris. Circulation 75:1192–1199
25. de Zwaan CH, Bär FW, Janssen J et al. (1988) Effects of thrombolytic therapy in unstable angina: clinical and angiographic results. J Am Coll Cardiol 12:301–309
26. Gotoh K, Minamino T, Katoh O et al. (1988) The role of intracoronary thrombus in unstable angina: angiographic assessment and thrombolytic therapy during ongoing anginal attacks. Circulation 77:526–534
27. Topol EJ, Nicklas JM, Kander NH et al. (1988) Coronary revascularization after intravenous tissue plasminogen activator for unstable angina pectoris: results of a randomized double-blind, placebo-controlled trial. Am J Cardiol 62:368–371
28. Meyer J, Bär FW, Barth H et al. (1989) Randomised double-blind trial of intravenous recombinant pro-urokinase (rscu-PA) VS streptokinase in acute myocardial infarction (PRIMI trial). Lancet i:863–867
29. Cornier B, Vahanian A, Conard J et al. (1988) Is thrombosis really safe? Coronary thrombolysis: current answers to critical questions. Current Medical Literature, London, p 122–127

Coronary Angioplasty in Unstable Angina

J. MEYER, H.-J. RUPPRECHT, R. BRENNECKE, M. KOTTMEYER, R. ERBEL, and T. POP [1]

Introduction

When Grüntzig introduced the revolutionary method of percutaneous transluminal coronary angioplasty (PTCA) for the treatment of coronary artery stenoses, he initially devoted this technique only to patients with stable angina pectoris [8]. Very soon, however, it was discovered simultaneously by Williams et al. [19] and by our group [12] that this method can also be used in patients with unstable angina pectoris. The earliest experiences with PTCA in 1980 were published by our two groups (Table 1). In these series the average

Table 1. Earliest experiences 1978–1980 with PTCA in unstable angina pectoris

	Williams et al. [19]	Meyer et al. [12]
Degree of stenosis	80% ± 16%	76% ± 11%
Degree of stenosis after	34% ± 13%	37% ± 11%
Success rate	13/17	14/23
Death rate	0%	0%
Infarction	3%	0%
Surgery	1%	1%

degree of stenosis was somewhat lower than that today, while the residual stenosis after treatment was slightly higher. The very rough balloons and guiding catheters available in those days and the inability to move the guide at the top of the catheter were responsible for the low success rates. Both groups, however, were able to demonstrate that the PTCA technique can be applied to patients with unstable angina pectoris with a remarkably low complication rate. Further results also by other groups have since confirmed the indication and contributed to further success [2, 6, 13, 15, 16].

Since 1978 we have used PTCA to treat patients with stable and with unstable angina as well as those immediately after thrombolytic therapy [4, 14]. In patients with unstable angina we always try to stabilize the patient's

[1] II. Medizinische Klinik und Poliklinik der Universität, Langenbeckstrasse 1, 6500 Mainz, West Germany

W. Bleifeld et al. (Eds.)
Unstable Angina

condition in the coronary care unit. Preferentially we schedule the coronary arteriography in cooperation with the cardiac surgeons in order to perform diagnostic arteriography and PTCA in the same procedure. By this combined diagnostic-therapeutic approach we save time, avoid a second exposure of the patient to the catheterization laboratory, save contrast material and other expenses, and lower the costs for personnel.

This chapter reports the results of our 11 years of experience in the Medical College of the RWTH in Aachen and the Medical College of the Johannes Gutenberg University in Mainz.

Methods

All patients with unstable angina had either experienced worsening in frequency, severity, or duration of episodes of chest pain or presented with recent onset angina or pain at rest within the past 2 months. In all patients transient changes in the ST-segment and/or T-waves were documented. PTCA was performed in these patients after initial medical treatment including intravenous nitrates, beta-blockers, calcium antagonists, acetylsalicylic acid, and intravenous heparin. Acute myocardial infarction was excluded by serial electrocardiograms and enzyme evaluations. Patients with left main disease and severe diffuse disease were not considered for PTCA. In patients with multivessel disease only the most severe lesion or in the case of ST-segment changes the ischemia-related lesions were dilated. Informed consent was obtained in all patients. During the procedure a surgical team was available in case of emergency. All patients received 20 mg nifedipine and 500 mg aspirin three times on the day before the procedure. During the procedure, intravenous heparin in a dose of 10000–15000 U as well as a continuous drip of low molecular weight dextran was given. A Swan-Ganz catheter was placed into the pulmonary artery. Immediately after the procedure, heparin (3000 U) and nitroglycerin (0.2 mg) was given in the diseased coronary artery to prevent thrombus formation and coronary spasm. Control angiography was performed in multiple projections to confirm the result.

The angioplasty procedure was considered successful if it resulted in at least a 20% reduction of luminal diameter narrowing and a luminal diameter narrowing of less than 50% without the patient undergoing major complications (death, myocardial infarction, emergency CABG). After the PTCA procedure, the femoral sheath was left in the groin and removed after 24 h. During this period, all patients were on intravenous heparin. The patients were usually discharged 3 days after the procedure. They continued to receive treatment with nifedipine (60 mg daily) and aspirin (500 mg daily) for 6 months. Control arteriography was recommended routinely, and if indicated, a second PTCA was performed 6 months after the initial PTCA procedure.

Results

Early Results

Between 1978 and 1984 only balloons with a fixed guide wire at the tip of the balloon catheter were available. In those days the immediate results were not entirely satisfying (Fig. 1). In the years 1986–1988 the degree of stenoses which could be passed with the balloon and subsequently dilated rose slightly. Especially the residual degree of stenoses after the whole PTCA procedure dropped significantly to 35.8% ± 16.6%. Thus, the improvement of luminal diameter at this time was 46.8 ± 17.6%.

In some patients with unstable angina pectoris a total occlusion of the culprit vessel was found at diagnostic angiography. In most cases these occlusions had occurred quite recently. The collateral perfusion was very limited. In 24 of 38 patients (Fig. 2) we were able to pass the occlusion and to dilate the

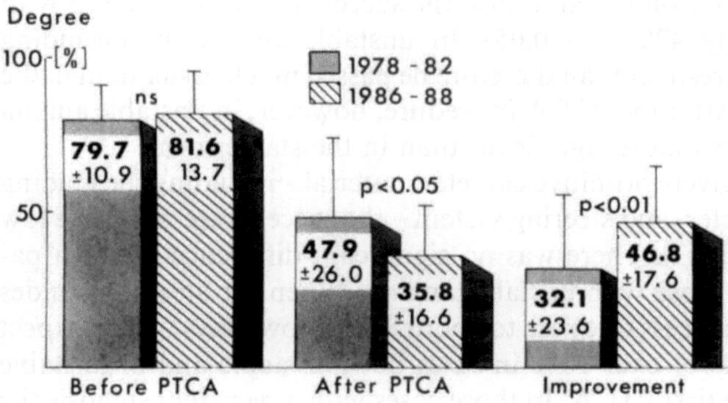

Fig. 1. Early results of PTCA in unstable angina pectoris. Comparison of the degree of stenoses 1978–1982 and 1986–1988

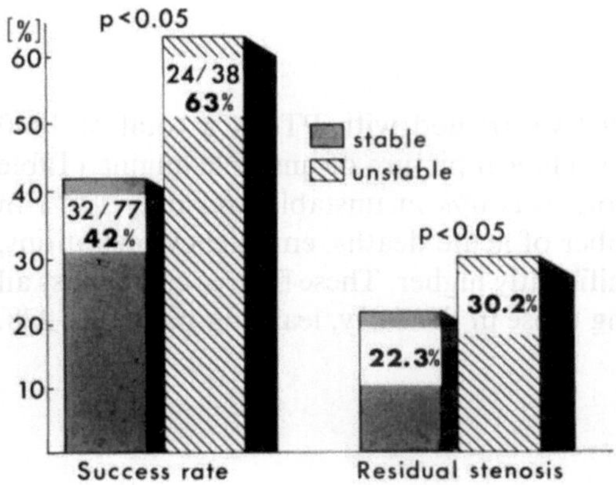

Fig. 2. Comparison of PTCA in patients with totally occluded coronary arteries. Stable versus unstable angina pectoris

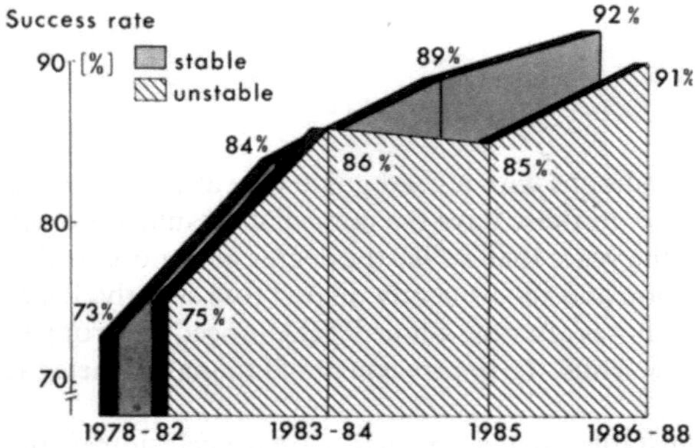

Fig. 3. Development of the success rate in early PTCA maneuvers. Comparison of stable and unstable angina pectoris over the period 1978–1988

residual stenosis (63%). Compared to this, the success rate in 77 patients with stable angina was only 42% ($p < 0.05$). In unstable angina the occluding thrombus is generally fresh and can therefore be passed much easier than in the stable form [5, 7, 10]. After the PTCA procedure, however, in unstable angina the residual stenosis was more significant than in the stable form.

Because of the relatively primitive catheter material – including the guiding catheter, balloon catheter, and steering system – the success rate was quite low from 1978 to 1982 (Fig. 3). There was no significant difference between patients with stable and those with unstable angina. When the steerable guides became available, the success rate rose to about 85%. Nowadays we can expect an average success rate of over 90% in cases both of stable and of unstable angina undergoing the first PTCA. In those cases with a recurrent stenosis the success rate in repeated PTCA is usually higher, probably because of the somewhat smoothed vessel lumen.

Complication Rates

In the 10 years from 1978 to 1988 we treated with PTCA a total of 1840 patients, 29% of whom showed the clinical picture of unstable angina (Table 2). The rate of major complications was 6% in unstable and only 1.5% in stable angina ($p < 0.01$). The number of acute deaths, emergency operations, and acute infarctions was also significantly higher. These figures encompass all patients receiving PTCA, including those in the early, learning phase in 1978.

Late Results

As with the initial success rate, there were differences between patients treated for the first time and those in whom a second or third PTCA was performed at the same vessel site. For reasons of comparison we therefore report only those patients with the first PTCA attempt.

In 185 patients with unstable angina and 500 patients with stable angina we were able to perform a repeat coronary arteriography 6 months after the procedure (Fig. 4). The degree of stenoses before PTCA did not differ between the group with stable and that with unstable angina. After treatment there were only very small residual narrowings, below 25% of luminal diameter. At follow-up, however, patients with unstable angina showed a significantly higher degree of restenoses than did those with previously stable angina. Restenosis was defined as (a) loss of over 50% of the initial gain in luminal diameter and (b) a luminal diameter narrowing of over 50%. Not only the degree of vessel stenosis was higher in patients with unstable angina but also the proportion of patients showing a significant restenosis (Fig. 5).

Although the initial degree of stenosis may be equal in patients with stable and unstable angina, early and late results are quite different. Patients with unstable angina are apparently in another phase of their coronary artery disease. The endothelium of the vessel is often broken up and covered with fresh thrombotic material [5, 7, 10]. Even if we are able to compress this thrombus, and even if we treat these patients with heparin intracoronarily and

Table 2. Total number of PTCA complications 1978–1988 ($n=1840$)

	Unstable angina ($n=534$)	Stable angina ($n=1306$)
Death	6 (1.1%)	1 (0.08%)
Emergency operation	15 (2.8%)	8 (0.6%)
Infarction	11 (2.1%)	10 (0.8%)
Total major events	32 (6.0%)	19 (1.5%)

$p<0.01$

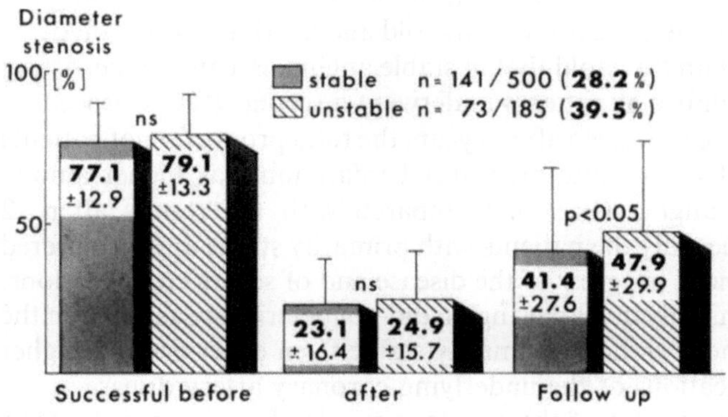

Fig. 4. Comparison of early results and those at 6-month follow-up after the first PTCA procedure in patients with stable and unstable angina

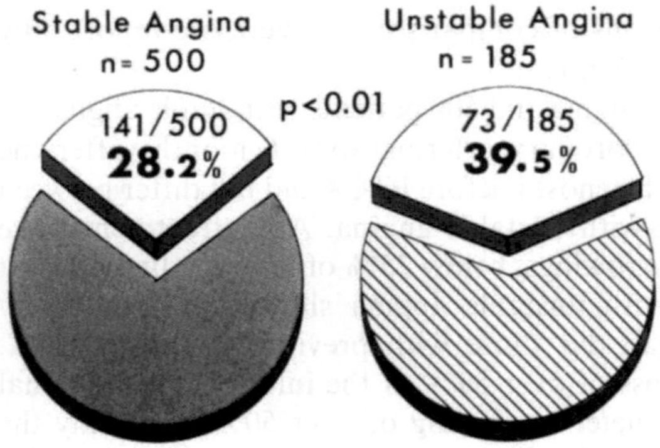

Fig. 5. Angiographical relapse rates at 6-month follow-up in patients with stable and unstable angina pectoris (1983–1988)

with aspirin and calcium antagonists, there is a remarkably high rate of early restenoses. Additional contributing factors such as increased vasomotor tone and localized spasm may be found [1, 3, 5, 10, 11, 17]. In a multivariate analysis on 453 cases of stable and unstable angina pectoris we identified the following factors responsible for restenoses: initial degree of stenosis before PTCA ($p<0.02$), residual stenosis after PTCA ($p<0.0001$), maximal inflation time ($p<0.005$), and the condition in unstable state ($p<0.01$).

Long-Term Results

Although the status of a patient with unstable angina may become quiescent initially, the outlook for the following year, even that for the subsequent days or weeks, remains unknown [16–18]. We therefore followed a large number of patients by means of written questionnaires and telephone interviews both with the patients and with the referring physicians. Within the first 12 months after an attempted PTCA (Fig. 6) there was a highly significant difference between patients with initially stable and those with initially unstable angina. In unstable angina the rate of death was ninefold and the rate of acute myocardial infarction more than threefold that in stable angina. Because of persisting instability a larger number of patients underwent a second PTCA procedure or bypass surgery ($p<0.05$). Even after 3 years the total proportion of patients who died or suffered from acute myocardial infarction was higher among those with unstable angina (Fig. 7). Compared with the results after 12 months, however, especially the patients with primarily stable angina suffered from a more pronounced progress of the disease and of severe complications. While patients with initially unstable angina did not deteriorate as much in the 2nd and 3rd years, those with the primarily stable form experienced a higher rate of severe complications of the underlying coronary artery disease.

Regarding the time course of these serious events after attempted PTCA (Fig. 8) we found that acute complications could generally be attributed to the

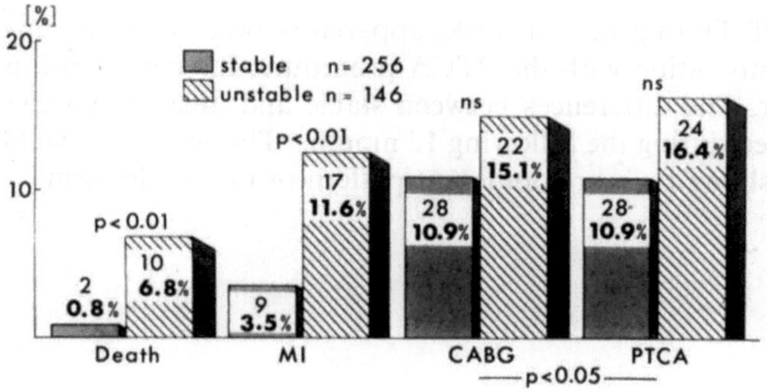

Fig. 6. Cumulative rates of major events during the first 12 months after attempted PTCA. Comparison of patients with initially unstable and stable angina. *MI*, Myocardial infarction; *CABG*, coronary artery bypass graft

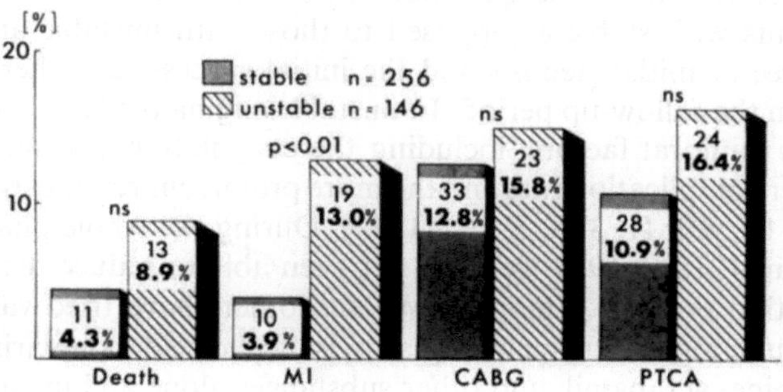

Fig. 7. Cumulative 3-year event rate of cardiovascular complications after attempted PTCA. Comparison of patients with initially stable and unstable angina

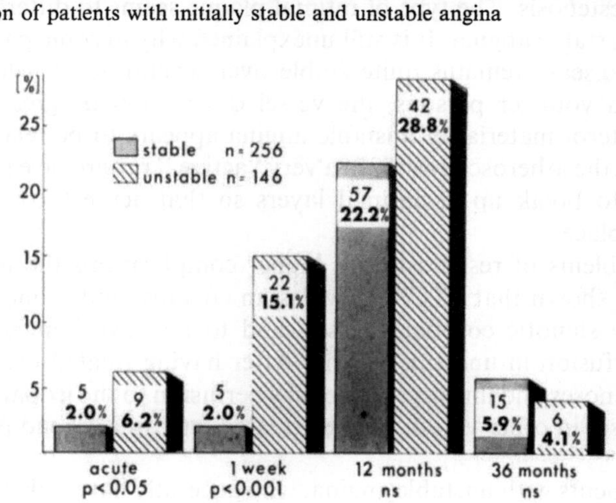

Fig. 8. Time course over 36 months of serious events after attempted PTCA procedure. Comparison of patients with initially stable and unstable angina

PTCA procedure itself. During the 1st week, apparently because of the unstable situation in combination with the PTCA procedure, the complication rate was much higher. The differences between stable and unstable angina became less pronounced during the following 12 months. The very late results beyond the 2nd year showed a more dominant pattern of the stable form.

Discussion

Form more than a decade the clinical syndrome of unstable angina has attracted great interest with respect to diagnosis, prognosis, and medical and surgical treatment. After the initial results of Williams et al. [19] and our group [12], several other groups have adopted this technique and have reported their results [2, 6, 13, 15, 16, 18]. Although there is no difference in the PTCA treatment of patients with stable as opposed to those with unstable angina regarding the degree of initial stenosis and the initial success rate, there are major differences in the follow-up period. In unstable angina the large variety of endothelial and humoral factors, including the coagulation system, contribute to the higher complication rate and the more prominent restenosis rate, at least within the 1st year [1, 3, 5, 7, 10, 11, 17]. During the whole phase of our experience from 1978 to 1989 we have not been able to reduce the high recurrence rate within the first 6 months. We and others have tried various additional therapeutic regiments, including acetylsalicylic acid, coumarin, nitroglycerin, nifedipine, verapamil, and other substances alone and in various combinations. Up to now no satisfying therapeutic approach has been found to the problem of restenosis. The type of intimal plaque seems to differ from that in patients with stable angina. It is still unexplained why in some patients the atherosclerotic disease remains quite stable over several years, while in others, especially in younger persons, the vessel destruction progresses so rapidly. The cholesterol material in unstable angina appears to be relatively soft, suggesting that the atherosclerosis is in a very "active," progressive phase. It has a tendency to break up its intimal layers so that acute thrombotic reactions can take place.

Despite the problems of restenosis and higher complications the results over the years have shown that PTCA provides an effective and economical way to treat highly stenotic coronary vessels and to improve immediately coronary artery perfusion in unstable angina. After having treated the most serious coronary stenoses and improved coronary perfusion to the jeopardized myocardium, stenoses in other vessels may be treated later in a second procedure.

Especially in patients with unstable angina, who generally have only few or no angiographically visible collaterals, we feel that a cautious and relatively conservative approach is advisable. PTCA can postpone the time of bypass graft surgery, while in some critical situation it may provide time until bypass surgery is available. Finally, since the costs for equipment, material, and personnel, including those for hospital stay, are approximately only one-quarter of those required for bypass surgery, considerable economic advantages are offered [9].

References

1. Davies MJ, Thomas AC (1985) Plaque fissuring – the cause of acute myocardial infarction, sudden ischemic death and crescendo angina. Br Heart J 53:363–373
2. De Feyter PJ, Serruys PW, van den Brand M, Soward AL, Hugenholtz PG (1985) Percutaneous transluminal coronary angioplasty in unstable angina pectoris: the Rotterdam experience. In: Hugenholtz PG, Goldman BS (eds) Unstable angina – current concepts and management. Schattauer, Stuttgart, pp 229–237
3. Epstein SE, Talbot TL (1981) Dynamic coronary tone in precipitation, exacerbation and relief of angina pectoris. Am J Cardiol 48:797–803
4. Erbel R, Pop T, Henrichs KJ, von Olshausen K, Schuster CJ, Rupprecht HJ, Steuernagel C, Meyer J (1986) Percutaneous transluminal coronary angioplasty after thrombolytic therapy: a prospective controlled randomized trial. J Am Coll Cardiol 8:485–495
5. Falk E (1985) Unstable angina with fatal outcome: dynamic coronary thrombosis leading to infarction and/or sudden death. Circulation 71:699–708
6. Faxon DP, Detre KM, McGabe CH et al. (1983) Role of percutaneous transluminal coronary angioplasty in the treatment of unstable angina: report from the National Heart, Lung, and Blood Institute Percutaneous Transluminal Coronary Angioplasty and Coronary Artery Surgery Study Registries. Am J Cardiol 53 (12):131C–135C
7. Fitzgerald DJ, Roy L, Catelle F, Fitzgerald GA (1986) Platelet activation in unstable coronary disease. N Engl J Med 315:913
8. Grüntzig AR, Senning A, Siegenthaler WE (1979) Nonoperative dilatation of coronary-artery stenosis: percutaneous transluminal coronary angioplasty. N Engl J Med 301:61–67
9. Jang GC, Block PC, Cowley MJ, Grüntzig AR, Dorros G, Holmes DR, Kent KM, Leatherman LL, Myler RK, Sjolander SME, Stertzer SH, Vetrovec GW, Willis WH, Williams DO (1984) Relative cost of coronary angioplasty and bypass surgery in a one-vessel disease model. Am J Cardiol 53:52–55
10. Mandelkorn JB, Wolf NM, Singh S et al. (1983) Intracoronary thrombus in non-transmural myocardial infarction and in unstable angina pectoris. Am J Cardiol 52:1–6
11. Maseri A, L'Abbate A, Baroldi G et al. (1978) Coronary vasospasm as a possible cause of myocardial infarction: a conclusion derived from the study of "preinfarction" angina. N Engl J Med 299:1271–1277
12. Meyer J, Böcker B, Erbel R, Bardos P, Messmer BJ, Effert S (1980) Treatment of unstable angina with percutaneous transluminal coronary angioplasty. Circulation 62:III-160
13. Meyer J, Schmitz H, Erbel R, Kiesslich T, Böcker-Josephs B, Krebs W, Braun PC, Bardos P, Minale C, Messmer BJ, Effert S (1981) Treatment of unstable angina pectoris with percutaneous transluminal coronary angioplasty. Cathet Cardiovasc Diagn 7:361
14. Meyer J, Merx W, Schmitz H, Erbel R, Kiesslich T, Dörr R, Lambertz H, Bethge C, Krebs W, Bardos P, Minale C, Messmer BJ, Effert S (1982) Percutaneous transluminal coronary angioplasty immediate after intracoronary streptolysis of transmural myocardial infarction. Circulation 66:905–913
15. Meyer J, Schmitz HJ, Kiesslich R, Erbel R, Krebs W, Schulz W, Bardos P, Minale C, Messmer BJ, Effert S (1983) Percutaneous transluminal coronary angioplasty in patients with stable and unstable angina pectoris. Analysis of early and late results. Am Heart J 106:973
16. Rupprecht HJ, Erbel R, Brennecke R, Pop T, Jung D, Kottmeyer M, Hering R, Meyer J (1988) Aktuelle Komplikationsrate der perkutanen transluminalen Koronarangioplastie bei stabiler und unstabiler Angina. Dtsch Med Wochenschr 113:409–413

17. Serruys PW, Steward R, Booman F, Michels R, Reiber JHC, Hugenholtz PG (1980) Can unstable angina pectoris be due to increased coronary vasomotor tone? Eur Heart J 1: B 71–85
18. Steffenino G, Meier B, Finci L, Rutishauser W (1987) Follow up results of treatment of unstable angina by coronary angioplasty. Br Heart J 57:416–419
19. Williams DO, Riley RS, Singh AK, Gewirtz H, Most AS (1981) Evaluation of the role of coronary angioplasty in patients with unstable angina pectoris. Am Heart J 102:1–9

Surgical Treatment of Unstable Angina

B. J. MESSMER [1]

Introduction

True unstable angina represents a serious threat to the coronary patient. Immediate and aggressive treatment is mandatory. Unfortunately, the clinical definition of unstable angina has become less and less clear, so that results from different studies are not necessarily comparable.

The term unstable angina, introduced by Fowler in 1971 [6], was defined by Conti et al. in 1973 [3] as either new-onset angina, crescendo angina, or angina at rest together with ST-segment or T-wave changes during the attacks but without new Q-wave formation in the ECG and without successive elevation of the serum enzyme levels. Bashour et al. [1] include under unstable angina also postmyocardial infarction angina, silent ischemia during the periinfarction period, and non-Q-wave myocardial infarction. In the CASS Registry unstable angina was defined as angina that occurs within 1 week of enrollment together with either new-onset angina, angina at rest, acute coronary insufficiency with pain longer than 30 min and ST-T or T-wave changes, or a changing pattern of angina [8].

Due to this wide spectrum of different symptoms with various possibilities in interpretation it is not surprising that almost 5400 patients enrolled in the CASS Registry were thought to have had unstable angina, and that 3311 of them underwent coronary bypass surgery [8]. In another surgical study Rahimtoola et al. [14] reported an incidence of 28.5%. For the present study patient selection was more strict, taking into consideration that unstable angina leading to invasive treatment should represent an emergency situation.

Clinical Material

Definition of Unstable Angina for Patient Selection

In this study a patient was defined as being in unstable condition when he suffered severe anginal attacks combined with transient ischemic ECG

[1] Abteilung für Thorax-, Herz- und Gefäßchirurgie, Klinikum der RWTH, 5100 Aachen, West Germany

W. Bleifeld et al. (Eds.)
Unstable Angina

changes but without significant enzyme elevation. The attacks either were of new origin or underwent a substantially changing pattern to the worse but had to be refractory to medical treatment. This restrictive definition excluded patients with simple increase in symptoms as well as patients with no or insufficient medical treatment. It also excluded patients with simple angina at rest or nocturnal angina, who belong to functional class IV (CCS) but should not necessarily be classified unstable.

Patient Population

During the 5-year period between 1983 and 1987, 128 out of 3326 coronary bypass patients (3.8%) met the requirements for true unstable angina. The yearly proportion varied between 2.7% and 5% (Fig. 1). Patient data are given in Table 1. Of the 128 patients 91 (70%) were men and 37 (30%) were women. As expected, the duration of acute or crescendo symptoms was short and

Table 1. Basic patient data

Number of patients	128
Men : woman	91 (70%) : 37 (30%)
Age (years)	59 ± 8
Duration of crescendo angina (months)	1.25 ± 1.47
Previous stable angina	91 (71%)
Previous myocardial infarct	34 (26.5%)
Recent (< 4 weeks) myocardial infarct	25 (19%)
Previous PTCA	15
Previous CAB surgery	3

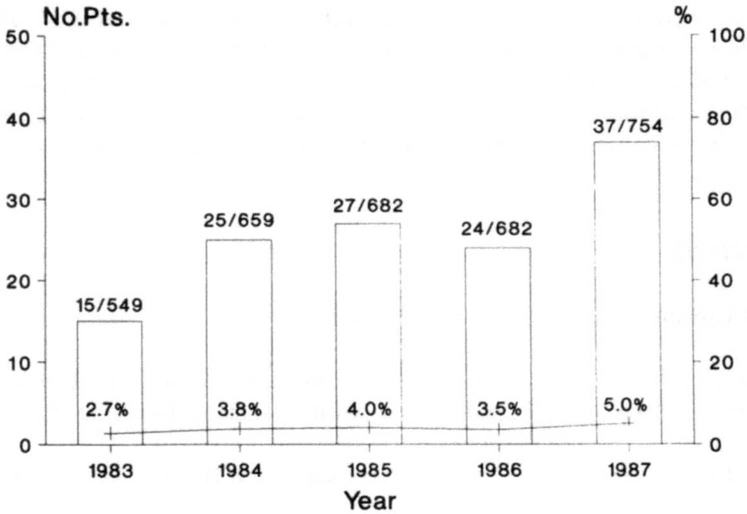

Fig. 1. Number of patients operated upon for unstable angina 1983–1987

averaged 6 weeks. The mean age of patients was 59±8 years (range, 38–77 years) with a majority between the ages of 50 and 69. Only one patient was below 40, but 12 were over 70 years of age.

All patients came to the hospital as emergencies and were incapacitated by the severity of their symptoms. Transient stabilization was possible, however, by complete bed rest and vigorous antianginal treatment using intravenous nitroglycerin, heparin, and nifedipine or a combination of these. Previous history revealed an old myocardial infarction in 34 patients (26.5%); two of them underwent thrombolysis combined with PTCA. Earlier stable angina was reported by 91 patients (71%). Of major interest is the fact that 25 patients (19%) had a recent nontransmural infarction with unstable postinfarct angina. Almost half of these patients were treated by thrombolysis, but only two had also had PTCA. Altogether 15 patients had previous PTCA, but this was initially successful in only five while it failed in ten, with acute complications in six patients. Three patients had had previous coronary bypass surgery (Table 1).

Isolated left main stem stenosis was present in three patients (2.3%), but another 15 patients with double- or triple-vessel disease had additional significant left main stenosis, for a total of 14% (18 patients) with significant left main stenosis. Single-vessel disease was present in 15.6%, and the LAD was involved in all but one patient who had acute dissection of a dominant RCA during PTCA. Double-vessel disease was found in 33 patients (25.8%), and, again, in all of them the LAD was involved. More than half of the patients (56.3%) had triple-vessel disease (Table 2). In all, significant (>75%) proximal LAD stenosis or occlusion was found in 100 out of 128 patients (84%; Table 2).

All surviving patients have been followed for a minimum of 1 and a maximum of 6 years. Actuarial survival was calculated according to the method of Kaplan-Meier.

Table 2. Distribution of coronary stenoses

	n	Percentage
Isolated LM stenosis[a]	3	2.3
Single-vessel disease	20	15.6
LAD	19	
RCA	1	
CX	0	
Double-vessel disease	33	25.8
LAD+RCA	20	
LAD+CX	13	
RCA+CX	0	
Triple-vessel disease	72	56.3
LAD+CX+RCA	68	
LM+RCA	4	

[a] Total patients with LM stenosis, 18 (14%).

Surgical Considerations

The majority of patients (73.5%) came to operation with continuous nitroglycerin and heparin infusion, often combined with intravenous nifedipine. It is of great importance not to stop this therapy prior to operation and to administer sufficient sedatives before taking such patients to the operating room. Smooth induction of anesthesia is necessary to prevent ischemic reactions and myocardial damage. Prior to surgery the intraaortic balloon pump is never used, and prophylactic insertion of the balloon is not advisible. It is helpful, however to insert a catheter into the femoral artery, which later can be used as a guide for the intraaortic balloon if necessary.

Surgery was performed in all cases using extracorporeal circulation, moderate hypothermia of 28 °C and myocardial protection with cristalloid cardioplegic solution. Complete revascularization is mandatory, as in all coronary bypass patients. In the present series an average of three anastomoses per patient was performed. This is one anastomosis less than our average for patients operated upon for stable angina. The difference is due to the higher proportion of patients with single- and double-vessel disease. Two-thirds of the patients had three or more bypasses inserted. Unlike in patients with stable angina, internal mammary grafts were not used in the present series.

Results

Ten patients died within the 1st month after surgery, which means a hospital mortality of 7.8%. Intraoperative or early postoperative myocardial failure was responsible for death in eight patients and severe intraoperative hypoxemia of unknown origin in one. Lower limb necrosis resulting from the intraaortic balloon followed by severe renal failure was the cause of death in one patient suffering from additional peripheral arteriosclerotic disease. Circulatory support with the intraaortic balloon pump was necessary in 16 patients (12.5%); half of these died while the others recovered.

Early nonfatal complications are listed in Table 3. Significant congestive heart failure confirmed peri- or early postoperative myocardial infarction, and

Table 3. Nonfatal complications

	n	IABP
Significant CHF	7	6
Peri-/postoperative infarct	3	1
Electrical instability	3	1
Bleeding	3	0
Transient ischemic attack	1	0
Pneumonia	1	0

IABP, Intraaortic balloon pump; CHF, congestive heart failure.

electrical instability probably due to localized subendocardial damage represented the most frequent nonfatal complications. Bleeding, transient ischemic attacks, and pneumonia occurred with a frequency not different from the average in open heart surgery patients.

Long-term follow-up in the present series was 100% and covered a minimum of 1 and a maximum of 6 years with an average of 3 years. During this time 11 patients died (Table 4). Myocardial infarction (three), congestive heart failure (three), and cardiac reoperation (one) were responsible for cardiac death in seven patients while four patients died of noncardiac causes. It should be noted that four of the cardiac deaths occurred in patients belonging to the older age group. Overall actuarial survival at 5 years was 80% (Fig. 2). During

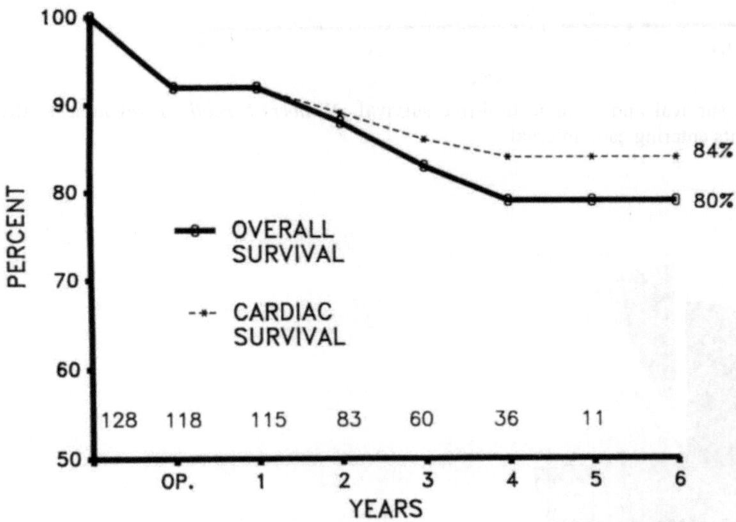

Fig. 2. Actuarial survival for patients with unstable angina. Overall survival includes death from all causes; cardiac survival includes cardiac-related deaths only

Table 4. Late deaths after surgery for unstable angina

Cause of late death	*n*	Age at operation (years)	Interval (months)
Cardiac death			
Myocardial infarct	3	63, 72, 73	13, 30, 27
Congestive heart failure	3	45, 71, 72	19, 13, 30
Cardiac reoperation	1	56	39
Noncardiac death			
Cerebral hemorrhage	2	67, 68	43, 13
Pulmonary embolism	1	56	30
Cancer	1	71	21
Total	11	65	27

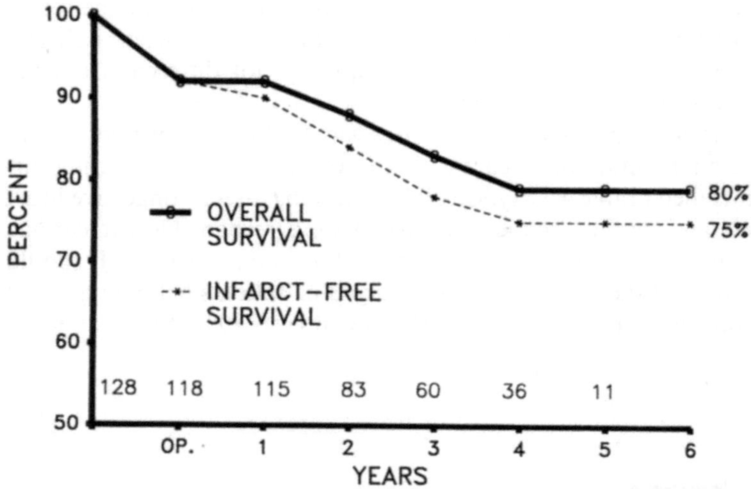

Fig. 3. Actuarial survival and complication-free survival. *Numbers beneath curves* indicate the number of patients entering each interval

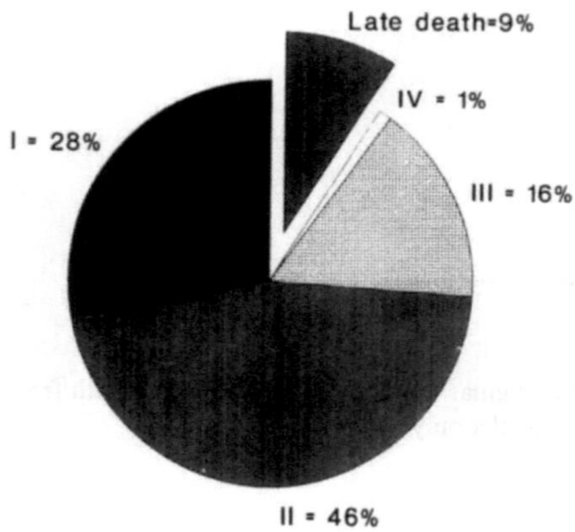

Fig. 4. Distribution of postoperational functional class in 111 patients at mean follow-up of 36 ± 16 months

the follow-up period six patients suffered from a nonfatal myocardial infarction, which results in a complication-free survival rate of 75% at 5 years (Fig. 3). At the last control, 28% of surviving patients were in functional class I, 56% in class II, 16% in class III, and one patient was in class IV (Fig. 4). The functional status of the surviving patients was quite similar regardless of whether the follow-up was 1, 2, 3, 4, or 5 years. In all five groups 70%–80% of patients were in either functional class I or II (Fig. 5).

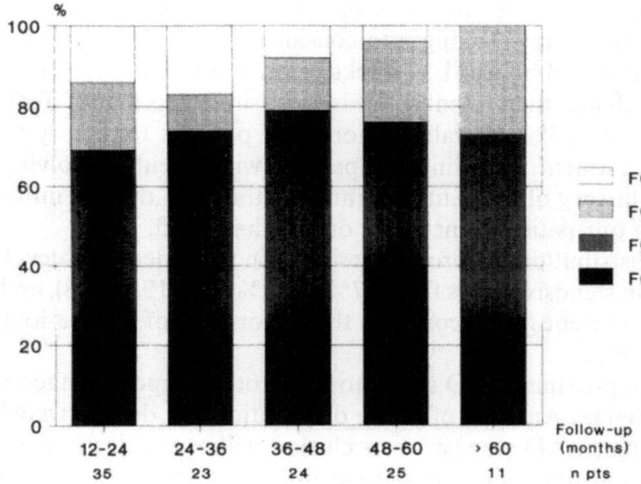

Fig. 5. Functional class (CCS) according to the length of follow-up

Discussion

When dealing with unstable angina, a major disadvantage is the lack of a clear and standardized definition. It is therefore not amazing that the incidence of patients with unstable angina varies enormously among different reported series. In the present study the overall incidence was 3.8%, with a variance between 2.7% in 1983 and 5% in 1987, but without significantly increasing tendency to date. This may change, however, since early catheterization and consecutive bypass grafting in suitable cases have become the method of choice after previous vigorous antianginal treatment.

Unstable angina represents an emergency or at least an urgent situation which cannot be handled without invasive treatment either by surgery or by PTCA. All our patients initially had to be treated by intravenous administration of nitroglycerin, combined with heparin; intravenous nifedipine often had to be given in addition. Even though stabilization of the acute situation was often possible, especially under strict bed rest, 73.5% of our patients were still dependent on intravenous medication at the time of surgery. Using similar selection criteria, Naunheim et al. [12] reported an incidence of 7.1%, which is quite comparable to that in our experience and is certainly more reliable than the high figures reported by others [8, 14].

At first glance, operative mortality of 7.8% seems rather high, especially when compared with the first United States National Cooperative Study on treatment of unstable angina, in which an operative mortality of 3% was reported [16]. This was found unacceptable by Jones et al. [7], who had a rate of only 1.2% in a series of 78 patients. The latter series is, however, not necessarily representative because only 36% of the patients were in need of intravenous antianginal therapy. Taking into consideration that 90% of our patients had a nontransmural infarct 1–4 weeks prior to surgery, often combined with signs of evolving, the present series is most similar to that of Teoh et al. [18], who found an 8.5% mortality among 224 patients refractory to intravenous medical treatment, including also patients with recent or evolving infarction. However, history of a recent nontransmural infarct did not influence mortality among our patients since only one of them died.

Of interest is the distribution of coronary lesions. The reported prevalence for significant left main stenosis ranges from 17% to 36% [2, 5, 12, 15, 18], and the 14% found in the present group confirms the importance of such lesions for the unstable situation.

Involvement of the proximal LAD seems to be an other important factor leading to unstable angina. Analysis of lesion distribution has demonstrated that significant proximal LAD stenosis or occlusion without major impairment of left anterior wall function was present in 84%, and in all but two patients with either single- or double-vessel disease the LAD was involved. It seems obvious that high-grade proximal LAD stenosis represents indeed a strong trigger mechanism for unstable angina. Due to lack of analysis of the ECG during the preoperative ischemic attacks it cannot be confirmed that the LAD stenosis was also the culprit lesion in all these patients, but earlier observations [11] support this assumption.

The relatively high proportion of single- and double-vessel disease selected for surgical treatment raises the question of PTCA in such patients. Meyer et al. [9, 10] initiated PTCA for unstable angina over 10 years ago, and similar good immediate results as in patients dilated for stable angina have been obtained. Yet, the 6-month control showed a slightly worse clinical and angiographic picture [11]. More recently De Feyter et al. [4] confirmed these findings in a group of 200 patients, demonstrating a good initial result but also a considerably high procedure-related complication rate of 10.5% and a restenosis rate of 32% within a 2-year follow-up period.

Due to the rather modest long-term results of PTCA in unstable angina it has become our policy to favor coronary bypass grafting except in patients with single-vessel disease. But even here surgery is preferred when a LAD stenoses involves a major diagonal branch. Complete revascularization is a major goal also in emergency patients, and the simple dilatation of the culprit lesion in multiple-vessel disease as advocated by De Feyter et al. [4] must result in a higher recurrence rate of angina and in a reduced maximal work capacity.

In spite of every possible protective precaution patients with true unstable angina remain a high-risk group for surgery. Immediate and optimal blood supply is mandatory especially to the jeopardized area, which in the vast majority is the territory of the LAD. This consideration leads to the use of a vein graft rather than that of the internal mammary artery. Due to its often small caliber and its hard to control spastic reactions the otherwise ideal internal mammary artery cannot guarentee full flow from the very beginning. Although the use of conventional vein grafts seemed to us more favorable during the present study, the internal mammary artery has also been used in unstable patients more recently and so far without negative effects.

Long-term results after surgery for unstable angina are scarce in the literature. Rahimtoola et al. [14] reported an overall survival of 92% at 5 and 83% at 10 years. Similar results were reported by McCormick et al. [8] for patients from the CASS registry, whose overall survival was 87% at 5 and 79% at 7 years. In this CASS Registry study, late survival was highly dependent upon the left ventricular wall motion score, the degree of congestive heart failure, and the presence or absence of associated illness such as diabetes, hypertension, and peripheral vascular disease. On the other hand, survival was not different for patients with single- and double-vessel involvement but was significantly lower for these with triple-vessel disease. Similar risk parameters have been found by Scott et al. and Parisi et al. [13, 17] in the randomized study of the Veterans Administration for treatment of patients with unstable angina.

Taking into consideration that early mortality in the present study was 7.8% for these critically ill patients, long-term survival after successful surgery does not differ substantially from that in patients operated upon for stable angina. Similarly the functional status of surviving patients is more than satisfactory, with three-quarters of patients either in functional class I or II and without major deterioration during the first 5 years. Analysis of the 20 class III and IV patients demonstrates that in almost half of them noncoronary causes such as additional valvular heart disease, far advanced age, endogenous depression, extreme obesity and difficulty in maintaining monthly social security payment were basically responsible for the patient indicating an unsatisfactory result which could not be confirmed by objective tests.

In our experience unstable angina is not as frequent as often indicated. Coronary bypass surgery represents a valuable treatment, and surgery is certainly the method of choice in patients with multiple-vessel disease to achieve complete revascularization. Indication for emergency or urgent surgery is given in patients who can live only on continuous infusion of nitroglycerin, heparin, and/or nifedipine, but one must be aware that this patient population represents a high-risk group with a significantly higher surgical mortality and a higher peri- and postoperative infarction rate. The long-term expectations in these patients are, however, not different from patients operated upon for stable angina.

References

1. Bashour TT, Myler RK, Andreae GE, Stertzer SH, Clark DA, Ryan CJ (1988) Current concepts in unstable myocardial ischemia. Am Heart J 115:850–861
2. Christakis GT, Fremes SE, Weisel RD et al. (1986) Reducing the risk of urgent revascularization for unstable angina: a randomizied clinical trial. J Vasc Surg 3:764–772
3. Conti CR, Brawley RK, Griffith LS, Pitt B, Humphries JO, Gott VL, Ross RS (1973) Unstable angina pectoris: morbidity and mortality in 57 consecutive patients evaluated angiographically. Am J Cardiol 32:745–750

4. De Feyter PJ, Suryapranata H, Serruys PW, Beatt K, van Domburg R, van den Brand M, Tijssen JJ, Azar AJ, Hugenholtz PG (1988) Coronary angioplasty for unstable angina: immediate and late results in 200 consecutive patients with identification of risk factors for unfavorable early and late outcome. J Am Coll Cardiol 12:324–333
5. Eugene J, Ott RA, Piters KM, Stemmer EA (1985) Operative risk factors associated with unstable angina pectoris. Arch Surg 120:279–282
6. Fowler NO (1971) Preinfarction angina. Circulation 44:755–758
7. Jones EL, Waites TF, Craver JM, Bone DK, Hatcher CR Jr, Thompkins T (1982) Unstable angina pectoris: comparison with the National Cooperative Study. Ann Thorac Surg 34:427–434
8. McCormick JR, Schick EC, McCabe CH, Kronmal RA, Ryan TJ (1985) Determinants of operative mortality and long-term survival in patients with unstable angina. J Thorac Cardiovasc Surg 89:683–688
9. Meyer J, Böcker B, Erbel R, Bardos P, Messmer BJ, Effert S (1980) Treatment of unstable angina with percutaneous transluminal coronary angioplasty (PTCA). Circulation 62:III-160
10. Meyer R, Schmitz H, Erbel R, Böcker-Josephs B, Krebs W, Braun PC, Bardos P, Minale C, Messmer BJ, Effert S (1981) Treatment of unstable angina pectoris with percutaneous transluminal coronary angioplasty (PTCA). Cathet Cardiovasc Diagn 7:361
11. Meyer J, Schmitz HJ, Kiesslich T, Erbel R, Krebs W, Schulz W, Bardos P, Minale C, Messmer BJ, Effert S (1983) Percutaneous transluminal coronary angioplasty in patients with stable and unstable angina pectoris: analysis of early and late results. Am Heart J 106:973–980
12. Naunheim KS, Fiore AC, Arango DC, Pennington DG, Barner HB, McBride LR, Harris HH, Willman VL, Kaiser GC (1989) Coronary artery bypass grafting for unstable angina pectoris: risk analysis. Ann Thorac Surg 47:569–574
13. Parisi AF, Khuri S, Deupree R, Sharma GV, Scott S, Luchi R (1989) Medical compared with surgical management for unstable angina. Circulation 80:1176–1189
14. Rahimtoola SH, Nunley D, Grunkemeier G, Tepley J, Lambert L, Starr A (1983) Ten-year survival after coronary bypass surgery for unstable angina. N Engl J Med 308:676–681
15. Rankin JS, Newton JR Jr, Califf RM, Jones RH, Wechsler AS, Oldhamm HN Jr, Wolfe WG, Lowe JE (1984) Clinical characteristics and current management of medically refractory unstable angina. Ann Surg 200:457–465
16. Russell RO, Resnekov K, Wolk M (1978) Unstable angina pectoris: National Cooperative Study group to compare surgical and medical therapy. II. In-hospital experience and initial follow-up results in patients with one, two and three vessel disease. Am J Cardiol 42:839–848
17. Scott SM, Luchi RJ, Deupree RH and the Veterans Administration Unstable Angina Cooperative Study Group (1988) Veterans Administration Cooperative Study for Treatment of Patients with Unstable Angina. Results in patients with abnormal left ventricular function. Circulation 78 [Suppl I]:113–121
18. Teoh KH, Christakis GT, Weisel RD, Katz AM, Tong CP, Mickleborough LL, Scully HE, Baird RJ, Goldman BS (1987) Increased risk of urgent revascularization. J Thorac Cardiovasc Surg 93:291–299

The Endangered Elephant Enters Cardiology: Lessons for Unstable Angina

L. H. Opie [1]

Introduction

The elephant, we are told, is an endangered species, the males being hunted for their tusks and rapidly diminishing in numbers. While real elephants might be disappearing, figurative elephants have become popular in cardiology. We owe to Packer the idea that our various views of congestive heart failure were like six blind men trying to describe the elephant. In a lecture to the Department of Medicine of the University of Montreal in February 1988, I dragged the elephant into unstable angina. The six blind men crowded around the elephant were looking at six different definitions of unstable angina (Table 1), and according to each different definition different therapeutic options could be obtained.

Table 1. The elephant and unstable angina: the six different views of the six blind men

Rest angina, relatively stable
Mixed angina
Silent ischemia in mixed angina
Episodic rest angina
True unstable angina with risk of infarction
Prinzmetal's angina
Pre-infarction angina
Unstable angina at rest

It might be useful to divide these views of the blind men into the 'rear' views that can relatively easily be distinguished from the three 'frontal' views. The former include three types of angina at rest which are not truly unstable and need to be distinguished from three types of truly unstable angina at rest. The common denominator to all six conditions is the angina at rest, and it has in the past been supposed that a rest component to angina automatically makes

[1] Heart Research Unit and Hypertension Clinic, University of Cape Town, Observatory 7925, South Africa

W. Bleifeld et al. (Eds.)
Unstable Angina

it a more severely threatening condition than purely effort angina. Despite this seeming confusion, I shall argue that the therapeutic lessons learned from studies with beta-blockers, calcium antagonists and antithrombotic agents have given sufficient insight into these various conditions to eliminate the irrelevant 'rear' views to focus on the 'frontal' views and among the 'frontal' views to leave one residual essential condition, about which a good degree of unanimity has been achieved when it comes to understanding the aetiology and therapy. In the end, what is it about the elephant that makes it so distinctive? It is the trunk. Therefore of the six views it is the view of the trunk, namely true unstable angina at rest, that is most relevant to this update. Each of these six conditions will be examined in order.

Mixed Angina

Patients with mixed angina have both an effort component and a rest component. In the past, it was supposed that the rest component would respond better to therapy with calcium antagonists than with beta-blockade, because it was thought on theoretical grounds to be caused by coronary spasm. However, theory yielded to fact as hard studies came to be undertaken. A surprise emerged. In the few studies of mixed angina in which there has been a combination of chest pain at rest and effort angina, the therapy of choice turned out to be not calcium antagonists but beta-blockade (Table 2). Therefore, the simple concept that the rest pain was due to spasm added to organic obstruction did not seem to hold. It follows that another aetiology for the rest component of mixed angina must be sought. The studies leading to this conclusion are now reviewed.

Nifedipine therapy, known to be strikingly effective in Prinzmetal's angina, was less helpful in mixed angina; the variable clinical benefit could be matched by a correspondingly variable effect on the diameter of the critical stenoses [6]. In about half of the cases studied, the critical stenoses increased in diameter in response to nifedipine, and nifedipine improved the rest component, as defined by De Cesare et al. [6]. It might be supposed that beta-blockade was acting on the rest component by reducing the heart rate and therefore the oxygen demand. Again, unexpectedly, the benefits of beta-blockade on the silent component of angina were actually more marked on those episodes of ECG changes *not* preceded by an increase in heart rate [3]. Thus, there is no evidence that beta-blockade is ineffective in mixed angina, nor that nifedipine is the therapy of choice as is still so commonly assumed. It follows that coronary artery spasm is not the sole cause of the anginal pain occurring at rest in this type of unstable angina.

Silent Ischemia in Mixed Angina

Increasingly, transient silent ischemia is being detected in patients with angina pectoris (effort and/or rest) by continuous ST monitoring techniques. Such ST changes are now thought to be another expression of the anginal syndrome, just as is the pain. In simplified and somewhat contradictory terms, it is angina without anginal pain. It is supposed that there may be a spectrum of manifestations of angina in which mild or moderately severe episodes may be silent, in contrast to the more severe or prolonged episodes which actually reach the threshold for pain [34]. This threshold varies from patient to patient. Some patients feel pain less acutely than others, and for example there is defective pain perception in hypertensive patients. Thus the severity of the actual underlying ischemia is not the only factor at work [13]. Data starting to emerge suggest that these silent ischemic episodes in patients with either effort angina or rest angina respond both to beta-blockers and to calcium antagonists [34] and possibly even better to beta-blockade [3].

ST Deviations in Mixed Angina. The concept of preferential calcium antagonist therapy for mixed angina is also not supported by the data of Andre-Fouet et al. [1]. Although diltiazem was much better than propranolol in episodes of rest pain (duration not stated), in patients with combined effort and rest angina diltiazem was as good as propranolol but no better. It is only when true coronary spasm is thought to be the cause of spontaneous angina in a patient also with effort angina, that it is logical to prefer calcium antagonists to beta-blockade as first-line therapy.

Episodic Rest Angina

In patients with angina at rest but with short-lived attacks of chest pain, less than 10 min in duration, several studies attest to the benefit of calcium antagonists [24, 25, 31]. Transient ST deviations (60% silent, 83% ST depression) responded better to nifedipine (120 mg daily) or verapamil (480 mg daily) than to isosorbide dinitrate (120 mg daily) according to Rizzon et al. [31]. In the study of Parodi et al. [25], over 1600 ischemic episodes of ST-segment shift were studied, and 43% were silent. The mean duration of pain was 6 min, whereas the mean duration of the silent episodes was about 3 min. In a careful study interspersed with three placebo periods, verapamil 400 mg daily was considerably better than propranolol 300 mg daily.

The aetiology of these very short-lived attacks of chest pain is not known. However, the fact that so many attacks both of overt chest pain and of silent ischemia occurred predictably over several days suggests that the condition as a whole is stable and an example of stable rest angina. Because the brief attacks respond so much better to calcium antagonists and to nitrates than to beta-

Table 2. Effects of calcium antagonists alone or compared with beta-adrenergic blockers in Prinzmetal's angina, angina at rest, unstable angina, threatened myocardial infarction. (From [23])

	Type of angina	Calcium antagonist or beta-blocker doses and effects	Conclusion
Prinzmetal's angina			
Previtali et al. [26]	Short-lived attacks of rest pain or of silent ischemia promptly relieved by NG	N 60–120 mg daily; four-hourly doses; episodes of ischemia fell from 21 to 1 per 48 h	N $\gg$ placebo
Kimura and Kishida [16]	Prinzmetal's angina (rest pain with ST elevation)	V 240 mg (about), N 40 mg, D 160 mg; all reduced chest pain	N = D = V. Response rates 94%, 91% and 86%
Feldman et al. [8]	Prinzmetal's angina (rest pain with ST elevation); decreasing incidence with time	D 120 or 240 mg/day, both effective; 6 patients pain free, two no change	D > placebo
Rest angina, non-Prinzmetal			
Parodi et al. [24, 25]	Up to 180 episodes of ECG ischemia per 24 h, mostly silent; Attacks of chest pain <15 min	V 400 mg daily reduced painful and silent episodes by about 80%; P 300 mg daily no effect	V 400 $\gg$ P 300; note highly selected population (10/167 patients with unstable angina at rest)
Andre-Fouet et al. [1]	Recent onset of rest pain	D (titrated to 540 mg daily, mean 280) much better than P (titrated to 360 mg, mean 160) in patients with rest but no effort angina	D 280 $\gg$ P 360
Mixed angina			
Andre-Fouet et al. [1]	Effort and rest angina	D (titrated as above) versus P (titrated)	D = P
De Cesare et al. [6]	Effort and rest angina	N 40–80 mg daily exacerbated 19/22 patients and reduced stenotic lumen in 12/29	N had no overall benefit; slightly over half of patients may improve
Quyyumi et al. [27]	Effort and nocturnal angina	N 30–60 mg daily, A 100 mg daily; A better as judged by pain relief and lessened nocturnal ST changes on Holter	A 100 > N 60; A also better for effort component

'True' unstable angina			
Capucci et al. [2]	Variety from short-lived pain to pre-infarction state	V (480 mg/day) reduced anginal attacks from 3 to 0.2/day ($p<0.01$). P (240 mg/day) reduced attacks to 1.6/day ($p<0.01$)	V 480 ≫ P 240 in recurrent rest angina mostly with severe CAD
Theroux et al. [35]	Unstable angina at rest; Prinzmetal's excluded	D (360 mg/day titrated) equal to P (240 mg/day titrated)	D 360 = P 240 in unstable angina with threatened infarction
Muller et al. [20]	Angina <45 min; ECG changes or documented CAD; about three anginal attacks per day	N (80–120 mg daily), P 80–240 mg daily (added to background P in 67 patients, mean dose 115 mg), isosorbide dinitrate 40–80 mg daily	If prior BB, N addition better than increased dose of BB and/or nitrates; if no prior BB, N less effective
HINT Study [14]	Unstable, defined as angina at rest with variable ST-segment changes or pain >15 min with ST-segment changes	N 60 mg daily seemed harmful, trial stopped; M 200 mg seemed beneficial	N alone probably contraindicated in unstable angina; BB or N + BB better; in patients not already on a BB, BB treatment of first choice; in patients already on BB, N improves
Mauritson et al. [19]	Recurrent angina up to five attacks per day with added silent ST deviations	V 320–480 mg/day; V 320 mg in five patients on 1st day reduced anginal episodes from 5.4 to 2.2 per day ($p<0.01$)	V 320 initially highly effective; by 3rd day only 6 of 10 patients pain free despite V 480 dose
Mauri et al. [18]	Worsening angina, changing effort angina, chest pain <20 min	Intravenous D or V, 0.002 mg/kg per minute; both reduced silent ischemic episodes	D = V, both better than intravenous nitrates
Threatened myocardial infarction			
Muller et al. [21]	Threatened myocardial infarction chest pain >45 min	N (120 mg daily) similar to placebo; 75% developed AMI in both groups; possible increase in early 2nd week mortality with N	N ineffective in threatened infarction; N also ineffective in limiting infarct size (enzyme release)

A, atenolol; D, diltiazem; M, metoprolol; N, nifedipine; P, propranolol; V, verapamil; NG, nitroglycerin; BB, beta-blockade; Prinzmetal's, variant anginal pain with ST-segment elevation; CAD, coronary artery disease; AMI, acute myocardial infarction blockade, it is reasonable to assume that coronary spasm is at work, as also argued by Maseri et al. [17].

More difficult to categorize are the studies of Andre Fouet et al. [1] who made the observations on patients with recent onset of rest angina, some of whom would appear to have true unstable angina because myocardial infarction developed. None of the patients had effort angina. Diltiazem was much better than propranolol in these patients, suggesting that there was a true component of vasospastic angina, even though the duration of the chest pain is not clearly stated in this study.

Prinzmetal's Angina

Prinzmetal's angina, although now thought to be rather rare, is truly an example of unstable angina because, and this is sometimes forgotten, several of Prinzmetal's original patients went on to develop myocardial infarction. Prinzmetal's angina is generally thought to respond better to therapy with calcium antagonists than with beta-blockade. Is this view justified?

Can Beta-Blockade Really Increase Coronary Spasm? In animal experiments, alpha-receptor mediated vasoconstriction of superficial vessels can be promoted by beta-blockade. Yet during alpha-mediated vasoconstriction endocardial blood flow may improve by the transmural anti-steal mechanism [7]. In patients, the possibility that beta-blockade might set the stage for coronary artery spasm by unopposed coronary $alpha_1$-adrenergic activity cannot be disputed, although the number studied have been small, so that this complication of beta-blockade has been established only in a limited number of patients with true Prinzmetal's variant angina [32]. Even when the spectrum of coronary spasm is enlarged to the wider syndrome described by Maseri et al. [17], in which the ECG changes may vary from major ST-segment elevation or depression to minor changes in the T-wave, there is again no specific proof that beta-blockade is harmful to such lesser degrees of vasospasm.

Calcium Antagonists and Vasospastic Angina. Therapy with all three calcium antagonists is highly effective in Prinzmetal's angina. The three first-generation agents appear to be approximately equi-effective (Table 2). However, strict double-blind comparisons between these agents are not available. Nifedipine 60–80 mg daily is the rough equivalent of isosorbide dinitrate 60–80 mg daily. Nifedipine or verapamil (but not diltiazem) has been successfully combined with isosorbide dinitrate. Whereas the role of large vessel spasm in this condition is not under dispute, the actual trigger to the spasm has been much more difficult to define and is probably complex in aetiology.

Prolonged Chest Pain at Rest: True Pre-infarction Angina

The next entity is that of prolonged chest pain, with genuinely impending infarction, for example, when pain lasts more than 45 min. The data of Muller et al. in Boston [20] show that beta-blockade is better than is fixed dose nifedipine. This category of prolonged chest pain is clearly an extension of chest pain of shorter periods of duration. For example, the recent influential Dutch HINT Study [14] defined unstable angina as chest pain at rest with variable ST-T changes or anginal pains lasting more than 15 min with a documented history of infarction or unstable angina (note the circular definition) or of coronary artery disease as proven by angiography. Pain relief had to be achievable by nitrates or by a single dose of a narcotic analgesic. Early infarction was a frequent end-point, so that as a group these patients indeed had pre-infarction unstable angina, although they would constitute patients we currently define simply as unstable angina at rest.

Unstable Angina at Rest: The Condition as we now Know It

The sixth and final blind man is looking at that variety of rest angina which is true unstable angina, as currently understood by most cardiologists and authors, being a chest pain lasting for longer than 15 min and arbitrarily less than 45 min (the longer the pain lasts, the higher the chances of infarction) and accompanied by ischemic ECG changes but not by an increase in blood enzyme levels. Some other definitions need assessment.

Rahimtoola et al. [28] have defined unstable angina as one of the following: (a) crescendo angina, being anginal pain with a recent increase in frequency, intensity and duration despite medical therapy; (b) prolonged rest anginal pain, sufficiently severe to warrant admission to the coronary care unit without, however, ECG or enzyme evidence of acute myocardial infarction; or (c) spontaneous angina 3–30 days after the onset of acute myocardial infarction. This definition would include patients with longer episodes of chest pain which may go onto myocardial infarction as end-point [9, 12].

Recent Onset Effort Angina. Conti et al. [4] regarded such patients as also having unstable angina. In practice, these patients are included in other groups. Thus 51 of the 57 patients of Conti et al. [4] presented with multiple daily episodes of ischemic cardiac pain; all but one had angina at rest. Of the 57 two died, and of the remaining 55 patients 40 were treated surgically; of the 15 given medical therapy, 10 were potential candidates for surgery. Thus there seems little to be gained in regarding these patients as a special sub-category. It is this condition of unstable angina that is now known to be due to incipient thrombus formation with possibly the addition of spasm or at least changes in vasomotor tone, in which the major aetiological role is now ascribed to platelet aggregation and the initiation of the thrombolytic process, all thought to follow plaque rupture. The condition is distinguished from acute myocardial infarction by the absence of total coronary occlusion, the absence of blood enzyme changes, and the absence of ECG changes characteristic of infarction.

Pathophysiology of Unstable Angina at Rest. The heterogeneous nature of the pathophysiology of unstable angina is now becoming apparent. For example, both Stone [34] and Forrester et al. [10] propose that unstable angina may be due to a dynamic interaction between several major mechanisms. Four critical factors in the mechanism of unstable angina are the atherosclerotic plaque, the platelets, a partial thrombus and coronary vasospasm. A ruptured or fissured or ulcerated atherosclerotic plaque may lead to a nidus for platelet aggregation and partial thrombosis, usually reversible in unstable angina [5]. The plaque could, for example, act as a trigger for spasm-induced dynamic stenosis, possibly by an interaction between platelets and the damaged endothelium. The result could be release of vasoconstrictive substances including thromboxane-A_2. Heterogeneous aetiological factors demand a more complex approach to therapy, especially when it is considered that prolonged pain and left ventricular failure, as found in some patients with unstable angina, may lead to catecholamine release with consequences such as tachycardia and a metabolically based increased myocardial oxygen demand [22]. Each patient warrants individual assessment. Hugenholtz [15] states that: "There will never be one therapy for every case of unstable angina pectoris, nor will there ever be the best therapy for unstable angina. There will only be an optimal therapy for that particular stage of the syndrome at that particular moment in time for that patient."

Beta-Blockade Versus Calcium Antagonist Therapy for Unstable Angina. The closer the patient is to threatened infarction, the stronger is the case for beta-blockade. On the other hand, the closer the patient is to Prinzmetal's vasospastic angina, the stronger is the case for calcium antagonists. These potential differences appear to be particularly important in the case of nifedipine. In true unstable angina, where infarction is treatened, nifedipine is usually contraindicated unless used together with beta-blockade [14, 20]. It follows that it would be preferable to use diltiazem or verapamil if calcium antagonist monotherapy is desired [18]; no strict comparisons between these two agents and nifedipine exist. In choosing between beta-blockade and diltiazem therapy, there appears to be no real difference in the one study [35], whereas the other study with a greater number of patients corresponding more to angina at rest than to true unstable angina showed greater benefit for diltiazem [1]. Verapamil was better than propranolol when a number of patients were also included who did not appear to have true pre-infarction angina [2]. Thus which of these agents is best in unstable angina at rest is to some extent determined by the exact sub-category of the angina, the duration of the chest pain, and how 'pre-infarction' it is.

Therapies in Evolution. As I have discussed in detail previously, antithrombotic therapy is not only under evaluation but accepted. Thus aspirin and anticoagulation are standard in the management of unstable angina at rest. Thrombolytic therapy works in certain patients, specifically those with a major thrombosis as a cause for their unstable angina (see the chapter by Commerford et al., this Volume). Thromboxane-A_2 receptor antagonists are already under trial. A host of vasoconstrictors can be therapeutically opposed, and vasodilators acting at the level of the endothelium can be introduced. The role of the recently defined substance endothelin is under active study. Endothelin appears to be an important vasoconstrictor, and its effects could respond to therapy with anti-endothelin antibodies or peptides reacting with the active chains of endothelin.

Role of Endothelium: Therapeutic Implications. In the genesis of dynamic obstruction, a critical interaction is that between the endothelium, platelets, and vasoconstrictors released from the platelets such as serotonin and thromboxane-A_2. When the endothelium is damaged, certain vasodilator stimuli are blunted [29, 30], and vasoconstrictor stimuli predominate. The endothelial relaxing factor [11] is of crucial importance. Certain agents which are vasoconstrictors in vascular tissue denuded of endothelium can, in the presence of endothelium, cause vasodilation. Such factors include histamine, serotonin and some prostaglandins [33]. For example, serotonin, released from damaged platelets, becomes a vasoconstrictor when the endothelium is removed. Vasodilators may accordingly be divided into those which require the endothelium for their activity and those which do not, such as the nitrates [29]. In conditions where there is endothelial damage, as in atheroma, stimuli which are normally vasodilatory may become vasoconstrictive. Maintenance of endothelial integrity may be critical in avoiding coronary artery spasm. At present no therapeutic agents are available to restore endothelial integrity. Surgeons can now layer coronary grafts with endothelial cells. It is not too fanciful to guess that in the further future angioscopic layering of new endothelial cells could help to protect the damaged endothelium.

Conclusions

The seemingly confusing area of angina at rest is becoming clarified, in so small part due to our better understanding of what two major therapeutic agents, namely calcium antagonists and beta-blockade, can and cannot do. For example, the theory that coronary spasm plays a major role in unstable angina has not been discredited but appears unlikely in view of the relative failure of the calcium antagonist nifedipine to be powerfully active in unstable angina. On the other hand, the relative success of beta-blockade suggests that there is a non-spastic source of the obstruction. Further success with agents modifying the clotting mechanism such as aspirin has supported the concept of Davies and others that unstable angina represents a condition in which there is partial coronary obstruction on an organic basis. The partial success of thrombolytic agents supports the concept of partial thrombosis as a causative factor in unstable angina.

Thus, the six blind men are no longer puzzled by their different views of the same elephant. Five views of the elephant can be eliminated and one, the head-on view of the trunk, is left: the trunk is true unstable angina at rest, and there is an increasing unanimity concerning its definition and treatment. Nonetheless, even with this view limited to the trunk of the elephant, there are many unsolved problems particularly in the area of the dynamic component of the thrombotic process, the interaction between the thrombotic and dynamic elements, the role of spasm if any, the role of the endothelium, and the possibility of new types of therapy acting at the level of the endothelium.

References

1. Andre-Fouet X, Usdin JP, Gayet C et al. (1983) Comparison of short-term efficacy of diltiazem and propranolol in unstable angina at rest – randomized trial in 70 patients. Eur Heart J 4:691–698
2. Capucci A, Bassein L, Bracchetti D et al. (1983) Propranolol v. verapamil in the treatment of unstable angina. A double-blind cross-over study. Eur Heart J 4:148–154
3. Chierchia S, Glazier JJ, Gerosa S (1987) A single-blind, placebo-controlled study of effects of atenolol on transient ischemia in 'mixed' angina. Am J Cardiol 60:36A–40A
4. Conti CR, Brawley RK, Griffith LSC et al. (1973) Unstable angina pectoris: morbidity and mortality in 57 consecutive patients evaluated angiographically. Am J Cardiol 32:745–750
5. Davies MJ (1989) The pathological basis of angina pectoris. Cardiovasc Drugs Ther 3:249–255
6. De Cesare N, Bartorelli A, Fabbiocchi F et al. (1988) Nifedipine and angina pectoris. Short-term changes in quantitative coronary angiography with nifedipine and clinical response to treatment in effort-induced, mixed and spontaneous angina pectoris. Chest 93:485–492
7. Feigl EO (1987) The paradox of adrenergic coronary vasoconstriction. Circulation 76:737–745
8. Feldman RL, Pepine CJ, Whittle J, Conti CR (1982) Short- and long-term responses to diltiazem in patients with variant angina. Am J Cardiol 49:554–559
9. Fischl SJ, Herman MV, Gorlin R (1973) The intermediate coronary syndrome. Clinical, angiographic and therapeutic aspects. N Engl J Med 288:1193–1198
10. Forrester JS, Litvack F, Grundfest W et al. (1987) A perspective of coronary disease seen through the arteries of living man. Circulation 75:505–513
11. Furchgott RF (1983) Role of endothelium in responses of vascular smooth muscle. Circ Res 53:557–573
12. Gazes PC, Mobley EM, Faris HM et al. (1973) Preinfarctional (unstable) angina – a prospective study – ten year follow-up. Prognostic significance of electrocardiographic changes. Circulation 48:331–337
13. Glazier JJ, Chierchia S, Brown MJ et al. (1986) Importance of generalized defective perception of painful stimuli as a cause of silent myocardial ischemia in chronic stable angina pectoris. Am J Cardiol 58:667–672
14. Holland Interuniversity Nifedipine/Metoprolol Trial (HINT) Research Group (1986) Early treatment of unstable angina in the coronary care unit: a randomised double-blind placebo-controlled comparison of recurrent ischaemia in patients treated with nifedipine or metoprolol or both. Br Heart J 56:400–413
15. Hugenholtz PG (1986) Unstable angina pectoris. In: Krebs R (ed) Treatment of cardiovascular diseases by Adalat® (nifedipine). Schattauer, Stuttgart, pp 187–229
16. Kimura E, Kishida H (1981) Treatment of variant angina with drugs: a survey of 11 cardiology institutes in Japan. Circulation 63:844–848

17. Maseri A, Severi S, De Nes M et al. (1978) "Variant" angina: one aspect of a continuous spectrum of vasospastic myocardial ischemia. Pathogenetic mechanisms, estimated incidence and clinical and coronary arteriographic findings in 138 patients. Am J Cardiol 42:1019–1035
18. Mauri F, Mafrici A, Biraghi M, Cerri P, De Biase AM (1989) Effectiveness of calcium antagonist drugs in patients with unstable angina and proven coronary artery disease. Eur Heart J 9 [Suppl N]:158–163
19. Mauritson DR, Johnson SM, Winniford MD et al. (1983) Verapamil for unstable angina at rest: a short-term randomized, double-blind study. Am Heart J 106:652–658
20. Muller J, Morrison J, Stone PH et al. (1984) Nifedipine therapy for patients with threatened and acute myocardial infarction: a randomized double-blind placebo-controlled comparison. Circulation 69:740–747
21. Muller JE, Turi ZG, Pearle DL et al. (1984) Nifedipine and conventional therapy for unstable angina pectoris: a randomized, double-blind comparison. Circulation 69:728–739
22. Opie LH (1975) Metabolism of free fatty acids, glucose and catecholamines in acute myocardial infarction. Relation to myocardial ischemia and infarct size. Am J Cardiol 36:938–953
23. Opie LH (1988) Calcium channel antagonists. II. Use and comparative properties of the three prototypical calcium antagonists in ischemic heart disease, including recommendations based on an analysis of 41 trials. Cardiovasc Drugs Ther 1:461–491
24. Parodi O, Simonetti I, L'Abbate A et al. (1982) Verapamil versus propranolol for angina at rest. Am J Cardiol 50:923–928
25. Parodi O, Simonetti I, Michelassi C et al. (1986) Comparison of verapamil and propranolol therapy for angina pectoris at rest: a randomized, multiple crossover, controlled trial in the coronary care unit. Am J Cardiol 57:899–906
26. Previtali M, Salerno JA, Tavazzi L et al. (1980) Treatment of angina at rest with nifedipine: a short-term controlled study. Am J Cardiol 45:825–830
27. Quyyumi AA, Crake R, Wright OM et al. (1987) Medical treatment of patients with severe exertional and rest angina: double-blind comparison of beta-blocker, calcium antagonist and nitrate. Br Heart J 57:505–511
28. Rahimtoola SH, Nunley D, Grunkemeier G et al. (1983) Ten year survival after coronary artery bypass surgery for unstable angina. N Engl J Med 308:676–681
29. Rapaport RM, Murad F (1983) Endothelium-dependent and nitrovasodilator-induced relaxation of vascular smooth muscle: role of cyclic GMP. J Cyclic Nucleotide Prot Phosphoryl Res 9:281–296
30. Rapaport RM, Draznin MB, Murad F (1983) Endothelium-dependent relaxation in rat aorta may be mediated through cyclic GMP-dependent protein dephosphorylation. Nature 306:174–176
31. Rizzon P, Scrutinio D, Mangini SG et al. (1986) Randomized placebo-controlled comparative study of nifedipine, verapamil and isosorbide dinitrate in the treatment of angina at rest. Eur Heart J 7:67–76
32. Robertson RM, Wood AJ, Vaughan WK et al. (1982) Exacerbation of vasotonic angina pectoris by propranolol. Circulation 65:281–285
33. Rubanyi G, Vanhoutte PM (1985) Inhibitors of prostaglandin synthesis augment beta-adrenergic responsiveness in canine coronary arteries. Circ Res 56:117–125
34. Stone PH (1987) Calcium antagonists for Prinzmetal's variant angina, unstable angina and silent myocardial ischemia. Therapeutic tool and probe for identification of pathophysiologic mechanisms. Am J Cardiol 59:101B–115B
35. Theroux P, Taeymans Y, Morissette D et al. (1985) A randomized study comparing propranolol and diltiazem in the treatment of unstable angina. J Am Coll Cardiol 5:717–722

Subject Index

MIX
Papier aus verantwortungsvollen Quellen
Paper from responsible sources
FSC® C105338

If you have any concerns about our products,
you can contact us on
ProductSafety@springernature.com

In case Publisher is established outside the EU,
the EU authorized representative is:
Springer Nature Customer Service Center GmbH
Europaplatz 3, 69115 Heidelberg, Germany

Printed by Libri Plureos GmbH
in Hamburg, Germany